Essentials of
Paediatric Anaesthesia
and
Intensive Care

Essentials of
Paediatric Anaesthesia
and
Intensive Care

Editors

Sharmila Ahuja MD, DA
Former Professor
Department of Anaesthesiology and Critical Care
UCMS and Guru Tegh Bahadur Hospital
Delhi

Abhijit Bhattacharya MD, DAcp
Former Professor and Head
Department of Anaesthesiology and Critical Care
UCMS and Guru Tegh Bahadur Hospital
Delhi

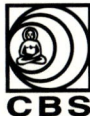

CBS Publishers & Distributors Pvt Ltd

New Delhi • Bengaluru • Chennai • Kochi • Kolkata • Mumbai
Hyderabad • Nagpur • Patna • Pune • Vijayawada

Essentials of
Paediatric Anaesthesia
and
Intensive Care

ISBN: 978-81-239-2940-8

Copyright © Editors and Publisher

First Edition: 2016

Published by Satish Kumar Jain and produced by Varun Jain for
CBS Publishers & Distributors Pvt Ltd
4819/XI Prahlad Street, 24 Ansari Road, Daryaganj, New Delhi 110 002, India.
Ph: 23289259, 23266861, 23266867   Fax: 011-23243014   Website: www.cbspd.com
e-mail: delhi@cbspd.com; cbspubs@airtelmail.in.

Corporate Office: 204 FIE, Industrial Area, Patparganj, Delhi 110 092
Ph: 4934 4934   Fax: 4934 4935   e-mail: publishing@cbspd.com; publicity@cbspd.com

Branches

• **Bengaluru:** Seema House 2975, 17th Cross, K.R. Road, Banasankari 2nd Stage, Bengaluru 560 070, Karnataka
  Ph: +91-80-26771678/79   Fax: +91-80-26771680   e-mail: bangalore@cbspd.com

• **Chennai:** 7, Subbaraya Street, Shenoy Nagar, Chennai 600 030, Tamil Nadu
  Ph: +91-44-26680620, 26681266   Fax: +91-44-42032115   e-mail: chennai@cbspd.com

• **Kochi:** Ashana House, 39/1904, AM Thomas Road, Valanjambalam, Eranakulam 682 018, Kochi, Kerala
  Ph: +91-484-4059061-62-64-65   Fax: +91-484-4059065   e-mail: kochi@cbspd.com

• **Kolkata:** No. 6/B, Ground Floor, Rameswar Shaw Road, Kolkata 700 014, West Bengal
  Ph: +91-33-2289-1126, 1127, 1128,   e-mail: Kolkata@cbspd.com

• **Mumbai:** 83-C, Dr E Moses Road, Worli, Mumbai-400018, Maharashtra
  Ph: +91-22-24902340/41   Fax: +91-22-24902342   e-mail: mumbai@cbspd.com

Representatives

• **Hyderabad**	0-9885175004	• **Nagpur**	0-9021734563	• **Patna**	0-9334159340
• **Pune**	0-9623451994	• **Vijayawada**	0-9000660880		

Printed at: HT Media Ltd. Noida

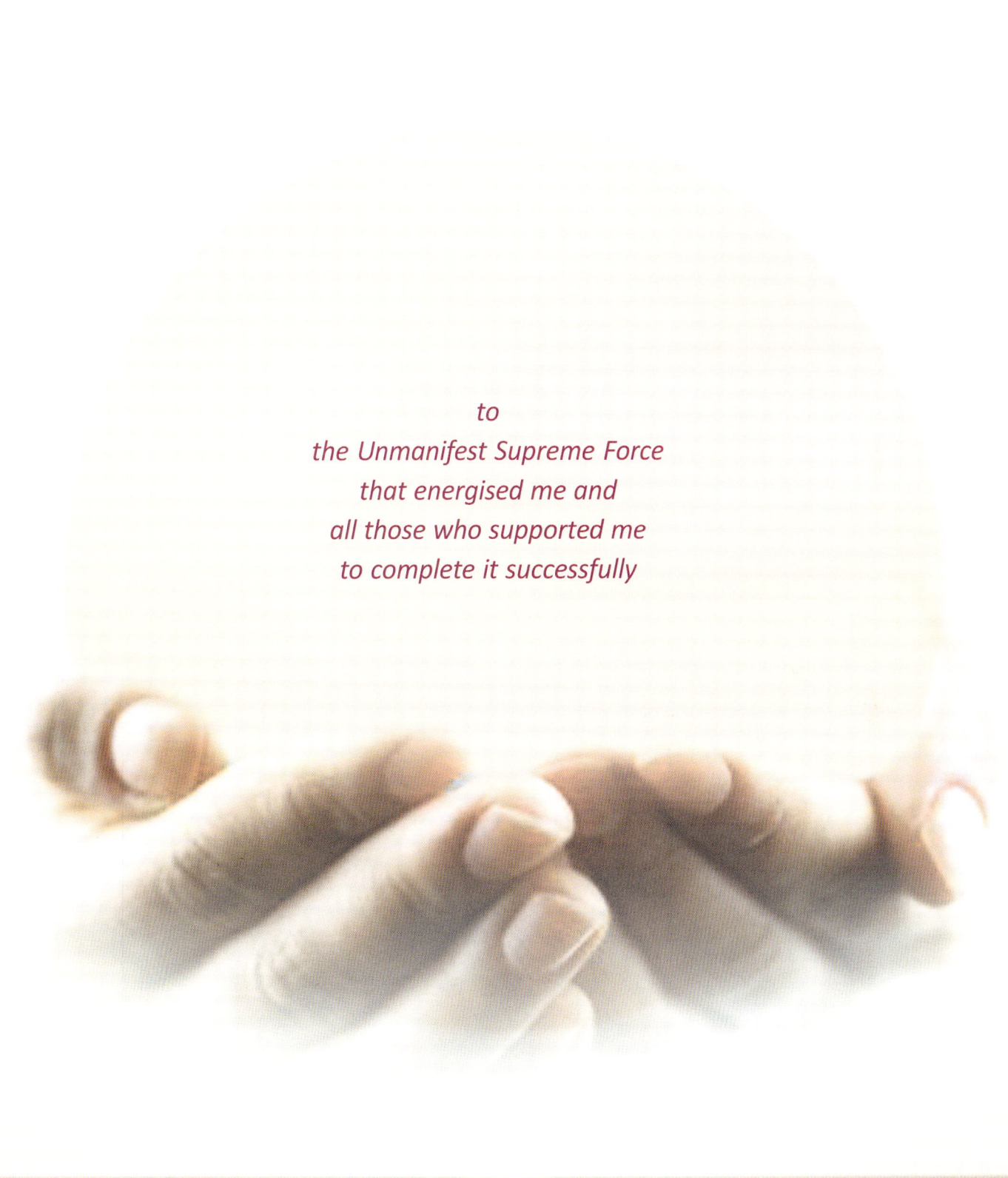

to
the Unmanifest Supreme Force
that energised me and
all those who supported me
to complete it successfully

Contributors

Deepti Agarwal MD
Specialist
Department of Anaesthesiology and Critical Care
UCMS and Guru Tegh Bahadur Hospital, Delhi

Sharmila Ahuja MD, DA
FormerProfessor
Department of Anaesthesiology and Critical Care
UCMS and Guru Tegh Bahadur Hospital, Delhi

Mahesh Kumar Arora MD
Professor and Head
Department of Anesthesia and Intensive Care
All India Institute of Medical Sciences (AIIMS), New Delhi

Balakrishnan Ashokka MD, FANZCA, MHPE
Clinical Lecturer
National University of Singapore

Dalim Kumar Baidya MD
Assistant Professor
Department of Anaesthesiology and Intensive Care
All India Institute of Medical Sciences (AIIMS), New Delhi

Abhijit Bhattacharya MD, DAcp
Former Professor and Head
Department of Anaesthesiology and Critical Care
UCMS and Guru Tegh Bahadur Hospital, Delhi

Sujata Chaudhary MD, MNAMS
Director Professor
Department of Anaesthesiology and Critical Care
UCMS and Guru Tegh Bahadur Hospital, Delhi

Purnima Dhar MD
Senior Consultant
Department of Anaesthesia
Apollo Hospital, New Delhi

Namita Kalra BDS, MDS
Professor and Head
Department of Paedodontics and Preventive Dentistry
UCMS and Guru Tegh Bahadur Hospital, Delhi

Amit Khatri BDS, MDS
Assistant Professor
Department of Paedodontics and Preventive Dentistry
UCMS and Guru Tegh Bahadur Hospital, Delhi

Priyanka Khurana MD
Specialist
Department of Anaesthesiology and Critical Care
UCMS and Guru Tegh Bahadur Hospital, Delhi

Anurag Krishna MCh, FAMS
Director
Paediatrics and Paediatric Surgery
Max Institute of Paediatrics
Max Healthcare Institute, New Delhi

Chetan Mehra DNB
Consultant
Department of Anaesthesia
Apollo Hospital, New Delhi

Anup Mohta MS, MCh (Paediatric Surgery), MAMS
Professor and Head
Department of Paediatric Surgery
Director
Chacha Nehru Bal Chikitsalaya (CNBC), New Delhi

Medha Mohta MD, MAMS
Reader
Department of Anaesthesiology and Critical Care
UCMS and Guru Tegh Bahadur Hospital, Delhi

Poonam Motiani MD, DNB, MNAMS
Assistant Professor
Department of Anaesthesia and Critical Care
Delhi State Cancer Institute (DSCI), New Delhi

V Muralidhar MD, MNAMS, FICCM (Fellow, Indian College of Critical Care
Medicine)
Senior Consultant
Department of Anaesthesia
Apollo Hospital, New Delhi

Dilip Pawar MD, DA, FAMS
Former Professor
Department of Anaesthesiology and Intensive Care
All India Institute of Medical Sciences (AIIMS), New Delhi

Hemkumar Pushparajan MD
Senior Resident
Department of Anaesthesiology and Intensive Care
All India Institute of Medical Sciences (AIIMS), New Delhi

Rashmi Salhotra MD
Assistant Professor
Department of Anaesthesiology and Crical Care
UCMS and Guru Tegh Bahadur Hospital, Delhi

Raminder Sehgal MD, DA, FICA
Former Director Professor
Maulana Azad Medical College, New Delhi

Former Senior Consultant
Department of Anaesthesiology, Pain and
Perioperative Medicine
Sir Ganga Ram Hospital, New Delhi

AK Sethi DA, MD
Director Professor and Head
Department of Anaesthesiology and Critical Care
UCMS and Guru Tegh Bahadur Hospital, Delhi

Aparna Sinha MD
Associate Director, Senior Consultant
Department of Anaesthesiology
Institute of Minimal Access, Metabolic and
Bariatric Surgery (MAMBS)
Max Superspecialty Hospital, New Delhi

Renu Sinha MD
Additional Professor
Department of Anaesthesiology and Intensive Care
All India Institute of Medical Sciences (AIIMS), New Delhi

Jayashree Sood MD, FFARCS, PGDHHM, FICA
Senior Consultant and Chairperson
Department of Anaesthesiology, Pain and
Perioperative Medicine
Sir Ganga Ram Hospital, New Delhi

Rajeshwari Subramaniam MD
Professor
Department of Anaesthesiology and Intensive Care
All India Institute of Medical Sciences (AIIMS), New Delhi

Karuna Taneja MD
Former Associate Professor
Department of Radiodiagnosis
All India Institute of Medical Sciences (AIIMS), New Delhi

Senior Consultant
Radiology
Max Superspecialty Hospital, New Delhi

Asha Tyagi MD, DNB, MNAMS
Reader
Department of Anaesthesiology and Critical Care
UCMS and Guru Tegh Bahadur Hospital, Delhi

Rachna Wadhwa MD, MNAMS
Associate Professor
Department of Anaesthesia
Dr BS Ambedkar Medical College, New Delhi

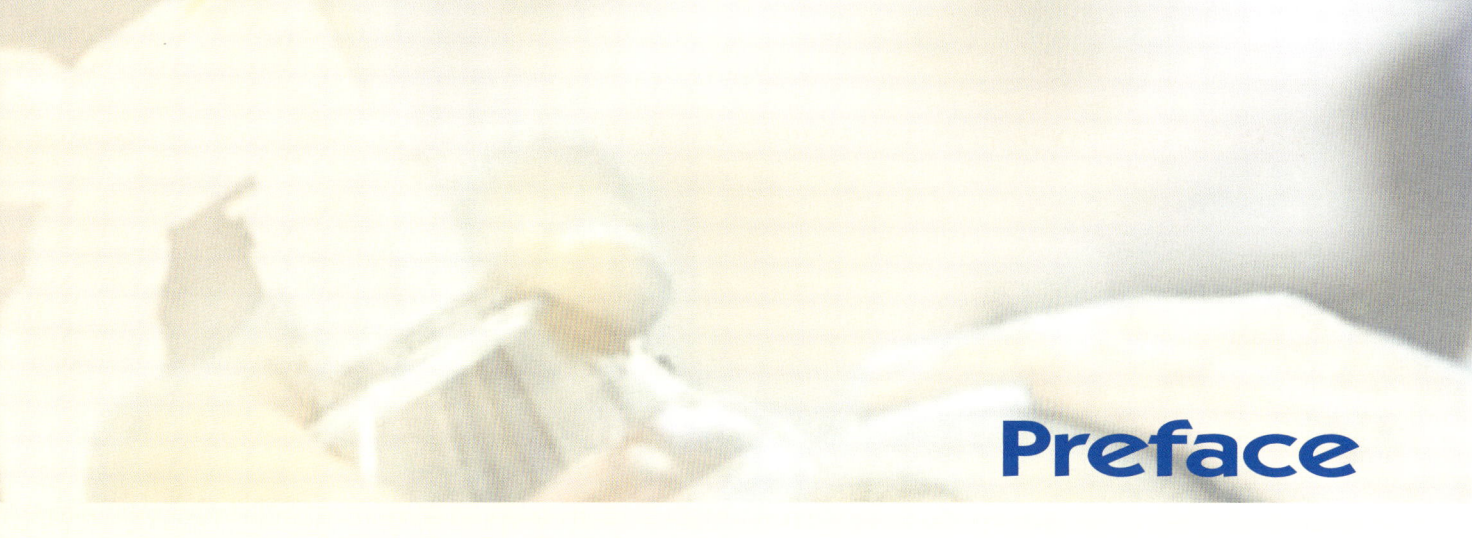

Preface

Providing anaesthesia for children is a well-established and recognized area of anaesthesia practice today. The speciality of paediatric anaesthesia has been steadily evolving to be a superspecialty, with the distinct realization that special knowledge and skills are required in order to provide safe anaesthesia service to this special subset of population, viz. neonates, infants and children.

Globally, more so in India, the paediatric population forms a large chunk of patients requiring surgery and anaesthesia. Paediatric anaesthesia, therefore, forms an integral component of curriculum for postgraduate trainees in anaesthesia, continuing towards higher training and specialization in this field. However, there are only a few centres with dedicated paediatric anaesthesiologists, and it is common to find an anaesthetist who is an occasional paediatric anaesthesiologist. There is thus a need for continuing medical education in the field of paediatric anaesthesia textbooks form an important media for this purpose. Though there are formal textbooks and chapters in books available in the market, we feel that there is a space for a comprehensive, yet holistic guide to safe anaesthesia practice in children. It has been a dream to fill this void, our special interest being the field of paediatric anaesthesia from the very beginning.

This book, *Essentials of Paediatric Anaesthesia and Intensive Care*, addresses not only the basic considerations for a child undergoing surgery, but progresses to some interesting newer areas of anaesthesia giving in children, such as laparoscopic surgery, foetal surgery, child with malignancy, and the child presenting for radiological and dental procedures. A particular section is dedicated to certain aspects of intensive care including organisation of paediatric ICU, the septic child, and the child who has consumed poison.

Certain emergent situations which pose a challenge and require special knowledge and skills, such as neonatal and paediatric resuscitation, child with burns and the child with trauma, form a separate section. All chapters have been contributed by experts in the field of paediatric surgery and anaesthesia, and it has been a privilege and unique experience to compile and edit a book on the subject.

We sincerely hope that this book, will benefit the postgraduate trainees, as also provide an easy guide to the practising anaesthesiologists and teachers in the field.

Sharmila Ahuja
Abhijit Bhattacharya

Acknowledgements

We are immensely grateful to all the contributing authors, most of whom are friends and colleagues with expertise in the field of paediatric anaesthesia, who kindly agreed to extend support in this venture. Their valuable contribution has made the book achieve its present format.

We are very grateful to Prof Rajeshwari Subramaniam and Dr Purnima Dhar for devoting their precious time and support during the initial stages of planning. Both have contributed significant chapters in the section on Basic Considerations for the Child Undergoing Surgery and deserve a special thanks.

Sincere thanks go to Mr YN Arjuna and his team at CBS Publishers & Distributors for their patience, support and perseverance that made the publishing of this book possible; particularly, Mrs Ritu Chawla and her team—Mr Surendra Jha, Mr Ram Murti and Mrs Sunita Rautela, to mention a few.

We are grateful to our family and friends for their unconditional support and encouragement, particularly Dr Aruna Batra, for her guidance and help throughout, specially during the proofreading phase!

Finally, we would like to thank the members of the Department of Anaesthesiology and Critical Care at UCMS and Guru Tegh Bahadur Hospital, Delhi, for their unstinting support and co-operation.

Sharmila Ahuja
Abhijit Bhattacharya

Contents

Anaesthesia in Special Situations

Section 3: Emergent Clinical Situations

Section 4: Intensive Care

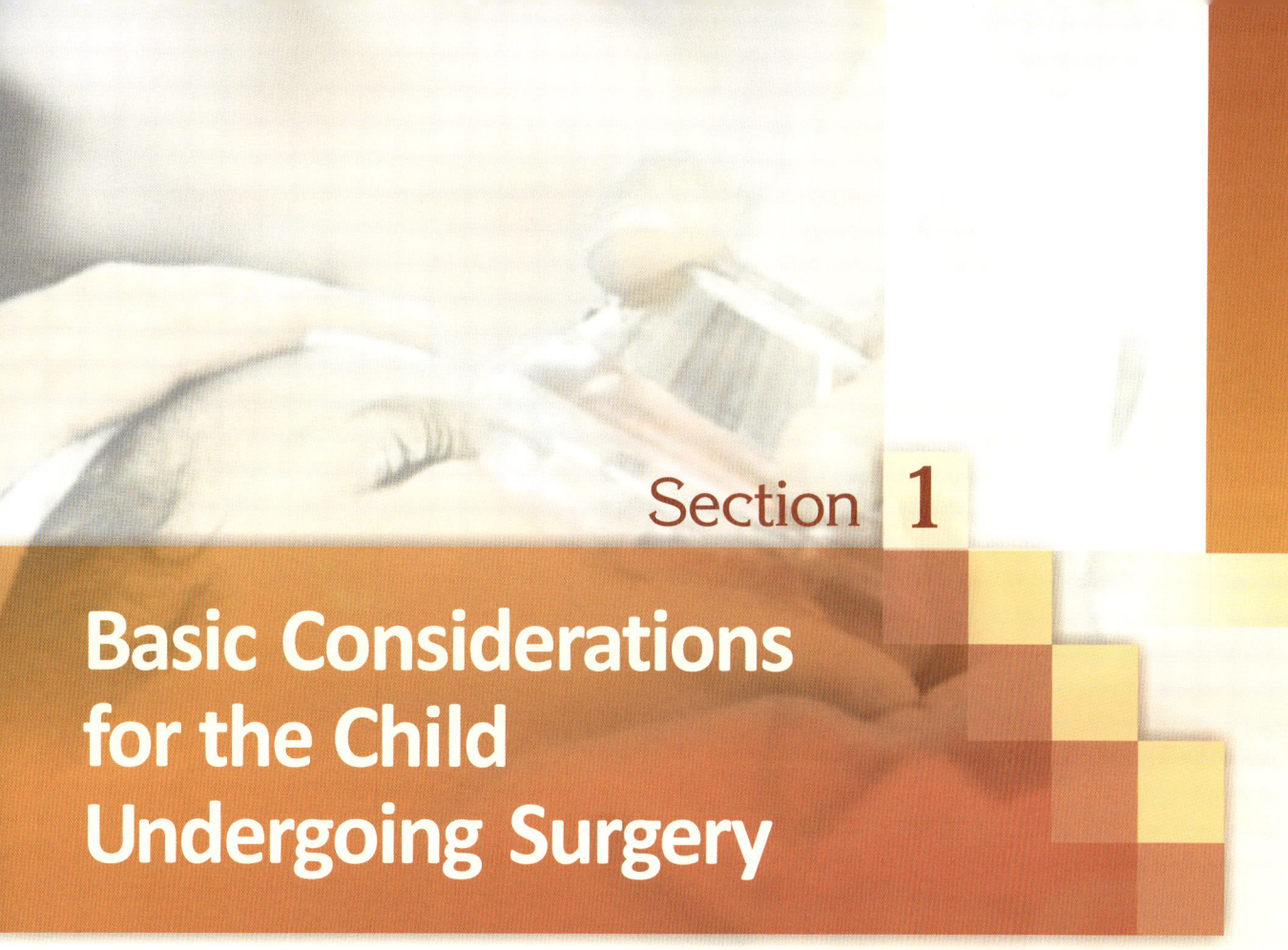

Section 1

Basic Considerations for the Child Undergoing Surgery

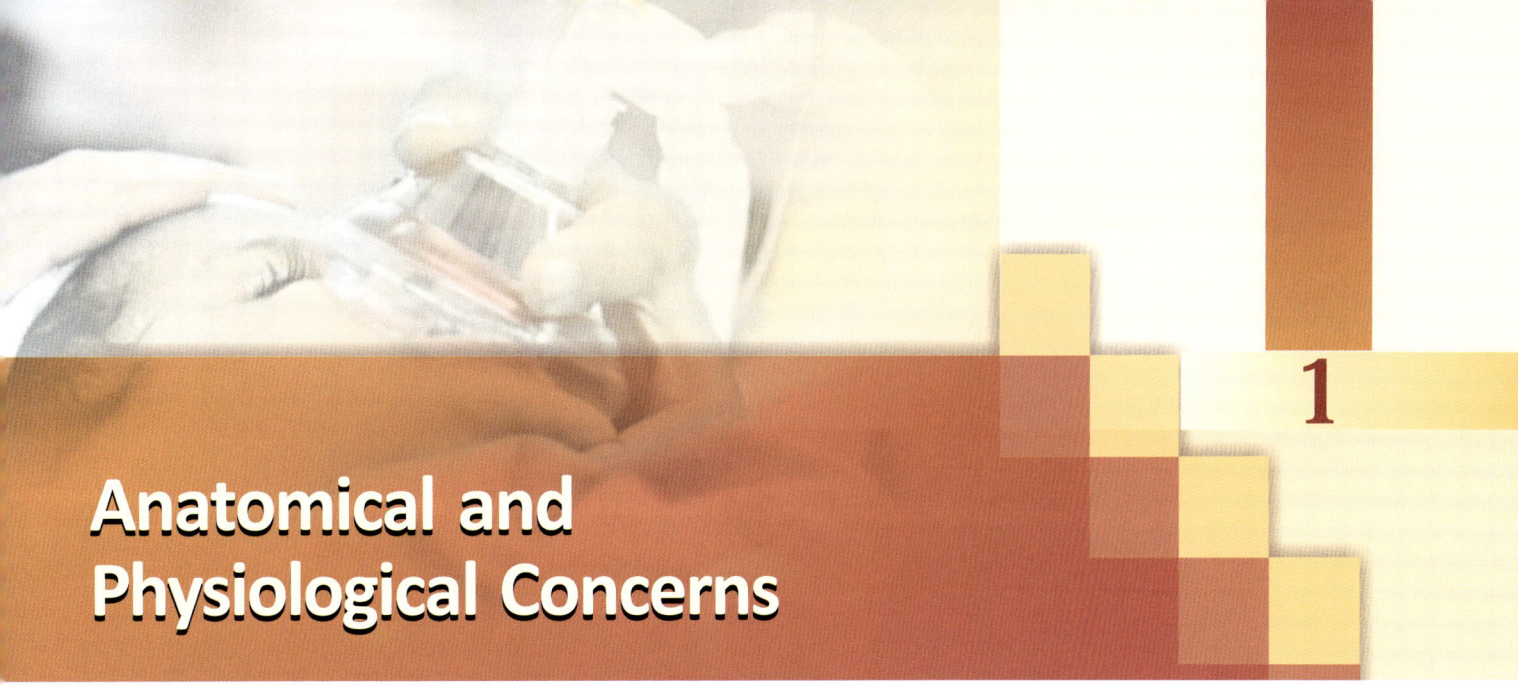

Anatomical and Physiological Concerns

Sharmila Ahuja, Deepti Agarwal

- Respiratory system
- Cardiovascular system
- Renal system
- Hepatobiliary system
- Gastrointestinal system
- Thermoregulation
- Relevant difference in relation to regional anaesthesia

INTRODUCTION

Paediatric anaesthesia requires a special understanding of anatomical, physiological and psychological differences especially in neonates and infants as they differ markedly from adolescents and adults. Apart from the most apparent difference in size, anatomical differences in the airway and physiological differences related to immature function of various organ systems are important factors to anaesthesiologist. Children are also more prone to develop psychological disturbances following hospitalization for anaesthesia and surgery.

These distinctive needs in paediatric patients have resulted in advances in technology leading to special airway devices and adjuncts, monitoring equipment and safer anaesthetics for paediatric anaesthesia safety and quality improvement. Pain services with regional anaesthesia techniques and measures to ease child's adaptation to hospitalization have also become an integral part of paediatric anaesthesia caregiving.

However, technology solely cannot replace continuing education and training for those wishing to be paediatric anaesthesiologist.

A thorough knowledge of the differences in anatomy and physiology is, therefore, an essential component of training for the anaesthesiologist providing anaesthesia services to neonates and children.

RESPIRATORY SYSTEM

Development of Lungs and Thorax

At birth the number of terminal air sacs are only one-tenth that of fully grown lungs. Development of alveoli takes place during first year of life and usually completed by 18 months of life.[1] Lung volumes in infants are small in relation to body size and increases with increase in height and weight. Normal values for lung functions at different ages are shown in Table 1.1.

Due to high metabolic requirement in infants, need for oxygen per unit body weight is higher than adults. Therefore, ventilatory requirement per unit of lung volume is markedly high and they desaturate faster during relatively short duration of apnoea.

In infants, lung compliance is high and so is chest wall compliance due to compliant cartilaginous rib cage. This makes them prone to marked decrease in functional residual capacity (FRC) leading to airway closure, atelectasis, ventilation–perfusion imbalance and hypoxaemia during general anaesthesia.[2]

Table 1.1	Normal values for lung function at various ages				
	Age				
	1 week	**1 year**	**5 years**	**12 years**	**Adult male**
Height (cm)	48	75	109	150	174
Weight (kg)	3.3	10	18	39	73
FRC (ml/kg)	25	26	36	48	42
VC (ml)	100	475	1100	2830	4620
V_T (ml)	17	78	130	260	500
f	30	24	20	16	12
V_D (ml)	75	21	49	105	150
C (ml/cm H_2O)	5	16	44	91	163
Peak flow rates (L/min)	10	–	136	325	457
R (cm H_2O/sec)	29	13	8	5	2
Cardiac output (L/min)	0.9	1.9	3.2	5.7	7.6

FRC–functional residual capacity; VC–vital capacity; V_T–tidal volume; f–respiratory frequency; V_D–dead space volume; C–compliance; R–airway resistance

(From Davis PJ, Cladis FP, Motoyama EK: Smith's Anesthesia for Infants and Children, 8th ed., p. 42. Philadelphia, Elsevier Mosby, 2011.)

A moderate decrease in FRC is seen in older infants more than 6 months of age and in older children. Infants lack adult type I muscle fibres in intercostal muscles and diaphragm and can achieve adult configuration by 2 years of age.[3] They are thus vulnerable to easy fatigability of respiratory muscles and apnoea in the event of increased work of breathing. Further, lack of adult muscle type also explains a higher respiratory rate in infants. Smaller sizes of airway from larynx to the bronchioles provide high airflow resistance, but when corrected for body size, airway size is larger and resistance is lower.[4] However, absolute small size of airway makes this group of patients susceptible to airway obstruction with relatively mild airway inflammation, oedema or secretions.

Because of a greater fall of FRC under anaesthesia in children, uneven distribution of ventilation and increased physiological dead space a tidal volume of 10 to 15 ml/kg is practical. Respiratory frequency of 20 to 30 breaths per minute in infants, 14 to 20 breaths per minute in children with a inspiratory to expiratory ratio of 1:2 aided by capnography is suggested. A low level of PEEP (positive end expiratory pressure) may help in preventing airway closure.

In neonates, affinity of haemoglobin to oxygen is high and P_{50} is low due to low 2,3-DPG and lower affinity of fetal haemoglobin for 2,3-DPG. After birth, total haemoglobin level decreases and P_{50} increases (highest at 10 months of age), therefore, lower haemoglobin levels are efficient in terms of oxygen delivery in infants and children.

Control of Breathing

The chemical and neural control of breathing in older infants and children are similar to adults. However, in premature infants and neonates, response to hypoxaemia and hypercapnia is not well developed as adults. Premature infants younger than 44 weeks postconceptual age are more prone to postoperative apnoea and postoperative hypoxaemia.[5]

Anatomical Differences in Upper Airway

Neonates have a relatively large-sized head, hypoplastic mandible and a large tongue. Size of tongue in relation to oropharynx can cause technical difficulty during laryngoscopy. Pharyngeal airway is protected from getting collapsed by the tonic activity of pharyngeal and laryngeal muscles. This tonic activity of the muscles, if depressed under sedation or paralysis, leads to airway narrowing and easy collapse of pharyngeal airway especially at the level of soft palate and base of tongue. In children, larynx is placed more cephalic in the neck; epiglottis is more angled over the laryngeal inlet, is large in size and difficult to manipulate; and vocal cords are placed at an angle (Fig. 1.1).[6,7] These differences cause difficulties in

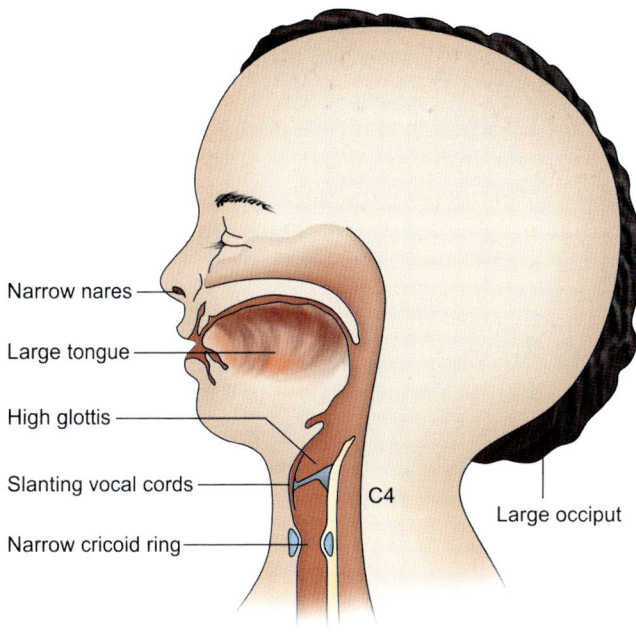

Fig. 1.1. Upper airway anatomical differences in paediatric patients

Narrow nares

Large tongue

High glottis

Slanting vocal cords

Narrow cricoid ring

C4

Large occiput

laryngoscopy and intubation and require special anatomical facemasks and laryngoscopes. Infants are considered obligate nasal breathers but most of them can convert to oral breathing after 5 months of age.

It was considered that paediatric larynx is funnel-shaped with the cricoid ring (laryngeal exit) being the narrowest point. It is in contrast to adult's larynx which is cylindrical in shape (Fig. 1.2).[6,7]

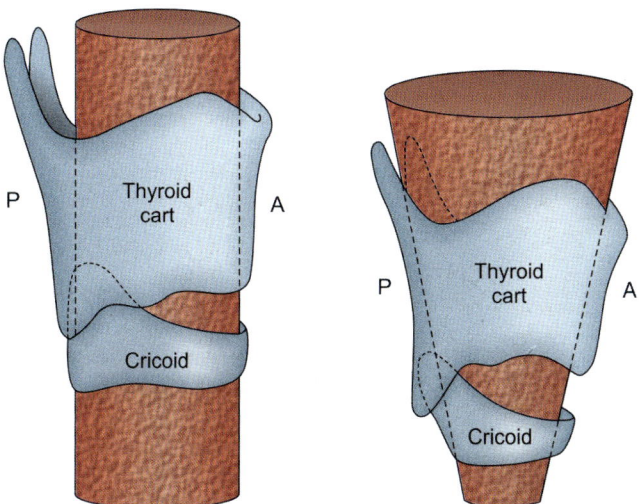

P

Thyroid cart

A

Cricoid

P

Thyroid cart

A

Cricoid

Fig. 1.2. Funnel-shaped larynx of infant on right compared to the cylindrical shape of the adult larynx on the left.

Recent studies have demonstrated that subglottis is the narrowest portion in majority of adults but it is so large that it is possible to pass a routine endotracheal tube beyond this.[8] In infants and children, however, due to greater proportional narrowing at cricoids, a tube may exert unwanted pressure on the mucosa of subglottic area. Thus uncuffed tubes were generally used in children younger than 6 years. Tubes with newer soft material and a more distally placed cuff which can pass beyond cricoid are available[9] and have allowed use of cuffed endotracheal tube possible even in infants.[10]

CARDIOVASCULAR SYSTEM

Transitional Circulation

At birth, lung inflation reduces pulmonary vascular resistance (PVR) and leads to increase in pulmonary blood flow. Cord clamping removes the low resistance placental circulation and results in increase in systemic vascular resistance. Alteration in the resistances in the cardiovascular system changes the pattern of blood flow through the three important shunts making fetal parallel type circulation to adult series type of circulation. Constriction and closure of ductus venosus occurs. Left atrial pressure exceeds the right atrial pressure closing the flap of tissue covering foramen ovale. Though functional closure of foramen ovale occurs at birth, anatomical closure occurs between 3 months and 1 year of age. Closure of ductus arteriosus proceeds slowly, functional closure takes place within 10–15 hours of birth but anatomically it takes 1–3 months to occlude. This postnatal circulation is a transitional circulation because closure of ductus arteriosus and foramen ovale is reversible during first days and weeks of life. Pain, crying and factors increasing pulmonary vascular resistance, like, hypoxia, hypercarbia, acidosis, hypothermia and lung diseases, increase right atrial pressure resulting in right to left shunting.

Pulmonary Vascular Resistance

Pulmonary vascular resistance decreases at birth after initiation of first breath. It reaches adult value by 2 months of age and remodelling process is complete by 6 months of age. PVR can be manipulated for therapeutic use in newborns with congenital heart diseases. Combination of a high inspired FiO_2, a PO_2 higher than 60 mm Hg, a $PaCO_2$ of 30 to 35 mm Hg, a pH of 7.50 to 7.60, and low inspiratory pressures without high levels of PEEP can produce decrease in PVR.

Myocardial Function

Myocardium in newborn is structurally and functionally immature. Ventricles are less compliant resulting in limited ability of neonatal heart to increase stroke volume by Frank–Starling law. Neonates have difficulty maintaining cardiac output with increased afterload and increase in preload causes little or no change in cardiac output.[11] By 6 months and certainly by 1 year of age, infants start responding to changes in preload, afterload, contractility and heart rate in adult manner. Increase in cardiac output remains rate-dependent during first 2 years of life[12] when myocardial remodelling occurs to reach adult configuration. Haemodynamic variables in children are shown in Table 1.2.

Newborn has a high cardiac output (180–240 ml/kg/minute) which is 2 to 3 times that of adult due to their high metabolic need. Autonomic innervation is incompletely developed at birth, though parasympathetic innervation is fully functional, sympathetic innervation is incompletely matured.

Baroreceptor sensitivity increases from birth to 6 weeks of age,[13] anaesthetic agents, like inhalational agents[14] or fentanyl,[15] can aggravate the relative insensitivity of the baroreceptor response in neonates.

RENAL SYSTEM

Kidney size and renal blood flow increases gradually after birth. GFR averages 40.6 ±14.8 ml/min per 1.73 m^2 in a full term neonate, by second postnatal week increases to 65.8 ±24.8 ml/min per 1.73 m^2 and reaches adult value by 2 years of age.[16]

At birth, kidney's ability to concentrate urine is not fully developed, even after water deprivation, neonates are not able to concentrate urine and urine osmolality achieved is less than adult values under similar condition. This has been attributed to immaturity and hypotonicity of medulla.[17] Also collecting ducts are less sensitive to antidiuretic hormone in neonates. Urine diluting capacity of neonatal kidneys matures by 3 to 5 weeks of birth.[17]

A term infant is able to conserve sodium despite a low GFR. However, a premature infant due to glomerulotubular imbalance is not able to do so and is prone to hyponatremia. Tubular function matures slowly by 12 to 18 months of age.[18]

HEPATOBILIARY SYSTEM

The neonate has less than 20% of the hepatocytes that are present in the adult liver, and liver growth continues until it reaches its mature size. It is roughly 4% of body weight at birth and when fully developed takes up 2.5–3.5% of body weight. As the infant grows, hepatic blood flow increases.

Liver is not functionally mature and is not capable to handle drugs in an adult manner. Some cytochrome P450 systems are mature at birth but others develop and are induced slowly after birth.[19,20] Phase II reactions are also impaired and may take a year to fully mature. Neonates have minimal glycogen stores and are prone to hypoglycaemia.

Table 1.2	Circulatory variables in infants and children				
Age	Heart rate (bpm)	Systolic blood pressure (mm Hg)	Diastolic blood pressure (mm Hg)	Cardiac index (L/min/m^2)	Oxygen consumption (ml/kg/min)
Preterm	150 ± 20	50 ± 3	30 ± 3	–	8 ± 1.4
Term	133 ± 18	73 ± 8	50 ± 8	2.5 ± 0.6	6 ± 1.0
6 months	120 ± 20	89 ± 29	60 ± 10	2.0 ± 0.5	5 ± 0.9
1 year	120 ± 20	96 ± 30	66 ± 25	2.5 ± 0.6	5.2 ± 0.1
2 years	105 ± 25	99 ± 25	64 ± 25	3.1 ± 0.7	6.4 ± 1.2
5 years	90 ± 10	94 ± 14	55 ± 9	3.7 ± 0.9	6.0 ± 1.1
12 years	70 ± 17	109 ± 16	58 ± 9	4.3 ± 1.1	3.3 ± 0.6
Young adult	75 ± 5	122 ± 30	75 ± 20	3.7 ± 0.3	3.4 ± 0.6

(From Katz J, Steward DJ: Anesthesia and Uncommon Diseases, 2nd edn., Philadelphia: W.B.Saunders,1993;p.5).

GASTROINTESTINAL SYSTEM

Gastric pH is alkalotic at birth. By the second day of life, pH is in the normal physiologic range as adults. The volume and acid concentration of the gastric fluid reaches the lower limit of adult value by 3 months of age and attains adult value by 2 years of age.[21] Peristalsis in the distal third of oesophagus is not as developed as in adults. Approximately, 40% of newborns will regurgitate and peristalsis may take several months to mature.[22] Newborns are thus susceptible to gastrointestinal reflux.

THERMOREGULATION

The combination of increase in heat loss from the body due to various factors, reduced efficacy of thermo-regulatory responses and less ability to produce heat make infants vulnerable to hypothermia. Large skin surface area to body mass ratio in preterm and term infants causes more heat loss than adults during anaesthesia. They have a thin layer of subcutaneous fat and reduced keratin content in skin, predisposing them to further heat loss through the process of conduction and evaporation. In addition, they have relatively large size of head, skin of the head makes up to 20% of total skin surface area.[23] This can account for up to 85% of body heat loss from the highly perfused brain through thin skull bones and sparse scalp hair.[24]

The ambient neutral temperature at which oxygen demand is minimal and temperature regulation can be done by physical process of vasoconstriction is 32°C to 35°C in neonates and 28°C in adults.[25] Thus active heat producing processes need to be invoked earlier as body temperature falls in infants than adults.

Heat generation is done by various processes, of which nonshivering thermogenesis is the main mechanism in infants while shivering thermogenesis by involuntary muscle activity is used in older children and adults. Nonshivering thermogenesis becomes less effective after first year of life when shivering thermogenesis takes over and becomes the most important mechanism of heat production. Nonshivering thermogenesis is metabolic heat production above basal metabolism in brown fat and to a lesser degree in white fat, by fatty acid metabolism and causes diversion of a high percentage of cardiac output through brown fat. This mechanism is active within hours after birth and can continue up to 2 years of age.[26] It can be inhibited by inhalational anaesthetics, intravenous agents, like propofol and fentanyl, β-receptor blockade or by sympathectomy.[27,28] Though it is the main source of heat production, the effects are restricted beyond a certain limit.

During anaesthesia and surgery, various factors predispose infants and children to hypothermia in addition to the fact that general anaesthesia also reduces the threshold for cold defence. Hypothermia can lead to hypoventilation or apnoea, anaesthetic overdose, metabolic acidosis, may exacerbate pre-existing cardiopulmonary pathology and can have adverse effects on immune function. Thus maintaining body temperature by active or passive warming, e.g. warming the operating room, placing the baby on warming mattress, keeping babies covered and use of humidified inspiratory gases, is vital part of anaesthetic management in children.

RELEVANT DIFFERENCE IN RELATION TO REGIONAL ANAESTHESIA

Regional anaesthesia is an integral part of peri-operative pain management in paediatric patients. With the advent of ultrasound imaging techniques, precise deposition of drug in the vicinity of nerve and reduced volume of local anaesthetic required, thereby reducing the toxicity, has further boosted the use of regional anaesthesia in this subset of patients.[29] Studies have shown that risk of complications with regional anaesthesia is low and preventable in children.[30,31]

General Considerations

Myelination of nerve fibres is incomplete at birth, thus local anaesthetics can easily penetrate nerve fibres and onset time for block is fast. Because of the same reason, dilute solutions of local anaesthetics produce same degree of block as undiluted solutions. Duration of action, however, is short due to greater vascular absorption of local anaesthetic.

Bones in neonates are mainly cartilaginous and ossification of nuclei can be easily damaged with sharp needles. Hence it is imperative to use short bevelled needles and avoid bone contact while performing a block.

Perineurovascular sheaths are loosely attached to underlying nerves, muscles, vessels, etc. This results in increased spread of small volume of local anaesthetic along the nerve path producing excellent blocks

Table 1.3	Some important factors influencing regional anaesthesia in children
Factors	**Implications**
Incomplete myelination of nerve fibres	Concentration of local anaesthetic needs to be adjusted
Termination of spinal cord at a lower level	Epidural blocks above L3 to be avoided
Projection of dural sac at lower level	Risk of inadvertent dural puncture Check for CSF reflux even during caudal block
Delayed fusion of sacral vertebrae	Sacral epidural more successful till age of 6–8 years
Increased fluidity of epidural fat	Large volume of local anaesthetic required as it diffuses along nerves
Delayed maturity of enzymatic pathways	Slower metabolism of local anaesthetics Risk of accumulation following repeat injections
Higher heart rate and cardiac output	Increased systemic absorption of local anaesthetic—shorter duration Higher efficacy of epinephrine
Sympathetic immaturity	Haemodynamic stability during regional blocks Fluid preloading and vasoconstrictors not required

but with the disadvantage of spreading to other anatomical spaces and distant nerves.

Central Neuraxial Blocks

At birth, there is single flexure of spine, cervical lordosis develops by 3 to 6 months and lumbar lordosis by 8 to 9 months. Thus orientation of epidural needle remains same for all epidural spaces till 6 months of age.

In a newborn, the spinal cord ends at the L3 or L4 level while dura mater ends at S3 or S4 vertebrae, they get placed to adult level of L1 and S2 respectively only after first year of life. Epidural should be avoided above L3 level to avoid injury to spinal cord and caudal epidural should be carefully attempted as there are high chances of dural puncture while performing it. Line joining anterior superior iliac spine passes at L5 or lower in infants instead of L4–L5 in adults.[32]

Because of delayed fusion of sacral vertebrae, sacral route for epidural block is possible in children. After the age of 6–8 years, identification of sacral hiatus becomes difficult, hence caudal blocks becomes less successful.

The fact that epidural fat is very fluid up to 6–7 years of life and local anaesthetics also spread and diffuse along the spinal nerves, large volume of local anaesthetic is required for desired level of epidural block.

Local Anaesthetics

Doses and volume of local anaesthetics should be carefully decided as immaturity of liver enzymes and low plasma protein content lead to drug toxicity and drug accumulation particularly after repeated or continuous injections.[33,34] Increased regional blood flow in children increases systemic absorption of local anaesthetics and increased efficacy of adrenaline in prolonging local anaesthetic duration. Sympathetic immaturity, however, maintains haemodynamic parameters in children during neuraxial blocks (Table 1.3).[35]

CONCLUSION

Differences in anatomy and physiology in various organ systems, particularly in the respiratory and cardiovascular systems, amongst patients in paediatric age group, particularly neonates, have been well recognised. The implications of these differences have been clearly outlined, leading to advances in technology and understanding of safe practices, thereby improving the level of care and safety while providing anaesthesia services to this subset of patients.

REFERENCES

1. Langston C, Kida K, Reed M, et al. Human lung growth in late gestation and in the neonate. Am Rev R Respir Dis 1984;129:607.

2. von Ungern-Sternberg BS, Hammer J, Schibler A, et al. Decrease of functional residual capacity and ventilation homogeneity after neuromuscular blockade in anesthetized young infants and preschool children. Anesthesiology 2006;105:670–675.

3. Keens TG, Bryan AC, Levison H, Ianzzo CD. Developmental pattern of muscle fibre types in human ventilator muscles. J Appl Physiol 1978;44:909–913.

4. Stocks J, Godfrey S. Specific airway conductance in relation to postconceptional age during infancy. J Appl Physiol 1977;43:144–154.

5. Cote CJ, Zaslavsky A, Downes JJ, et al. Postoperative apnea in former preterm infants after inguinal herniorrhaphy. Anesthesiology 1995;82:809–822.

6. Eckenhoff JE. Some anatomic considerations of the infant larynx influencing endotracheal anesthesia. Anesthesiology 1951;12:401–410.

7. Berry FA. Anatomy and physiology of the infant. In: Anaesthetic Management of Difficult and Routine Paediatric Patients, 2nd edn. New York: Churchill Livingstone, 1990; p127.

8. Seymour AH, Prakash N. A cadaver study to measure the adult glottis and subglottis: Defining a problem associated with the use of double- lumen tubes. J Cardiothorac Vasc Anesth 2002;16:196–198.

9. Ho AM, Aun CS, Karmakar MK. The margin of safety associated with the use of cuffed paediatric endotracheal tubes. Anaesthesia 2002;57:173–175.

10. Bernet V, Dullenkopf A, Maino P, Weiss M. Outer diameter and shape of paediatric tracheal tube cuffs at higher inflation pressures. Anaesthesia 2005;60:1123–1128.

11. Gilbert RD. Control of fetal cardiac output during changes in blood volume. Am J Physiol 1980;238:H80–H86.

12. Friedman W, George B. Treatment of congestive heart failure by altering loading conditions of heart. J Pediatr 1985;106:697–706.

13. Patton D, Hanna B. Postnatal maturation of baroreflex heart rate control in neonatal swine. Can J Cardiol 1994; 10:233–238.

14. Murat I, Lapeyre G, Saint-Maurice C. Isoflurane attenuates baroreflex control of heart rate in human neonates. Anesthesiology 1989;70:395–400.

15. Murat I, Levron J. Effects of fentanyl on baroreceptor reflex control of heart rate in newborn infants. Anesthesiology 1988;68:717–722.

16. Schwartz GJ, Brion LP, Spitzer A. The use of plasma creatinine concentration for estimating glomerular filtration rate in infants, children, and adolescents. Pediatr Clin North Am 1987;34:571–590.

17. Aperia A, Zetterstrom R. Renal control of fluid homeostasis in the newborn infant. Clin Perinatol 1982;9: 523–533.

18. Spitzer A. Renal physiology and functional development, In: Edelmann CM Jr, Boston, Little (Eds). Pediatric Kidney Disease, 1st edn. Brown and Co. 1978; p25–128.

19. Jacqz-Aigrain E, Cresteil T. Cytochrome P450- dependent metabolism of dextromethorphan: Fetal and adult studies. Dev Pharmacol Ther 1992;18:161–168.

20. Ward RM, Mirkin BL. Perinatal/neonatal pharmacology. In: Brody TM, Larner J, Minnerman KP (Eds). Human Pharmacology: Molecular-to-Clinical, 3rd edn. St Louis: Mosby-Year Book, 1998; p873–883.

21. Agunod M, Yomaguchi N, Lopez R, et al. Correlative study of hydrochloric acid, pepsin and intrinsic factor secretion in newborns and infants. Am J Dig Dis 1969;14:400–414.

22. Winter H, Grand R. Gastroesophageal reflux. Pediatrics 1981;68:134–136.

23. Anttonen H, Puhakka K, Niskanen J, Ryhanen P. Cutaneous heat loss in children during anaesthesia. Br J Anaesth 1995;74:306–310.

24. Fleming PJ, Azaz Y, Wiqfield R. Development of thermoregulation in infancy: possible implications for SIDS. J Clin Pathol 1992;45:17–19.

25. Hey EN. Thermal neutrality. Br Med Bull 1975;31:69–74.

26. Oya A, Asakura H, Koshino T, Araki T. Thermographic demonstration of non-shivering thermogenesisin human new-born after birth: its relation to umblical gases. J Pernatal Med 1997;25:447–454.

27. Ohlson KBE, Mohell N, Cannon B, et al. Thermogenesis in brown adipocytes is inhibited by volatile anesthtic agents. A factor contributing to hypothermia in infants? Anesthesiology 1994;81:176–183.

28. Plattner O, Semsroth M, Sessler DI, et al. Lack of nonshivering thermogenesis in infants anesthetized with fentanyl and propofol. Anesthesiology 1997;86:772–777.

29. Rubin K, Sullivan D, Sadhasivam S. Are peripheral and neuraxial blocks with ultrasound guidance more effective and safe in children? Paediatr Anaesth 2009;19:92–96.

30. Giaufre E, Dalens B, Gombert A. Epidemiology and morbidity of regional anesthesia in children: A one-year prospective survey of the French-language society of pediatric anesthesiologists. Anesth Analg 1996;83: 904–912.

31. Dalens BJ, Mazoit JX. Adverse effects of regional anaesthesia in children. Drug Saf 1998;19:251–268.

32. Busoni P, Messeri A. Spinal anesthesia in children: surface anatomy. Anesth Analg 1989;68:418–419.

33. Lerman J, Strong HA, LeDez KM, et al. Effects of age on the serum concentration of alpha-1 acid glycoprotein and the binding of lidocaine in pediatric patients. Clin Pharm Ther 1989;46:219–225.

34. Berde C. Convulsions associated with pediatric regional anesthesia. Anesth Analg 1992;75:164–166.

35. Dohi S, Seino H. Spinal anesthesia in premature infants: Dosage and effects of sympathectomy. Anesthesiology 1986;65:559–561.

2

Applied Pharmacology of Drugs Used in Perioperative Period

Sharmila Ahuja, Deepti Agarwal

- ■ **Factors affecting pharmacokinetics of drugs**
  - ● **Alteration in body composition**
  - ● **Protein binding**
  - ● **Hepatic and renal function maturity**
  - ● **Immature blood–brain barrier**
  - ● **Alterations in absorption of drugs by various routes**
- ■ **Intravenous anaesthetics**
- ■ **Inhalational agents**
- ■ **Neuromuscular blocking and reversal agents**
- ■ **Opioids**
- ■ **Sedatives and analgesics**
- ■ **Local anaesthetics and adjuvants**
- ■ **Miscellaneous drugs**

INTRODUCTION

In paediatric age group, pharmacological profile of drugs is different from adults. After birth, there are large changes in the physiological systems and they mature at varying rates during the initial years of life. The alterations occur in body weight and constitution, functioning and maturity of organ systems, and number, affinity and type of receptors. The variations in physiological processes are even more profound in premature neonates or in those with congenital malformations. These changes influence the pharmacokinetics and pharmacodynamics of a drug and hence the final achieved drug effect. Because of these physiological differences, pharmacological considerations applicable in adults or older children may not be appropriate for the younger patients and produce a need for age-dependent adjustments in doses.[1] Hence it is vital to understand the developmental pharmacology of neonates, infants and children.

The difference in pharmacokinetics, like absorption, distribution, metabolism and elimination of various drugs in paediatric patients, is influenced by body composition, protein binding, functional maturity of liver and kidney, cardiac output distribution, body temperature and maturation of blood–brain barrier. Apart from pharmacokinetic differences, changes at the receptor level cause age-related differences in pharmacodynamics.

FACTORS AFFECTING PHARMACOKINETICS OF DRUGS

Alteration in Body Composition

Paediatric patients have high total body water content especially in neonates which constitutes 85% of the body weight in the preterm neonate and 75% in term neonates. At five months of age, this decreases to approximately 60% and from this age onwards remains relatively constant.[4] Thus water-soluble drugs will have a greater volume of distribution in the neonate, so they may require a high initial loading dose per kilogram body weight to achieve effective plasma concentration compared to the older child.

Muscle and fat content as a proportion of total body mass is smaller in neonates as compared to older children. Fat contributes 3% of the body weight in a 1.5 kg premature neonate and 12% in a term neonate; this proportion doubles by 4–5 months of age. Protein mass increases from 20% in term neonate, to 50% in adult.

Therefore, anaesthetic drugs undergoing redistribution in adipose tissue and muscles have longer duration of action.

Protein Binding

Paediatric patients have low concentration of serum albumin and further, albumin has lower binding capacity and affinity for drugs in this subset of patients. Some substances found in plasma may further reduce protein binding in newborns, viz. bilirubin, fatty acids and maternal steroids. Neonates have low alpha one acid glycoprotein in blood to which basic drugs tend to bind. The reduced quantity and quality of protein binding has an effect on the concentration of 'free' active drug as well as its ability to cross membranes. It is of particular importance in those drugs given parenterally which are highly protein bound, have a high extraction ratio and a narrow therapeutic index.[5] The concentration of plasma protein and binding capacity reaches adult values by 1 year of age.

Hepatic and Renal Function Maturity

The cytochrome P450 system is responsible for phase I metabolism of drugs. Many cytochrome P450 isoforms are approximately 50% mature at birth thus reducing the ability of neonates to metabolize lipophilic drugs. However, some other cytochrome systems have been shown to be present at adult values at birth. Phase II metabolism is responsible for biotransformation to render the drug more polar for elimination through conjugation reactions, such as glucuronidation, sulfation and acetylation. Phase II reactions are often impaired in neonates resulting in longer half lives of drugs, like morphine and benzodiazepines. These reactions attain adult values by 1 year of age.[6]

Neonates and preterm infants have markedly diminished renal function due to immature glomerular and tubular function. Glomerular filtration rate reaches 80% of adult value by 6 months of age and proximal tubular secretion reaches adult levels by 7 months of age,[7] however, complete maturation of renal function takes place by 2 years of age. Therefore, neonates and preterm babies have a poor ability to handle water and solute loads. Drugs excreted via glomerular filtration will have longer half lives in neonates.

With maturity of end organ functions in older children and attainment of body composition similar to adults, with higher hepatic and renal blood flow, most medications have shortened half lives in children older than 2 years which lengthens as they approach adulthood.[8]

Immature Blood–Brain Barrier

The neonatal brain is relatively large and receives a higher percentage of the cardiac output (25%) compared to the adult. The blood–brain barrier (BBB) is the lipid membrane interface between the endothelial cells of the brain blood vessels and the extracellular fluid of the brain and is postulated to be immature in the neonate and premature babies. Therefore, drugs which are relatively water insoluble (e.g. morphine) can reach the central nervous system easily and cause respiratory depression even after small doses. Fentanyl on the other hand is more lipid-soluble and, therefore, the effect of a maturing BBB has less of an impact on its ability to reach the brain. However, respiratory depression caused by morphine has been attributed to other differences in pharmacokinetics also.[9] Developmental differences in BBB and drug transport, however, are not fully understood.

Alteration in Absorption of Drugs by Various Routes

Paediatric patients receive most anaesthetic drugs via intravenous route apart from other less common routes of administration, like oral, rectal, intramuscular and transdermal. Oral absorption of drugs is slower in neonates and infants up to 6–8 months of age due to delayed gastric emptying and slower intestinal motility.[10] Small, lipid-soluble unionized molecules with favourable dissolution characteristics in gastric fluid are better absorbed than larger ionized molecules. The gastric acid secretion is decreased and intragastric pH is elevated in neonates making absorption of many drugs variable in this group. In addition, the ability to solubilize and absorb lipophilic drugs can be influenced by age-dependent changes in biliary function.

Absorption through rectal route is also variable. Contents and formulation of rectal drug, rectal contractions and depth of rectal insertion, all affect absorption and relative bioavailability.

Factors, like reduced skeletal-muscle blood flow and inefficient muscular contractions, reduce rate of intramuscular absorption of drugs, this is offset by the relatively higher density of skeletal-muscle capillaries in infants than in older children resulting in increased absorption of intramuscular drugs in neonates and infants.

Neonates have a larger relative skin surface area, increased cutaneous perfusion and thinner stratum corneum which increase absorption of topically applied drugs. This can result in harm particularly with repeat dosing of drugs, like lidocaine-prilocaine cream (EMLA).[11] The higher ratio of total body surface area to body mass in infants and young children also affects drug absorption through these routes. Intrapulmonary route is sometimes used as an alternative emergency route for drug delivery in newborns. Drug deposition and systemic absorption after the intrapulmonary administration of a drug depends on developmental changes in the anatomy of the lung and its ventilatory capacity.

The bioavailability through transmucosal, oral or nasal routes has been found to be higher in children when compared to adults, e.g. fentanyl when given as lozenges is rapidly absorbed. The dose, therefore, needs to be adjusted accordingly.

In younger age groups, the greater fraction of the cardiac output distribution to the vessel-rich tissue group and the lower tissue/blood solubility affect the onset time of inhaled anaesthetic gases and vapours and is generally more rapid in infants than in adults. Solubility plays considerable role on the uptake of inhalational agents in children. The solubility in blood of inhalation agents is 18% less in neonates than in adults while the solubility in the vessel-rich tissue group is approximately one-half of those in adults[12] due to the greater water content and decreased protein and lipid concentration in neonatal tissues. Solubility of the less-soluble agents, such as nitrous oxide, is a little affected by age.

INTRAVENOUS ANAESTHETICS

Propofol

Propofol is a highly lipophilic drug, its rapid onset and short duration of action makes it a useful induction agent in paediatric age group. As compared to thiopentone, elimination half-life is shorter and clearance is faster, thereby resulting in faster and more clear-headed recovery after single induction dose.

In infants, the volume of distribution is high and clearance is in a maturing phase. Clearance is only 10% that of the mature value at 28 weeks gestation and 38% at term. Term neonates will achieve 90% of an adult clearance (1.83 L min^{-1} 70 kg^{-1}) by 30 weeks after birth.[13] Younger children have larger systemic clearance values than adult and older children. In children older than 3 years, volumes and clearance should be weight adjusted.[14]

Due to variation in pharmacokinetic variables, requirement of propofol in children is greater than adults and varies among children of different age. Induction dose of propofol in children less than 2 years is 2.9 mg/kg and 2.2 mg/kg for children aged 6–12 years. Introduction of elaborate delivery systems, advances in microprocessor technology and increased complexity of pharmacokinetic modelling have resulted in use of propofol especially in children for total intravenous anaesthesia (TIVA) and further to target controlled infusions (TCI).

Propofol is useful for brief and repeated sedation in children undergoing radiological procedures, radiotherapy and during transport from one care giving unit to another. It should be used with caution in children with defects in lipid metabolism as it may cause propofol infusion syndrome[15] and in children with history of egg allergy.[16]

Thiopentone

In neonates, there is a reduced requirement of thiopentone as compared to infants 1 to 6 months of age due to lower body fat and muscle content, decreased protein binding and greater penetration in brain despite a large volume of distribution. Elimination half-life is also longer as compared to older children. Children have a significantly high cardiac output and a rapid rate of total clearance of thiopentone, thus half-life is short as compared to adults.

Induction dose of thiopentone for infants is 7–8 mg/kg and for children is 5–6 mg/kg, however, dose should be reduced to 4–5 mg/kg in neonates and malnourished children. A 10% solution of thiopentone may be administered rectally in dose of 30 mg/kg.[8]

Ketamine

Ketamine, a phencyclidine, possesses potent analgesic property and unlike most induction agents usually does not depress cardiovascular and respiratory systems.[17] Ketamine is available as a mixture of two enantiomers—the S(+)-enantiomer has four times the potency of the R(–)-enantiomer. Clearance in the neonate is reduced while it becomes similar to adult rates within the first 6 months of life, when corrected for size using allometric models.

It produces number of adverse effects and hence indicated in specific situations. Ketamine is frequently chosen for anaesthetic induction in patients with cyanotic conditions, as it increases systemic vascular resistance and cardiac output and does not worsen right to left shunting. It is useful for induction of anaesthesia in hypovolemic children. Ketamine has also been commonly used in a dose of 2 mg/kg intravenously or 4–5 mg/kg intramuscularly in children undergoing various procedures. Emergence reactions are probably not affected by midazolam in children, but their incidence is low.[18] An anti-sialagogue may be required to diminish copious secretions.

INHALATIONAL AGENTS

Infants and toddlers have a high cardiac index, high respiratory rate, a greater proportion of cardiac output distribution to vessel-rich tissues and low tissue/blood solubility for inhalational agents. This results in faster uptake of volatile anaesthetics and a higher minimum alveolar concentration (MAC) requirement in children. On the other hand, young children, particularly neonates and infants, are also prone to overdose because of functional immaturity of cardiac development.[8] MAC requirement is lower in neonates as compared to infants and may be related to immaturity of brain.

Sevoflurane

Sevoflurane is useful for inhalational induction of anaesthesia and is considered better or equivalent to halothane for this purpose as it is less pungent. Sevoflurane has lower blood solubility than halothane, it produces rapid induction and recovery. It has a MAC of 3.3% for neonates, 3.2% for infants 6 months old and 2.5% for children older than 6 months of age.[19,20]

When compared with halothane, sevoflurane causes rapid induction and fewer incidences of coughing during induction. Sevoflurane produces lesser airway complications during induction compared to halothane but usually leads to higher incidence of excitement during emergence. It produces dose related respiratory depression; it decreases both tidal volume and respiratory rate and respiration needs to be assisted during sevoflurane induction. Sevoflurane causes increase in heart rate and little or no change in systolic blood pressure. Although it causes less myocardial depression than that by halothane,[21,22] a difference in safety has not been established.

Clinical implication of compound A, which is produced as a result of interaction of sevoflurane with carbon dioxide absorbent[23] is not clear in children.

Halothane

Before the use of sevoflurane, halothane was the induction agent of choice in children. In neonates, the MAC is 0.9%, it increases to 1.2% in infants aged 1 to 6 months, and declines gradually to 0.8% in the adults.

Halothane produces dose-dependent respiratory depression, it causes decrease in tidal volume and an increase in respiratory rate. It is a potent myocardial depressant and causes decrease in systolic pressures with no change in heart rate. Neonates and infants younger than 6 months of age are vulnerable to cardiac depressant effect of halothane. Concentration of halothane up to 1.5 MAC in children and up to 1 MAC in neonates affects haemodynamics similar to sevoflurane.[21] Given the number of cases where halothane has been used for induction, halothane hepatitis is considered to be not an important issue in this age group. Up to 10 µg/kg adrenaline can be administered with halothane with minimal risk of cardiac arrhythmias in children.[8]

Isoflurane

Major drawback of isoflurane is its pungent smell and high airway-related complications during induction, making it unacceptable for inhalational induction in children. MAC of isoflurane is 1.6% in neonates, 1.9% in infants aged 1 to 6 months and approaches adult value of 1.2% there on. It has a less myocardial depressant effect, maintains the heart rate, and thus may be useful for maintenance of anaesthesia in selected children.[8]

Desflurane

MAC requirement for desflurane is 9.2% for neonates, 9.4% for infants 1 to 6 months of age, 9.9% for infants 6 to 12 months of age, 8.7% for 1 to 3 years old and 8% for 5 to12 years old.[24] Desflurane has no hepatic metabolism unlike other volatile anaesthetics.

Desflurane causes high incidence of laryngospasm during inhalational induction in children.[25] Use of desflurane after induction for long surgical procedures is justified, however, because of rapid excretion and awakening.

NEUROMUSCULAR BLOCKING AND REVERSAL AGENTS

Depolarizing Muscle Relaxant

Succinylcholine is a water-soluble depolarizing muscle relaxant with rapid onset and offset. Its dose for intravenous administration in infants is twice (2 mg/kg) that for older children (1 mg/kg) due to larger volume of distribution. Intramuscular administration of a dose of 5 mg/kg body weight in infants and 4 mg/kg body weight in children will provide muscle relaxation in 3–4 minutes.

Succinylcholine has been implicated for causing malignant hyperthermia, masseter spasm and cardiac arrest in undiagnosed muscle dystrophies in children. Cardiac arrhythmias including cardiac sinus arrest can follow intravenous administration of succinylcholine, therefore, intravenous atropine is recommended even before the first dose of succinylcholine in children.[8] It is also suggested that its use in children should be reserved for emergency intubation or in instances where immediate securing of airway is necessary, like laryngospasm or difficult airway. Other issues, like myalgias and hyperkalemia with succinylcholine, are less important in children than adults. Availability of non-depolarizing blockers, such as mivacurium, rocuronium and rapacuronium with faster onset of action, further eliminates the need of using succinylcholine.[26]

Non-Depolarizing Muscle Relaxants

Neonates and infants have increased sensitivity to non-depolarizing neuromuscular blocking agents.

Extracellular fluid volume in which these polar drugs are mainly distributed is high in term neonates and start decreasing markedly during first year of life thereafter reaching adult values. Thus weight-based doses of neuromuscular agents yield smaller plasma concentration in neonates and infants than children and adults. This counterbalances the increased sensitivity observed in younger patients. However, immature clearance during infancy results in prolonged elimination half-lives due to larger volume of distribution.

Vecuronium, atracurium, rocuronium and cisatracurium are useful for short procedures and may be given by continuous infusion. Atracurium and cisatracurium being independent of hepatic and renal excretion are useful in newborns and children with impaired renal and hepatic function and same dose as adults can be used without much difference on the duration of action. Rocuronium can produce reliable muscle relaxation for tracheal intubation after 3–4 min of intramuscular administration (1 mg/kg for infants and 1.8 mg/kg body weight for children above 1 year of age) with a duration lasting for 1 hour. Rocuronium can also be used in place of succinylcholine in children where succinylcholine is contraindicated and can produce satisfactory intubating condition 45 seconds after intravenous dose of 1.2 mg/kg.[27] In addition, choice of non-depolarizing neuromuscular agent in children should also be based on their effects on cardiovascular system.

Neostigmine

Elimination half-life of neostigmine was found to be shorter for infants and children compared with adults.[28] The dose of neostigmine required to antagonize dTc-induced neuromuscular blockade is lower in infants and children than in adults.

In a dose of 50 μg/kg with atropine 20 μg/kg or glycopyrrolate 10 μg/kg, neostigmine antagonized neuromuscular block more predictably and with less variation than edrophonium (1 mg/kg) although edrophonium had a faster onset of effect.[29]

Sugammadex

Sugammadex is a cyclodextrin which forms covalent bond with rocuronium and antagonizes its effects. It can even reverse profound block of rocuronium, but reversal of other non-depolarizing muscle relaxant is to a lesser extent. This usefulness of sugammadex can obviate the need of succinylcholine requirement in children. In a study, sugammadex (2 mg/kg) was compared with neostigmine (0.03 mg/kg) for reversal of rocuronium (0.6 mg/kg) neuromuscular block in paediatric patients. Sugammadex provided safer extubation with a shorter recovery time than neostigmine.[30] Sugammadex is a promising future drug, however, present day use is limited by its high cost.

OPIOIDS

Morphine

Morphine, a commonly used opioid, is water-soluble but its lipid solubility is poor compared to other opioids. It is metabolized by hepatic pathways with the generation of inactive morphine-3-glucuronide (M3G) and active morphine-6-glucuronide (M6G). Approximately 20% of morphine is excreted unchanged via the renal system in neonates. M6G/M3G morphine ratios increase with age from 0.8 in neonates to 4.2 in children.[31] These ratio changes are attributed to the maturation of hepatic and renal clearance with age, but the clinical effect of these ratio changes is probably minimal in the neonate. Morphine clearance in term infants greater than 1 month old is comparable with children from 1 to 17 years old. In neonates aged 1–7 days, the clearance of morphine is one-third that of older infants and elimination half-life approximately 1.7 times longer.[32]

Other factors, like immature blood–brain barrier, reduced protein binding producing a higher free drug level, also contribute to altered response to morphine in neonates. However, there is no evidence to support age-related differences in respiratory sensitivity at equivalent plasma concentrations in neonates.

Morphine should be avoided in preterm infants and neonates and other short-acting opioids should be used. In nurse-controlled analgesia, background infusions should be omitted in neonates. A loading dose of 100 µg/kg followed by infusion of 10 to 30 µg/kg/minute can be used for children and infants older than 6 months. Infants receiving morphine should be nursed in an environment with extended monitoring facilities, trained staff, and access to ventilator equipment.[33]

Pethidine (Meperidine)

Pethidine, as it is more lipophilic, was considered to cause less respiratory depression in children. The fraction of drug entering the brain was also found to be similar to that in adults unlike morphine. However, it is not commonly used because of the adverse effects of its main metabolite, norpethidine.

Fentanyl

Fentanyl is a potent µ-receptor agonist with a potency 70–125 times that of morphine. Rapid onset and short duration of action makes fentanyl a commonly used opioid in paediatric patients. Like for other opioids, neonates exhibit a reduced rate of elimination of fentanyl because of immature metabolic mechanism including cytochrome P450 system. All metabolites are inactive and a small amount of fentanyl is eliminated unchanged through kidneys. Fentanyl clearance is 70–80% of adult values in term neonates and reaches adult values within the first 2 weeks of life.[34] Altered pharmacokinetics resulting in longer half-life of fentanyl is also seen in neonates undergoing abdominal surgery and during other conditions which alter hepatic blood flow, such as use of positive end expiratory pressure and vasopressors.[35]

Fentanyl has been used intravenously in a dose of 30–100 µg/kg for cardiac surgery when ventilation is controlled in postoperative period, otherwise much smaller dose of 2–10 µg/kg is advisable. Transdermal fentanyl is an alternative but use should be limited as high doses can be delivered due to increased permeability of neonatal skin.[36] Fentanyl induced bradycardia may require a vagolytic agent.

Remifentanil

A very short half-life and organ-independent elimination of remifentanil makes its pharmacokinetic profile predictable and useful for use in paediatric patients. The non-specific blood esterases that metabolise remifentanil are mature at birth and its clearance is greater in infants and neonates compared with older age groups with a reported terminal elimination half-life of between 10 and 35 minutes.[37] Because there is no drug accumulation, irrespective of the duration of infusion, the context-sensitive half-time remains constant. Remifentanil provides dose-dependent analgesia, while the adverse effects, e.g. respiratory depression, are also dose related. The occurrence of nausea and vomiting appears similar to other opioids. A bolus dose of 0.1 to 0.25 µg/kg should be used followed by an infusion of 0.25 µg/kg/min which can be increased or decreased at the rate of 0.05 to 0.1 µg/kg/min.[8]

In patients where reversal of respiratory depression effect of opioid is desired, naloxone in a dose of 0.01 to 0.03 mg/kg for children <5 years and 0.1 to 0.2 mg for older children is recommended. Since the duration of action is relatively short (30 to 45 min), repeat doses may be required.

SEDATIVES AND ANALGESICS

Benzodiazepines

Diazepam displays a very prolonged half-life in infants and particularly more in neonates. It has an active metabolite so not recommended for use in neonates and in infants up to 6 months of age.[8]

Midazolam is a water-soluble benzodiazepine with rapid onset of action and short duration of effect (elimination half-life is ~2 hours as compared to diazepam where half-life is ~18 hours). In healthy neonates, the half-life and the clearance are 3.3-fold longer and 3.7-fold smaller, respectively, than in adults. Midazolam is hydroxylated by CYP3A4 and CYP3A5; activities of these enzymes reaches adult value between 3 and 12 months of postnatal age, thus resulting in a half-life of 6–12 hours in neonates. When used intravenously a dose of 50 to 150 µg/kg of midazolam should be given over at least 5 min repeated 2–4 hourly, if required. Midazolam may also be administered orally (0.25–1 mg/kg, maximum of 20 mg), intramuscularly (0.1– 0.15 mg/kg, maximum of 7.5 mg), intranasally (0.2 mg/kg) and sublingually (0.2 mg/kg) and rectally (0.75 mg/kg, maximum of 20 mg). Dosage requirements are decreased by concurrent use of narcotics. For anticonvulsant therapy, it is given intravenously in a loading dose of 150 µg/kg over at least 5 min followed by a maintenance infusion dose of 60 to 400 µg/kg per hour (1 to 7 µg/kg per min).[38]

Oral midazolam is most commonly administered premedication in children, where it is given in a dose of 0.25–0.33 mg/kg, resulting in a very compliant child.

Dexmedetomidine

Dexmedetomidine is a selective alpha 2 adrenergic agonist with anxiolytic, sedative and analgesic properties. It has a quick onset and relatively short duration of action with minimal respiratory depression. With the increase in the dose of dexmedetomidine, it decreases both heart rate and systolic blood pressure in children in a similar fashion as in adults.[39] The pharmacokinetics of dexmedetomidine are similar in children compared to adults. However, clearance is reduced in neonates, which has been attributed to the immature enzymatic pathways in neonates. Clearance approaches adult values by about one year of age. To date, there are no FDA-approved indications for its use in children, but it has been found to be useful as a sole drug or has been combined with other sedatives for use in a number of procedures including radiological procedures, fibreoptic intubation and awake craniotomy.[40–42] Because large doses have been associated with severe bradycardia, an initial dose of 0.7 µg/kg over 10 minutes followed by an infusion of 0.5–1 µg/kg/hour is generally recommended. Intranasal dexmedetomidine in a premedication dose of 2 µg/kg has resulted in excellent sedation in children without causing adverse haemodynamic effects.[43]

Acetaminophen

Analgesic effect of paracetamol is mediated through inhibition of prostaglandin synthesis within the central nervous system. There are three major hepatic metabolic pathways: glucuronide conjugation, sulphate conjugation, and N-hydroxylation via the cytochrome P450 isozyme. The latter mechanism results in a highly reactive intermediate metabolite, N-acetyl-*p*-benzoquinone imine. Due to differences in the rate of development of metabolic enzymes, acetaminophen metabolism is different in neonates from adults, the major pathway being sulphate conjugation rather than glucuronidation. The normal adult ratio of glucuronidation to sulphation (2:1) is not achieved until 12 year of age. Immaturity of cytochrome isoenzyme in young children also results in less production of reactive metabolite, conferring protection against acetaminophen-induced hepatotoxicity.[44]

Neonates have the longest half-life of acetaminophen, infants have a shorter half-life while older children, adolescents, and adults had similar values.

Smaller doses and longer dosing interval are hence required in neonates and sick children. It is commonly used orally, rectally or intravenously in children. Bioavailability of rectal preparation is good in neonates as compared to older children and adults.[45] Intravenous paracetamol preparations are becoming widely popular and they have a higher analgesic potency than either the oral or rectal preparations though the time to peak analgesia is still 1–2 hours. Rectal dose in preterms aged 28–32 weeks is 20 mg/kg and from 28–32 weeks to 3 months of age is 30 mg/kg. Beyond the age of 3 months dose is 40 mg/kg. Intravenous dose should be administered according to postgestational age: 28–32 weeks, 10 mg/kg; 32–36 weeks, 12.5 mg/kg; and ≥ 36 weeks, 15 mg/kg.[46]

Non-Steroidal Anti-Inflammatory Drugs (NSAIDs)

NSAIDs are a heterogeneous group of compounds having antipyretic, analgesic and anti-inflammatory effects. NSAIDs act by reducing prostaglandin biosynthesis through inhibition of cyclo-oxygenase (COX) which exists as two major isoforms (COX-1 and COX-2). NSAIDs in children are effective analgesic adjuvant drugs that improves the quality of analgesia.

Pharmacokinetic studies of NSAIDs have showed a higher than expected dose requirement, if scaled by body weight from adult doses due to higher volume of distribution.[47] In neonates, clearance of NSAIDs is reduced and it increases with age. Use of NSAIDs is not recommended in infants less than 6 months of age as data for safe use is not available.[48]

They should be carefully used in children compromised by dehydration and hypovolaemia, with history of allergy to NSAIDs, with pre-existing renal diseases, liver diseases or coagulation disorders. Adverse gastrointestinal effects are significant as in adults. NSAIDs are useful for treatment of mild to moderate pain in paediatric patients. When used in combination with opioids, they have an opioid sparing effect of 30–40% and thus reduce opioid-related side effects.[49] They are also effective when combined with regional anaesthesia or nerve blocks.

The rate and extent of absorption after rectal administration of NSAIDs, such as ibuprofen, diclofenac, are less than oral routes. Dose of oral and rectal diclofenac is 1–3 mg/kg.

LOCAL ANAESTHETICS AND ADJUVANTS

Neonates demonstrate decreased clearance, decreased protein binding and high local absorption of local anaesthetic agents. Therefore, there is a risk of systemic toxicity and dosing schedules have to be adjusted accordingly. Safe doses of racaemic bupivacaine have been established in paediatric patients.[50] Use of ropivacaine has now largely replaced racaemic bupivacaine because of lower toxicity and lower risk of unwanted motor block.[51,52] Maximum dose of all the three local anaesthetics is 2 mg/kg in neonates and 2.5 mg/kg in children with maximum infusion of 0.2 mg/kg/hr and 0.4 mg/kg/hr in neonates and children, respectively. Ester local anaesthetics can be given to neonates as esterase systems are mature in early life.[53]

Topical cutaneous local anaesthesia, e.g. EMLA cream is an eutectic mixture of local anaesthetics containing lidocaine and prilocaine. When applied under an occlusive dressing it has an onset time of 60–90 min and duration of analgesia is 30–60 min. The maximum recommended dose in infants is 1 g because of the risk of methaemoglobinaemia. Amethocaine gel has a more rapid onset time of 30–60 min as it is more lipophilic and can be used safely in neonates as esterases are fully functional.

S(+)-ketamine 1 mg kg^{-1} as a sole agent in caudal has been found to be as effective as local anaesthetic[54] and clonidine 1–2 µg kg^{-1} as adjunct to caudal have been found to increase the duration of analgesia.[55] Routine use of opioids as additives to local anaesthetics for postoperative pain has not been shown to be effective[56] though neuraxial opioids have role in long duration extensive surgeries. Adjuvants should be carefully administered in neonates because of increased risk of sedation and apnoea.

MISCELLANEOUS DRUGS

Atropine and Glycopyrrolate

Atropine and glycopyrrolate are non-selective muscarinic receptor antagonists with fast onset of action. Glycopyrrolate has a quaternary amine and penetrates the biological membranes (blood–CNS, placental barriers) slowly and incompletely. Its oral absorption is slow and erratic, and hence it cannot be used as an oral premedicant. Nearly half of the atropine dose administered is excreted unchanged in the urine or as active metabolites and about 80% of glycopyrrolate is excreted as unchanged drug or active metabolites. There were no significant changes in the distribution volume or clearance of glycopyrrolate in children of different ages. The shortened elimination half-life in children between 1 and 3 years of age is of minor clinical importance.[57]

The recommended preanaesthetic dose of glyco-pyrrolate in infants and children is in a range of 0.004 to 0.006 mg/kg.[58] To reverse non-depolarizing neuromuscular blockade, the recommended paedia-tric dose is 0.2 mg given IV for every 1 mg of neostig-mine or 5 mg of pyridostigmine. Glycopyrrolate may be mixed in the same syringe as the anticholinesterase to allow for simultaneous administration.

Anticholinergics are frequently used to reduce the increase in oral secretions and bradycardia produced by anaesthetic agents. While widely accepted as beneficial by clinicians, controlled studies evaluating their efficacy have produced mixed results. In a study in children undergoing cardiac catheterization with sevoflurane-remifentanil anaesthesia, IV glyco-pyrrolate[59] 0.006 mg/kg was an effective adjunctive therapy to prevent bradycardia, and higher doses were not necessary. When atropine was compared with glycopyrrolate, both prevented bradycardia, however, tachycardia was more common in the atropine-treated patients and hypoxia was reported more frequently in the glycopyrrolate group (Table 2.1).[58]

CONCLUSION

A clear understanding of the pharmacological differences, dosages and routes of administration of various drugs and the differences in metabolism of drugs to be used is essential in order to provide safe and effective anaesthesia in neonates and children.

REFERENCES

1. Kearns GL, Abdel-Rahman SM, Alander SW, et al. Developmental pharmacology—drug disposition, action, and therapy in infants and children. N Engl J Med 2003;349:1157–1167.
2. Lack JA, Stuart Taylor ME. Calculation of drug dosage and body surface area of children. Br J Anaesth 1997;78:601–605.
3. Holford NHG. A size standard for pharmacokinetics. Clinical Pharmacokinet 1996;30:329–332.
4. Friis-Hansen B. Body water compartments in children: changes during growth and related changes in body composition. Pediatrics 1961;28:169–181.
5. Benet LZ, Hoener BA, et al. Changes in plasma protein binding have little clinical relevance. Clin Pharmacol Ther 2002; 71:115–121.

Table 2.1	Recommended dosages of anaesthetic agents in children	
Drug	**Bolus doses**	**Infusions**
Propofol	2.9 mg/kg (<2 yrs old) 2.2 mg/kg (6–12 yrs)	125–300 µg/kg/min
Thiopentone	4–5 mg/kg (neonates) 7–8 mg/kg (infants) 5–6 mg/kg (child)	
Ketamine	0.25-0.5 mg/kg (for analgesia) 2 mg/kg (induction) 10 mg/kg (rectally) 6–10 mg/kg (orally) 3–6 mg/kg (intranasally)	
Succinylcholine	2 mg/kg (infants) 1 mg/kg (children)	
Rocuronium	0.3 mg/kg, 0.6 mg/kg and 1.2 mg/kg 1 mg/kg (infants) intra-muscular 1.8 mg/kg (children >1 yr) intramuscular	
Cisatracurium	0.1 mg/kg	
Vecuronium	0.1 mg/kg	
Pancuronium	0.1 mg/kg	
Neostigmine	0.02–0.06 mg/kg+ atropine 0.02 mg/kg	
Edrophonium	0.3–1mg/kg	
Morphine	100 µg/kg or 50 µg kg^{-1} increments, repeated up to × 4 hrly	10 to 30µg/kg/min
Alfentanil	5–10 µg kg^{-1}	1–4 µg kg^{-1} min^{-1}
Fentanyl	2–10 µg kg^{-1}	0.1–0.2 µg kg^{-1}min^{-1}
Remifentanil	0.1–0.25 µg kg^{-1}	0.25–4 µg kg^{-1} min^{-1}
Sufentanil	0.025–0.05 µg kg^{-1}	
Midazolam	50 to 150 µg/kg repeated 2–4 hrly	
Dexmed	0.7µg/kg over 10 min.	0.5-1 µg/kg/hr
Acetaminophen	15 mg kg^{-1}	
Diclofenac	1–3 mg/kg	
Bupivacaine	2 mg/kg (neonates) 2.5 mg/kg (children)	0.2mg/kg/hr 0.4mg/kg/hr

6. Jacob R, Krishnan BS, Venkatesan T. Pharmacokinetics and pharmacodynamics of anaesthetic drugs in paediatrics. Indian J Anaesth 2004;48:340–346.

7. Arant BS Jr. Developmental patterns of renal functional maturation compared in the human neonate. J Pediatr 1978;92:705–712.

8. Cote CJ. Pediatric anaesthesia. In: Miller RD (Ed). Miller's Anesthesia, 8th edn. Philadelphia: Elsevier, 2015; pp 2757–2798.

9. Bouwmeester NJ, Anderson BJ, Tibboel D, et al. Developmental pharmacokinetics of morphine and its metabolites in neonates, infants and young children. Br J Anaesth 2004;92:208–217.

10. Liang J, Co E, Zhang M, et al. Development of gastric slow waves in preterm infants measured by electrogastrography. Am J Physiol 1998;274:G503–508.

11. Taddio A, Shennan AT, Stevens B, et al. Safety of lidocaine-prilocaine cream in the treatment of preterm neonates. J Pediatr 1995;127:1002–1005.

12. Lerman J, Schmitt Bantel BI, Gregory GA, et al. Effect of age on the solubility of volatile anesthetics in human tissues. Anesthesiology 1986;65:307–311.

13. Bouche MP, Versichelen LF, Struys MM, et al. No compound A formation with Superia during minimal-flow sevoflurane anesthesia: a comparison with Sofnolime. Anaesth Analg 2002;95:1680–1685.

14. Kataria BK, Ved SA, Nicodemus HF, et al. The pharmacokinetics of propofol in children using three different data analysis approaches. Anaesthesiology 1994;80:104–122.

15. Shipton EA, Prosser DO. Mitochondrial myopathies and anaesthesia. Eur J Anaesthesiol 2004;21:173–178.

16. Marik PE. Propofol. Therapeutic indications and side-effects. Curr Pharm Des 2004;10:3639–3649.

17. White PF, Way WL, Trevor AJ. Ketamine—its pharmacology and therapeutic uses. Anaesthesiology 1982;56:119–136.

18. Sussman DR. A comparative evaluation of ketamine anesthesia in children and adults. Anesthesiology 1974;40:459–464.

19. Kotah T, Ikeda K. Minimum alveolar concentration of sevoflurane in children. Br J Anaesth 1992;68:139–141.

20. Lerman J, Sikich N, kleinman S, Yentis S. The pharmacology of sevoflurane in infants and children. Anaesthesiology 1994;80:814–824.

21. Wodey E, Pladys P, Copin C, et al. Comparitive hemodynamic depression of sevoflurane versus halothane in infants: An echocardiographic study. Anaesthesiology 1997; 87:795–800.

22. Holzman RS, van der Velde ME, Kaus SJ, et al. Sevoflurane depresses myocardial contractility less than halothane during induction of anesthesia in children. Anaesthesiology 1996;85:1260–1267.

23. Fang ZX, Kandel L, Laster MJ, et al. Factors affecting production of compound A from the interaction of sevoflurane with Baralyme and soda lime. Anesth Analg 1996; 82: 775–781.

24. Taylor RH, Lerman J. Minimum alveolar concentration of desflurane and hemodynamic responses in neonates, infants, and children. Anesthesiology 1991;75:975–979.

25. Zwass MS, Fisher DM, Welborn LG, et al. Induction and maintenance characteristics of anesthesia with desflurane and nitrous oxide in infants and children. Anaesthesiology 1992;76:373–378.

26. Fisher DM. Neuromuscular blocking agent in paediatric anaesthesia. British J Anaesth 1999;83:58–64.

27. Mazurek AJ, Rae B, Hann S, et al. Rocuronium versus succinylcholine: Are they equally effective during rapid-sequence induction of anesthesia? Anesth Analg 1998;87: 1259–1262.

28. Fisher DM, Cronnelly R, Miller RD, et al. Neuromuscular pharmacology of neostigmine in infants and children. Anaesthesiology 1983;59:220–225.

29. Kirkegaard-Nielsen H, Meretoja OA, Wirtavuori K. Reversal of atracurium-induced neuromuscular block in paediatric patients. Acta Anaesthesia Scand 1995;39: 906–911.

30. Kara T, Ozbagriacik O, Sebnem H, et al. Sugammadex versus neostigmine in pediatric patients: a prospective randomized study Brazilian J Anesth 2014;64:400–405.

31. Barrett DA, Barker DP, Rutter N, et al. Morphine, morphine-6-glucuronide and morphine-3-glucuronide pharmacokinetics in newborn infants receiving diamorphine infusions. Br J Clin Pharmacol 1996;41:531–537.

32. Anderson BJ, Meakin GH. Scaling for size: some implications for paediatric anaesthesia dosing. Paediatr Anaesth 2002;12:205–219.

33. Haidon JL, Cunliffe M. Analgesia for neonates. Contin Education Care Pain 2010;10:123–127.

34. Anderson BJ, McKee AD, Holford NH. Size, myths and the clinical pharmacokinetics of analgesia in paediatric patients. Clin Pharmacokinet 1997;33:313–327.

35. Kuhls E, Gauntlett IS, Lau M, et al. Effect of increased intra-abdominal pressure on hepatic extraction and clearance of fentanyl in neonatal lambs. J Pharmacol Exp Ther 1995;274:115–119.

36. Barrett DA, Rutter N. Transdermal delivery and the premature neonate. Crit Rev Ther Drug Carrier Syst 1994; 11:31–59.

37. Davis PJ, Cladis FP. The use of ultra-short-acting opioids in paediatric anaesthesia: the role of remifentanil. Clin Pharmacokinet 2005;44:787–796.

38. Pacifici GM. Clinical pharmacology of midazolam in neonates and Children: Effect of disease—a review. International J Pediatrics, Vol 2014 (2014), Article ID. 309342, pp20.

39. Petroz GC, Sikich N, James M, et al. A phase I, two-center study of the pharmacokinetics of dexmedetomidine in children. Anaesthesiology 2006;105:1098–1110.

40. Koroglu A, Teksan H, Sagir O, et al. A comparison of the sedative, hemodynamic, and respiratory effects of dexmedetomidine and propofol in children undergoing magnetic resonance imaging. Anesth Analg 2006;103:63–67.

41. Jooste EH, Ohkawa S, Sun LS. Fibreoptic intubation with dexmedetomidine in two children with spinal cord impingements. Anesth Analg 2005;101:1248.

42. Everett LI, van Rooyen IF, Warner MH, et al. Use of dexmedetomidine in awake craniotomy in adolescents: Report of two cases. Paediatr Anaesth 2006;16:338–342.

43. Yuen VM, Hui TW, Irwin MG, et al. A randomised comparison of two intranasal dexmedetomidine doses for premedication in children. Anaesthesia 2012;11:1210–1216.

44. Roberts I, Robinson MJ, Mughal MZ, et al. Paracetamol metabolites in the neonate following maternal overdose. Br J Clin Pharmacol 1984;18:201–206.

45. Arana A, Morton NS, Hansen TG. Treatment with paracetamol in infants. Acta Anaesthesiol Scand 2001;45:20–29.

46. Palmer GM, Atkins M, Anderson BJ, et al. IV acetaminophen pharmacokinetics in neonates after multiple doses. Br J Anaesth 2008;1010:523–530.

47. Romsing J, Ostergaard D, Senderovitz T, et al. Pharmacokinetics of oral diclofenac and acetaminophen in children after surgery. Paediatric Anaesth 2001;11:205–213.

48. Kokki H. Nonsteroidal anti-inflammatory drugs for postoperative pain: a focus on children. Paediatric Drugs 2003;5:103–123.

49. Morton NS, O'Brien K. Analgesic efficacy of paracetamol and diclofenac in children receiving PCA morphine. Br J Anaesth 1999;83:715–717.

50. Berde CB. Toxicity of local anesthetics in infants and children. J Pediatr 1993;122:S14–20.

51. Bosenberg AT, Cronje L, Thomas J, et al. Ropivacaine plasma levels and postoperative analgesia in neonates and infants during 48–72 h continuous epidural infusion following major surgery. Paediatric Anaesth 2003;13:851–852.

52. Chalkiadis GA, Eyres RL, Cranswick N, et al. Pharmacokinetics of levobupivacaine 0.25% following caudal administration in children under 2 years of age. Br J Anaesth 2004;92:218–222.

53. Berde C. Local anaesthetics in infants and children: an update. Paediatric Anaesth 2004;14:387–393.

54. Marhofer P, Krenn CG, Plochl W, et al. S(+)-ketamine for caudal block in paediatric anaesthesia. Br J Anaesth 2000;84:341–345.

55. Lee JJ, Rubin AP. Comparison of a bupivacaine-clonidine mixture with plain bupivacaine for caudal analgesia in children. Br J Anaesth 1994;72:258–262.

56. Lerman J, Nolan J, Eyres R, et al. Efficacy, safety, and pharmacokinetics of levobupivacaine with and without fentanyl after continuous epidural infusion in children: a multicenter trial. Anesthesiology 2003;99:1166–1174.

57. Rautakorpi P, Ali-Melkkilä T, Kaila T, et al. Pharmacokinetics of glycopyrrolate in children. Journal of Clinical Anesthesia 1994;3:217–220.

58. Reyntjens K, Foubert L, De Wolf D, et al. Glycopyrrolate during sevoflurane-remifentanil-based anaesthesia for cardiac catheterization of children with congenital heart disease. Br J Anaesth 2005;95:680–684.

59. Desalu I, Kushimo OT, Bode CO. A comparative study of the hemodynamic effects of atropine and glycopyrrolate at induction of anesthesia in children. West Afr J Med 2005;24:115–119.

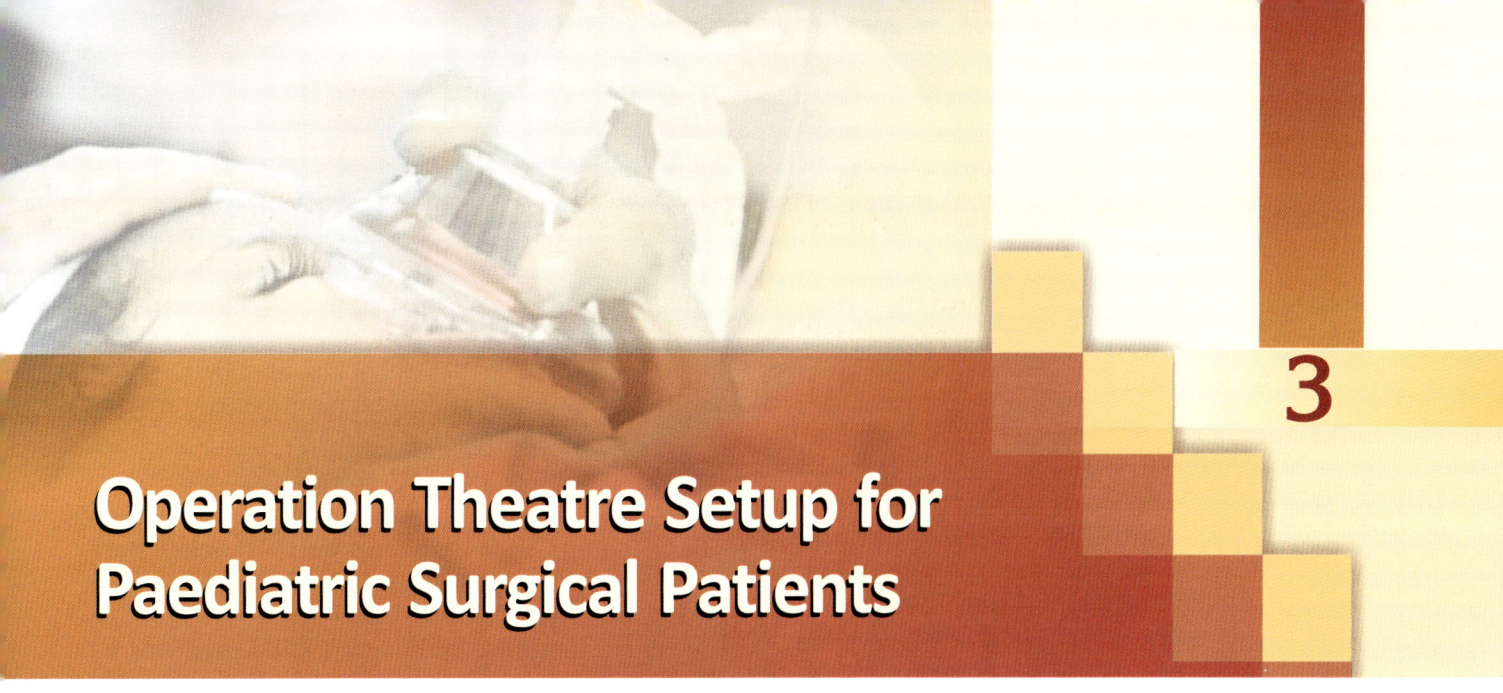

Operation Theatre Setup for Paediatric Surgical Patients

Anurag Krishna

…my purpose is here to doo theym good that have moste need, that is to save children: and to share the remedies that god hath created for the use of man…

Thomas Phaire
(*The Boke of Chyldren 1553*)

- **Safety considerations**
- **Infrastructure of a paediatric OR**
- **Baby-friendly, family-centred care**
- **Transfer to and from OR**

INTRODUCTION

As caregivers for sick children that need surgery, it is our responsibility to provide children with the best possible care in a safe operating room environment with best-in-class clinical outcomes. What will become a differentiator is that we do all this while giving our little patients and their anxious parents an experience that is pleasant and stress free. This chapter briefly touches upon the science of paediatric surgical operating room set up; and describes in some detail the art of caring for children.

The overarching principles for children's surgery[1] are that:

- Children are treated safely.
- They are treated in an environment that is suitable and responsive to their needs.

- Their parents are involved in the care and decision making.
- The care being delivered is of optimal quality.
- All involved in care are suitably trained and supported.

SAFETY CONSIDERATION

The elements that provide a safe environment are—personnel, processes and infrastructure.

Personnel

All children must be treated by appropriately trained professionals. Naturally, the surgeon must be qualified, credentialed and must hold the necessary privileges to perform the index surgical procedure. While it is accepted that some routine paediatric surgical procedures may be performed in general hospitals, it has been adequately demonstrated that for some index and complex procedures, best outcomes are achieved if the cases are done in high volume centers.[2–10] More recently, many paediatric surgical operations are done as day case surgeries. While these should be encouraged as much as possible, however, they place much more responsibility on the anaesthesia team. There are well-described guidelines[11] that must be strictly adhered to prevent complications. Anaesthesia in children should be undertaken or supervised by consultants with a substantial commitment to and appropriate training in paediatric anaesthesia.[1,2] In order to maintain core competencies, they should have a regular paediatric practice. Occasional practice is undesirable, particularly for elective surgery. The role of dedicated support staff (operating room assistants, anaesthetic nurses) with specific paediatric skills and training and an ability to respond to paediatric emergencies is paramount in creating a safe and efficient OR environment.

Processes

Clinical audits have clearly demonstrated that safety processes and aviation-style check lists have been able to drastically reduce adverse events and patient injuries.[12,13] These check lists must not be viewed merely as a chore but internalized to an extent that all team members believe in their value. Surgical and anaesthesia consents must be taken well before the

actual procedure by a team member senior enough to be able to answer all patient queries. Site marking must be done before the patient is shifted to the OR.[14] While in the OR, a surgical time-out helps the team focus on the procedure.

INFRASTRUCTURE OF A PAEDIATRIC OR

The OR equipment must be checked daily before start of the operating session. The American Society of Anesthesiologists Closed Claim study has found a greater incidence of equipment-related problems in paediatric patients in comparison to adults, with almost 50% in children aged less than 2 years.[15]

All emergency drugs for use in children must be available within the OR. The key monitoring systems include measuring temperature, heart rate, respiratory rate, oxygen saturation and end-tidal CO_2 levels. Adequate care must be taken to keep the baby warm during the procedure. Hypothermia set in rapidly in neonates and infants and is the most important factor contributing to post-surgical morbidity and mortality. In procedures where the operating time is expected to be long, or when the baby needs to be in a different position, care must be taken to ensure that all joints are in a neutral position and pressure points are comfortably padded to avoid position-related injuries (Figs 3.1 and 3.2). Corneal exposure must be prevented by securely shutting the eyelids and adequately padding the eyes, particularly if the baby is in prone position. Care must also be taken that the electro-cautery neutral plate is not wet. A malfunctioning

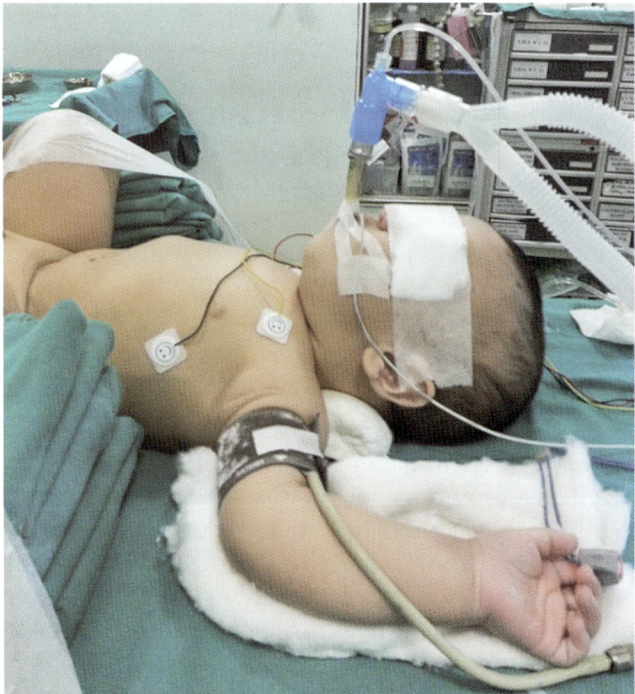

Fig. 3.1. Set-up before start of surgery. Note the monitoring that includes ECG recording, blood pressure recording, pulse oximetry, oral temperature probe and EtCO₂ monitor. Also note that eyes are protected and pressure areas are well padded with cotton wool

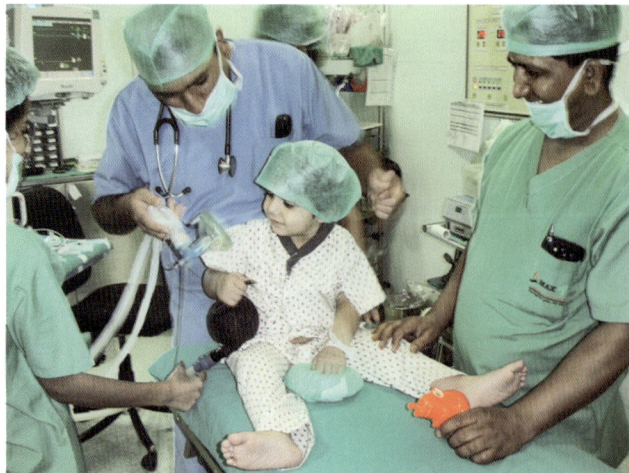

Fig. 3.2. The child playful during anaesthetic induction as helpful OR staff keeps the child engaged

electrocautery or a wet plate could result in serious burns.

The environment within the OR must be professional and efficient. Each member of the team must understand his role clearly. Only the necessary personnel need to be in the theatre and to-and-fro movement must be minimum. Safety drills must be rehearsed regularly. There is evidence that spontaneous noise during paediatric operations attains the magnitude of a lawn mower and peaks resembling a passing truck.[16] With specific interventions, this decibel level could be substantially reduced. This in turn reduces the surgeon's distress as well as intraoperative adverse events.

Operation Room Setup

The American Institute of Architects 2006 Guidelines for design and construction of healthcare facilities sets a minimum of 400 sq. ft. for a general OT and 600 sq. ft. for speciality OT. Ambulatory surgery OT can be of 150 sq. ft.[15] Additionally, storage space allocation for each OT must be at least 50 sq. ft. Temperature and humidity control and maintenance is one of the crucial elements of paediatric surgical care. Undetected, and often severe hypothermia is the most frequent thermal disturbance in the perioperative period. Children are particularly more prone to hypothermia since they have a larger body surface area to body weight ratio.[17] Typically, the OT ambient temperature is set for 19–21°C for the comfort of the OT personnel. It has been observed that at these temperatures nearly 50% of patients develop mild to severe hypothermia, depending on the duration and complexity of surgery.[18] This simply means that what is comfortable for you is too cold for the baby. Normothermia has been consistently shown in patients when the OT temperature has been set between 24–26°C. The same ambient temperature conditions must also be ensured in the pre- and postoperative areas.

A variety of equipment (for age and size) must be available to maintain normothermia, including warming lamps, circulating warm air devices, air humidifiers, and fluid warmers. There are not any controlled studies to suggest which works best. In our experience, we have used the following measures to good effect:

1. Wrapping the exposed parts in cotton wool for neonates and infants

2. Use of circulating warm air device—the Bair-Hugger blanket

3. Delivery of warm humidified anaesthetic gases using the HME device

4. Use of fluid warmers for prolonged surgeries

BABY-FRIENDLY, FAMILY-CENTRED CARE

A key differentiator in today's healthcare delivery is how well one manages the family during their stay in hospital for such a stressful event as their baby's surgery. The cornerstone to building this relation is honest and constant communication. Parents play crucial role in providing physical and psychological support to the child. Parents should be involved in all decisions affecting care. Involving them in the care of their child not only gives the child confidence and comfort but offers a more positive experience for all. We have seen parents often become experts in day-to-day management. However, inorder that they do this meaningfully, they need accurate, clearly understandable information and guidance.

Children and parents must be well prepared for the surgery well before hospitalization. Children who are unaware that they have to undergo surgery are extremely difficult to handle in the preoperative area. We and others[19,20] have seen that with the help of toys (Fig. 3.3) and a range of music and video clips, the preoperative handling of children and parents becomes very easy. These interventions minimise anxiety and reduce the requirements of anaesthetic agents.

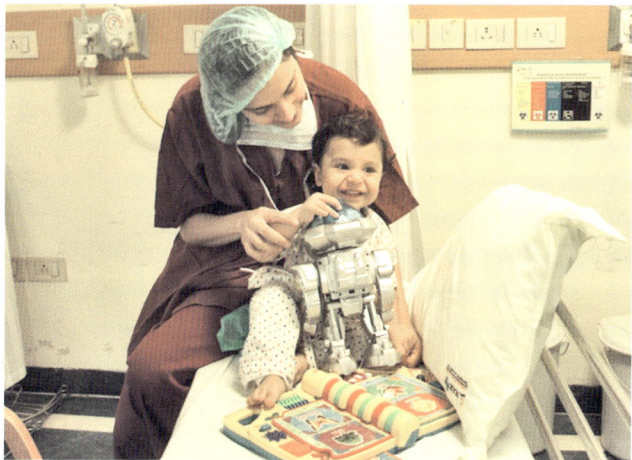

Fig. 3.3. A happy child playing with toys in the preoperative holding area as the mother looks on

It is our practice[21] as in other western countries[22] to allow one parent to be with the child at induction of anaesthesia. While there are studies[23] that suggest that parental presence does not reduce the child's overall anxiety, however, there is evidence to suggest that this practice improves the parental satisfaction with the separation process.[22] A dedicated OR assistant who can handle children well is invaluable as he can calm the child enough to have a smooth induction (Fig. 3.4).

After surgery, children must rest in a quiet recovery area that is separate from where adult patients are kept. It is helpful that parents are allowed to be with their child when they wake up. In order that the postoperative recovery experience is good, anaesthetic techniques should ensure that re-emergence from anaesthesia is smooth and the child is comfortably asleep. An agitated child in the recovery area can cause untold stress to the parents and can often result in dislodgement of intravenous lines or surgical drains. Pain assessment and effective pain management in infants and children is often given low priority. It has been amply demonstrated that even neonates and infants perceive pain. There should, therefore, be appropriate postoperative pain assessment and management policies, executed by a qualified pain management team.

TRANSFER TO AND FROM OR

Many adverse events can be avoided by ensuring a safe transfer of children undergoing surgery from ward to theatre and back. Several check lists and

protocols have been devised that can be used.[14] The intent of these check lists is to ensure that the right patient undergoes the right operation of the correct side each time.

SUMMARY

Children must undergo surgery in a safe, baby-friendly environment that ensures best outcomes.

1. Only trained professionals must give anaesthesia to or operate on children.
2. Children deserve to be treated with courtesy and dignity. Their privacy must be respected.
3. Parents must be intimately associated with the decision-making process and day-to-day management of their child.
4. The OR environment must be safe, efficient and must be fully equipped to handle any paediatric emergency.
5. Adherence to safety protocols and time spent on making the child comfortable improves outcomes and overall satisfaction level.

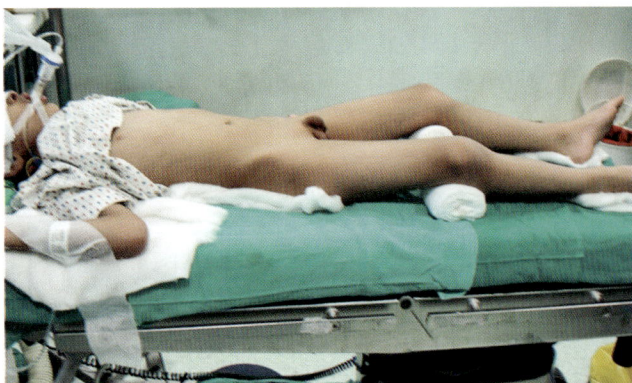

Fig. 3.4. Note the cotton rolls gently flexing the knee and padding the ankles. Note also the cotton on the sides preventing the cleaning solution from trickling on to the cautery pad

REFERENCES

1. The Children's Surgical Forum. Standards for children's surgery. 2013;www.rcseng.ac.uk/publications/docs/standards-in-childrens-surgery.
2. The Task Force for Children's Surgical Care. Optimal resources for children's surgical care in the United States. J Am Coll Surg 2014;218(3):479–487.
3. Report of the Children's Surgical Forum. Surgery for Children–delivering a world class service. 2007. https://www.rcseng.ac.uk/publications/docs/CSF.html/@@download/pdffile/CSF.pdf
4. Mamie C, Habre W, Delhumeau C, et al. Incidence and riskfactors of perioperative respiratory adverse events in childrenundergoing elective surgery. Paediatr Anaesth 2004;14:218e–224.
5. Chang RK, Klitzner TS. Can regionalization decrease thenumber of deaths for children who undergo cardiac surgery? Pediatrics 2002;109:173e–181.
6. Miller MR, Zhan C. Pediatric patient safety in hospitals: anational picture in 2000. Pediatrics.2004;113:1741e–1746.
7. Arul GS, Spicer RD. Where should paediatric surgery be performed?Arch Dis Child 1998;79:65e–70.
8. Hackel A, Badgwell JM, Binding RR, et al. Guidelines for the pediatric perioperative anesthesia environment. Pediatrics 1999;103:511e–516.
9. Ecoffey C. Paediatric perioperative anaesthesia environment. Curr Opin Anaesthesiol 2000;13:313e–315.

10. Cosper GH, Hamann MS, Stiles A. Hospital characteristics affect outcomes for common pediatric surgical conditions. Am Surg 2006;72:739e–745.

11. Royal College of Nursing. Children and young people in day surgery. 2013, https://www.rcn.org.uk/__data/assets/pdf_file/0009/78507/004_464.pdf.

12. Bellora E, Falzoni M. Surgery checklist implementation to reduce clinical risk in the pediatric operating room. Minerva Pediatr 2013;65(6):617–630.

13. Low DK, Reed MA, Geiduschek JM, Martin LD. Striving for a zero-error patient surgical journey through adoption of aviation-style challenge and response flow checklists: a quality improvement project. Paediatr Anaesth 2013;23:571–578.

14. Royal College of Nursing. Transferring children to and from theatre. 2011, https://www.rcn.org.uk/__data/assets/pdf_file/0003/395760/004127.pdf

15. Stjepanovic G. Pediatric Operating Rooms. In: Shine TSJ, Leone BJ, Martin DL (Eds.). Operating Room Design Manual. 2012. Available athttps://www.asahq.org/~/media/legacy/for%20members/practice%20management/ordm/or%20chapter%2013%20specialized%20operating%20rooms.pdf?la=en

16. Engelmann CR, Neis JP, Kirschbaum C, Grote G, Ure BM. A noise-reduction program in a pediatric operation theatre is associated with surgeon's benefits and a reduced rate of complications: a prospective controlled clinical trial. Ann Surg 2014;259:1025–1033.

17. Szmuk P, Rabb MF, Baumgartner JE, Berry JM, Sessler AM, Sesslaer DI. Body morphology and the speed of cutaneous rewarming. Anesthesiology 2001;95:18.

18. El-Gamal N, El-Kassabany N, Frank SM, et al. Age-related thermoregulatory differences in a warm operating room environment (approximately 26°C). Anesth Analg 2000;90:694.

19. Mifflin KA, Hackmann T, Chorney JM. Streamed video clips to reduce anxiety in children during inhaled induction of anesthesia. Anesth Analg 2012; 115:1162–1167.

20. Berghmans J, Weber F, van Akoleyen C, Utens E, Adriaenssens P, Klein J, Himpe D. Audiovisual aid viewing immediately before pediatric induction moderates the accompanying parents' anxiety. Paediatr Anaesth 2012; 22:386–392.

21. Lal P, Krishna A. Parental presence during anesthesia induction. Indian Pediatr 1997;34:331–334.

22. Tan L, Meakin GH. Anaesthesia for the uncooperative child. Continuing Education in Anaesthesia, Critical Care and Pain 2010;10:48–52.

23. Watson AT, Visram A. Children's preoperative anxiety and postoperative behavior. PaediatrAnaesthesia 2003; 13:188–204.

4

Equipment and Monitors Related to Paediatric Anaesthesia

Dilip Pawar

- Airway equipment
- Anaesthesia machine
- Warming equipment
- Airway cart

INTRODUCTION

Equipment and monitors form an integral part of anaesthesia practice. This is more so in paediatric anaesthesia practice, in order to ensure safe delivery and smooth conduction of anaesthesia devoid of complications or morbidity.

A thorough knowledge of airway equipment, anaesthesia machine, breathing systems, monitors and warming devices is essential for the anaesthesiologist who deals with routine or emergency anaesthesia in children.

AIRWAY EQUIPMENT

Masks

The important considerations are elimination or decrease of mechanical dead space and fitting the facial contour of the child, specially the younger ones. RBS (Rendell-Baker Soucek) mask has been developed from the moulds of facial contour of western children, however, it fits well with most of our children's face as well. Plastic masks with soft inflatable cuff around the periphery available nowadays are a good alternative, especially in children where normal mask application can be difficult (Fig. 4.1).[1]

The right way to put these masks is to put the lower margin of the mask between lower lip and chin and gently push to keep the mouth open while closing the mask over the nose, all the while providing a support to the mandible at the TM joint.

Airways

Oral airways should be readily available before starting any case as it could be life saving in difficult situation or inexperienced hand (Fig. 4.2). In my personal experience, have rarely used this piece of equipment.

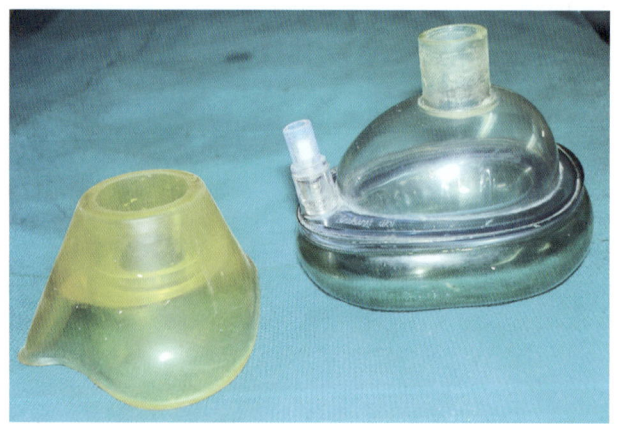

Fig. 4.1. Masks RBS and pneumatic cuff

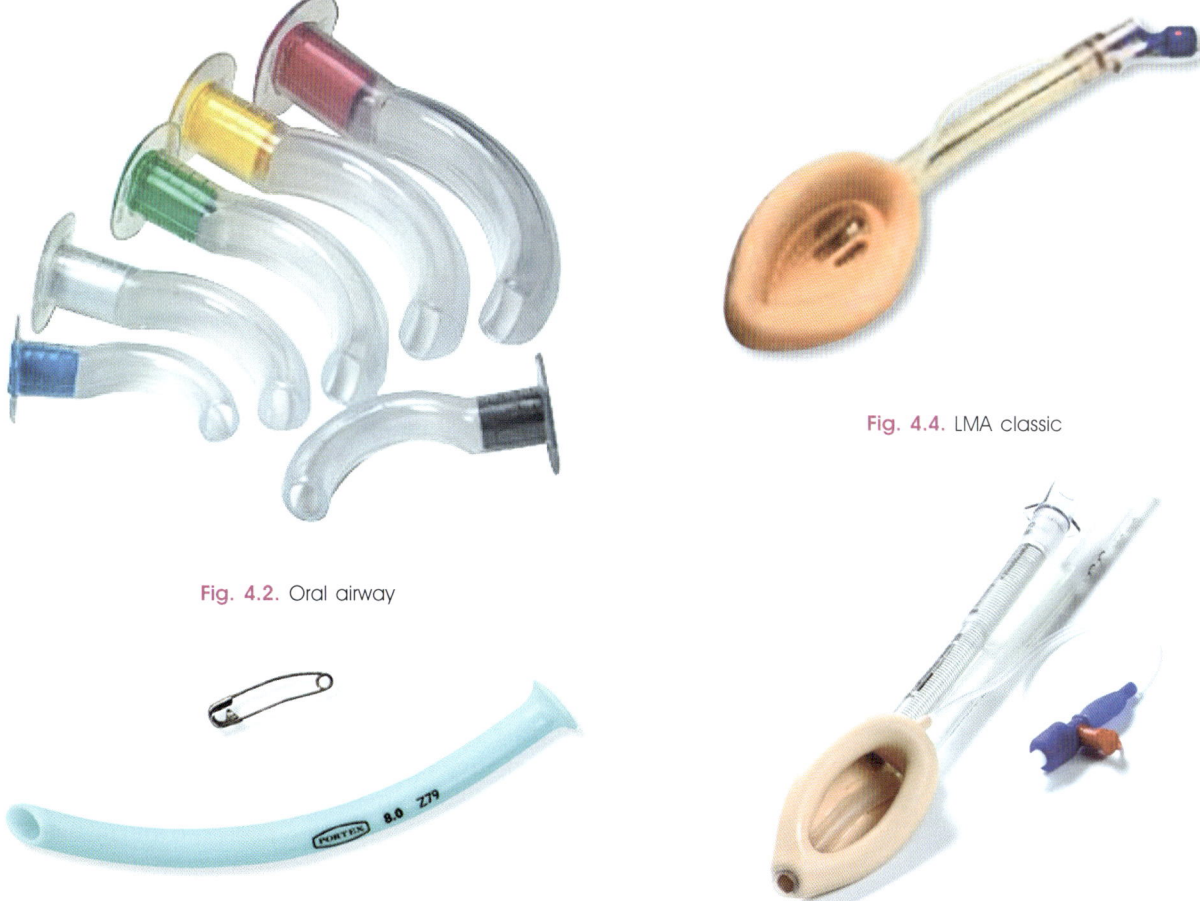

Fig. 4.2. Oral airway

Fig. 4.3. Nasopharyngeal airway

Fig. 4.4. LMA classic

Fig. 4.5. LMA Pro-Seal

It should be remembered that the top of the oral airway might push the tongue down to cause obstruction. When size is smaller the tongue might block the tip. Nasopharyngeal airway is less often used because of fear of injuring the enlarged adenoids except in cleft palate and pharyngoplasty cases. In older children and adolescents, when used is well tolerated in awake state. It should be firmly secured to prevent accidental passage to nasopharynx (Fig. 4.3).

LMA has brought a revolutionary change the way we manage airway now.[2,3] Though it was designed to be useful in abnormal airway, it is extensively used to manage normal airway, so much so that in many places, LMAs have replaced 50–80% of endotracheal intubation.

The paediatric size LMA classic (1,1.5 and 2,2.5) are smaller version of adult LMA and not designed for child anatomy. Hence, 1 and 1.5 sizes do not fit well and need to be secured manually in a particular position (Fig. 4.4). With 2nd generation LMA (Pro-Seal), where the stem is reinforced and flexible the situation has changed (Fig. 4.5). It provides a better seal and patients can be ventilated at a higher peak inspiratory pressure without significant leak. Certain makes, like Ambu, fit to the contour of the child's airway better and are easy to insert. Smaller sizes of supraglottic devices are also available in recent years and one should choose after practical evaluation for suitability in his/her environment.

Endotracheal Tubes (ETTs)

Though red rubber ETTs are still available and used in children, the PVC one has an advantage of offering a thin wall and wider internal diameter.

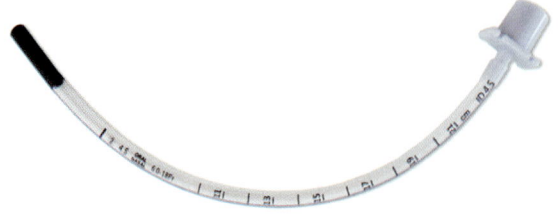

Fig. 4.6. Uncuffed ETT

Traditionally, non-cuffed tube has been used in children up to the size of 5.5, 6 and cuffed tube beyond that size[4,5] (Fig. 4.6). The advantage of cuffed tube is to minimize theatre pollution and decrease the cost of gases by reducing the fresh gas flow. Most of the cuff tubes available in the market are not specifically designed for children and are smaller version of adult tubes. Wess, et al. demonstrated how most of the contemporary available cuffed tubes have no

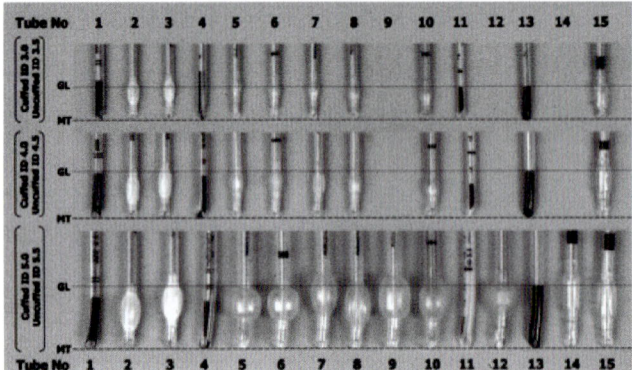

Fig. 4.7. Cuffed tubes (Wess et al) showing the non-standardized cuffs, marking and placement.

standardized approach to cuff size, the cuff placement, the laryngeal marker, etc. (Fig. 4.7).[6] They developed a Microcuff tube to avoid these shortcomings which is a polyurethane make, soft, gentle to tissue with a 10 cm H_2O pressure and placed close to the tip of the tube[7] (Fig. 4.8). However, the outer diameters at the cuff of these tubes are so wide (7.5 for a 3.5 ID tube) that one will choose a smaller size increasing resistance. The diameter of the cuff is wider than the ID of trachea so the cuff will get wrinkled and provide an uneven seal. It is about 7–8 times more expensive so cannot be used routinely in all cases.

With such development, it is tempting to change over to cuffed tube in all children including neonates and that is what has happened over last few years gradually. The other justification for not using non-cuff tube is that the traditional recommendation was not based on any scientific evidence. Safe use of the uncuffed tube for so many decades probably in millions of children is not real evidence!! Resulting in a case of irony of argument.

There is a large evidence of injury to larynx and subglottic region by the ETT especially a large size uncuffed tube or a cuffed tube. Often the cuff size is so wide (in some makes) that it partially remains in the larynx. So whenever a cuff tube is used for monitoring, the cuff pressure is mandatory. The size of the uncuffed tube should be determined by the formulae 3.5 + age in years.[8] An audible air leak around the ETT at a pressure of 20 cm H_2O should be looked for to choose the right tube.

Moulded preformed tubes, like RAE, and reinforced tubes, are especially useful in head and neck surgery (Figs 4.9 and 4.10).

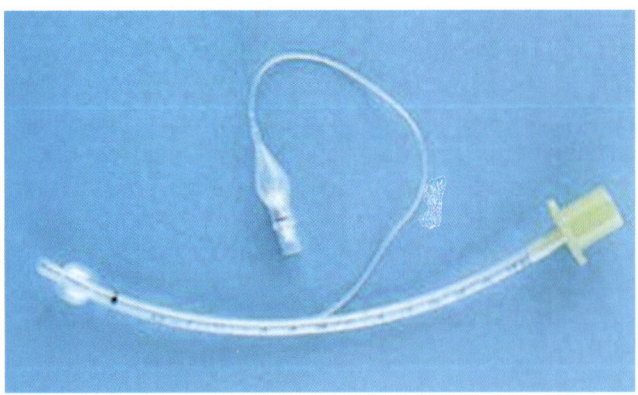

Fig. 4.8. Microcuff tube

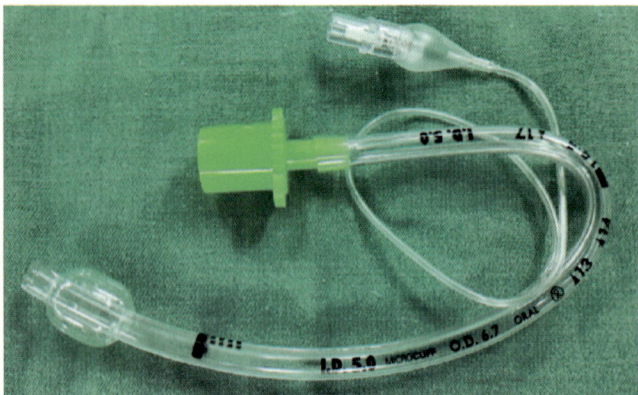

Fig. 4.9. RAE tube

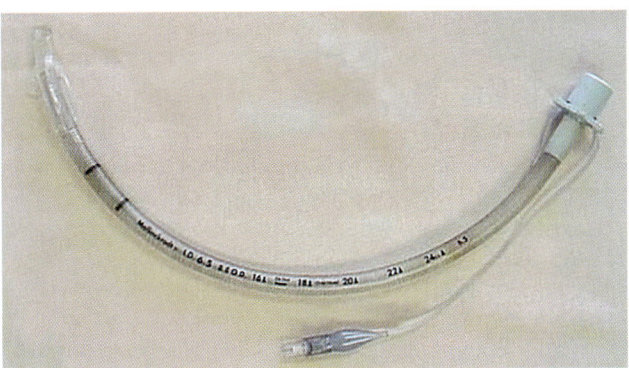

Fig. 4.10. Armoured ETT

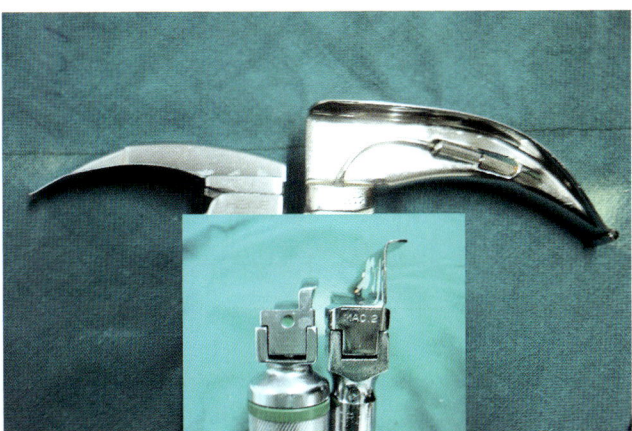

Fig. 4.12. Faulty deep spatula unsafe for infants

Laryngoscope

Laryngoscope with lightweight handle should be available with a variety of blades (Fig. 4.11). The infant laryngoscope available in our country is again a smaller version of adult blade with a deep spatula which might cause trauma to tissue while opening mouth (Fig. 4.12). The bulb is often seen protruding into the space meant to visualize the larynx and advance the tube, it deflects the tube laterally during advancement and might occlude the laryngeal vision (Fig. 4.13).

In infants and neonates, it is traditionally recommended to use straight blades (Magill) whereas curved blade (Mackintosh) is used in older children.[9]

However, there is no evidence to suggest the advantage of straight blade over the curved one. It depends on the traditional teaching and institutional practice. In my personal practice, I have rarely used straight blades even for neonates and knew some

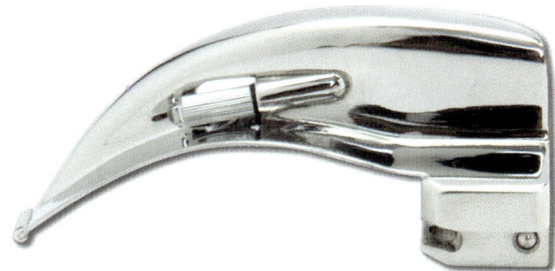

Fig. 4.13. Bulb protruding into the intubating space

eminent paediatric anaesthetist from Australia and Europe using mostly curved blade.

Fibreoptic flexible laryngoscope is the gold standard for any difficult intubation; small size of 1.8 is available for use in neonates.[10] In recent years, technology has changed the way we manage airway, especially in difficult situation. However, other devices available and can help difficult airway include: Bonfils fibrescopes (rigid), AirTraq disposable optical laryngoscope, C-MAC, GlideScope, TrueView, etc.[11] In paediatric group, the definite advantage of one device over other is not well reported.

Stylette

Soft maleable stylets should always be available for help change the shape of the ETT for ease of insertion (Fig. 4.14). It should be used only when a moulding of the curve of the tube is needed. Hardly have used it in my practice.

Lighted stylets are available for managing difficult airway but is much inferior to newer video-laryngoscopes.

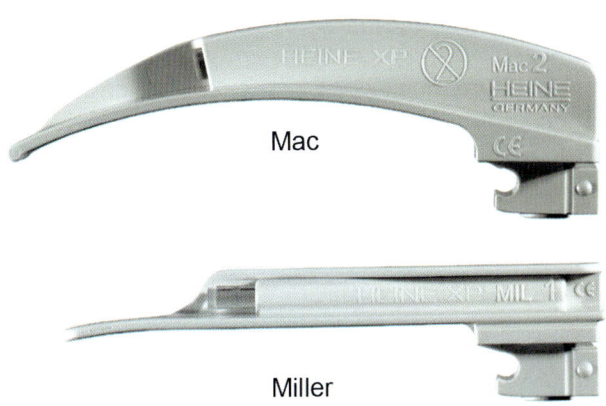

Mac

Miller

Fig. 4.11. Laryngoscope blades—Mackintosh and Miller

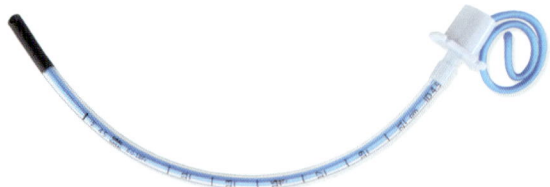

Fig. 4.14. Intubating stylette

Magill's forceps should always be available and is an useful tool in airway management. Be it packing the throat, or directing the ETT or removing tissue from oral cavity (Fig. 4.15). Gum elastic bougie is a simple but useful device. It can manage many moderately difficult situations easily. It can also be used as tube exchanges.

ANAESTHESIA MACHINE

No anaesthesia machine is marked presently for use in children alone. Adult anaesthesia machine is being used. We will discuss special features in these machines which can be helpful for paediatric use.

Breathing System (Circuits)

The work of brathing is important in spontaneously breathing infants that is the reason why the breathing systems used in children are designed to eliminate resistance and dead space. The Ayre's 'T' piece is valve less.[12] It was later modified by Jackson Rees to include the reservoir bag to the respiratory limb.[13] It has been popular all these years (Fig. 4.16). The only disadvange is that it uses higher fresh gas flow (FGF) leading to theatre pollution and cost. With introduction of costly inhalation agents, argument of using circle system holds good. A circle system allows lower FGF thereby cost-saving, maintain humidity and temperature,

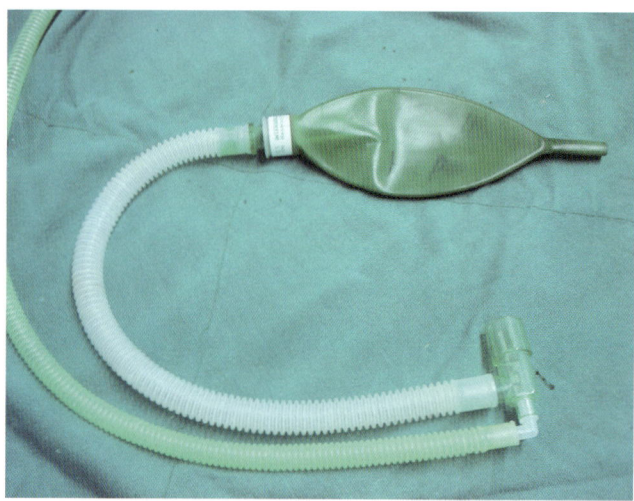

Fig. 4.16. Ayres 'T' piece with JR modification

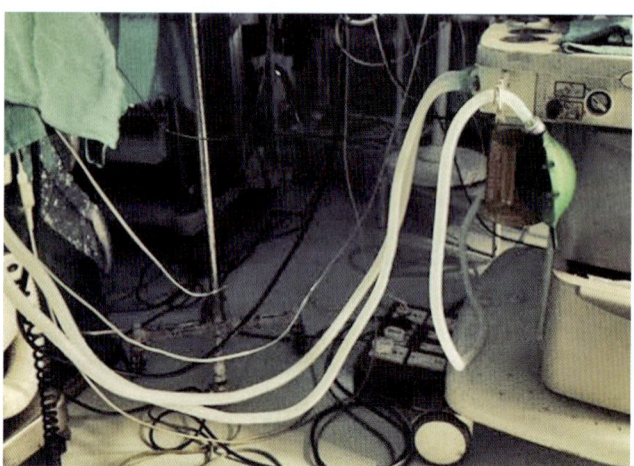

Fig. 4.17. Circle system with 15 mm tubing and small size Sodalime canister

which is important for children[14] (Fig. 4.17). In recent years, the usage of circle system with low flow has become more the norm. The use of 'T' piece is limited to neonatal induction, and transport of patient (Fig. 4.18). While using circle system, one has to ascertain certain features:

1. The total pneumatic volume of the system should be minimal.
2. There should be monitoring of inspired and expired oxygen and carbon dioxide
3. Offer less resistance with use of 15 mm tubings.
4. Small size sodalime canister.

Heated humidifier in the circle system provides heated humidified air and helps maintain mucocilliary

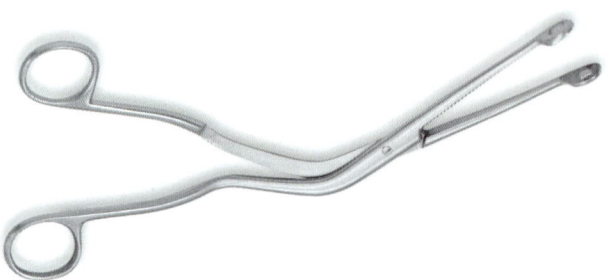

Fig. 4.15. Magill's forceps

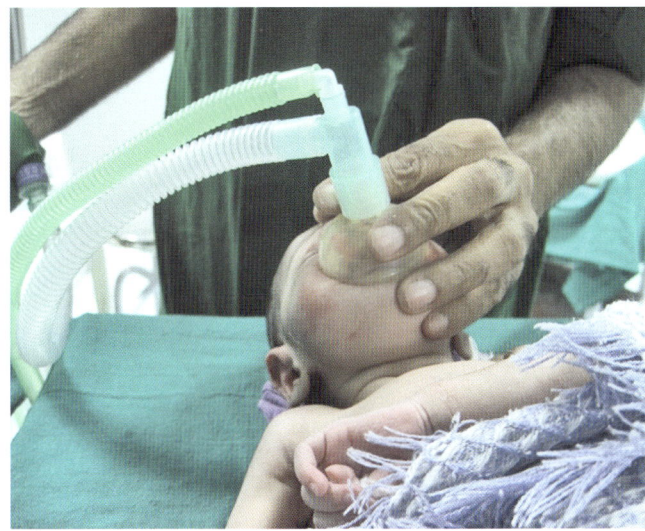

Fig. 4.18. Neonatal induction with "T" piece

activity. Its usage has decreased over the years and has been limited to neonates or infants less then 5 kg weight or those undergoing major prolonged surgery.

A bacterial filter with head and moisture exchange is commonly used in circle system and should be changed in every case to prevent contamination of the circuit. One should keep a watch that, in infants it might add to the mechanical dead space and consequent rise in $EtCO_2$.

Anaesthesia ventilator when used for children should have following features.

1. Ability to provide PEEP. As in infants, PEEP is an essential component of ventilatory strategy to maintain FRC over closing volume.

2. Ability to set age appropriate tidal volumes, inspiratory: expiratory ratio and rate from neonate to adolescent.

3. Volume guaranteed pressure regulated or controlled.

4. Provision for SIMV mode and PSV to assist spontaneously breathing children with varying trigger pressure.[15]

Monitor

Besides the standard monitoring of ECG, NIBP and pulse oxymeter, it should have, $EtCO_2$, temperature and inspired and expired gases and vapours[16] (Fig. 4.19).

A variety of oxymeter, probes for appropriate age should be available.[17–19] Spring-loaded probes are contraindicated in neonates and should be avoided in infants (Fig. 4.20); rather a wrap around probe should be used (Fig. 4.21). A variety of NIBP cuffs should also be available for different age group (Fig. 4.22).

Scavenge

The new generation machines come with scavenging systems for circle system. A device should be procured for 'T' piece scavenging.

Extra oxygen flow meter and airway pressure gases should be available for use of 'T' piece in neonates.

WARMING EQUIPMENT

It is important for surgery of neonates, infants and all major surgery. The OT temperature is important as

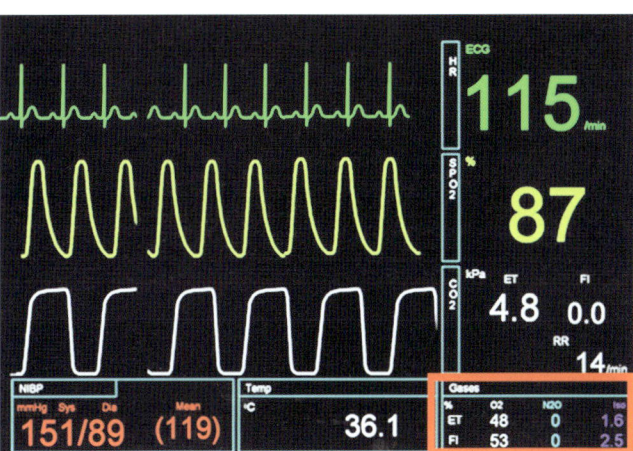

Fig. 4.19. Multiparameter monitor

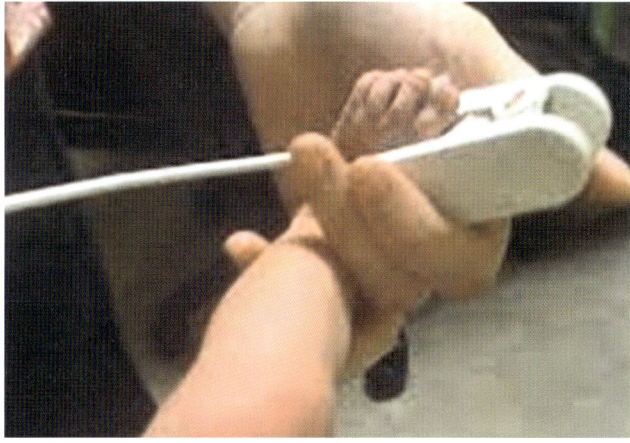

Fig. 4.20. Spring loaded probe should not be used in neonates

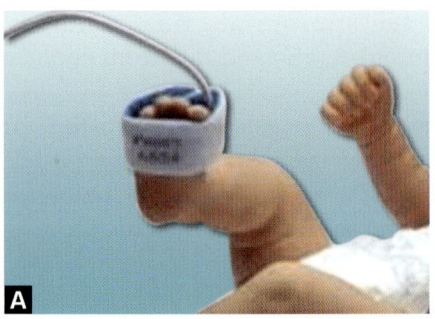 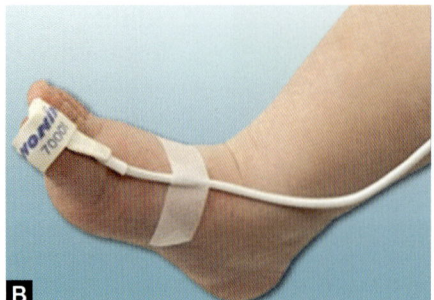 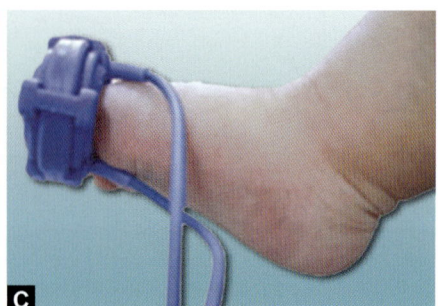

Fig. 4.21. Warp around probes

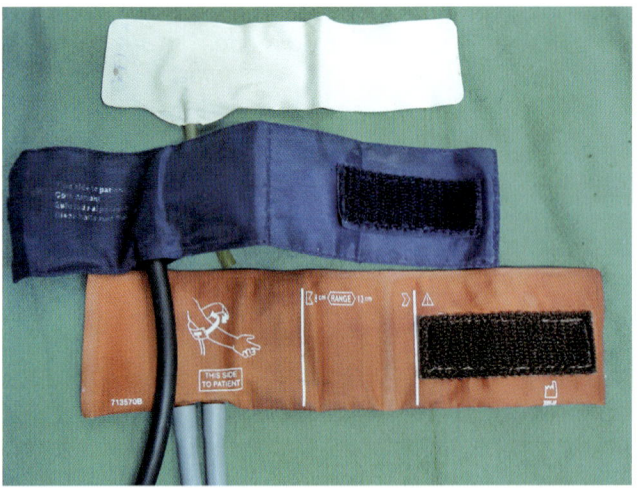

Fig. 4.22. BP cuff of various sizes

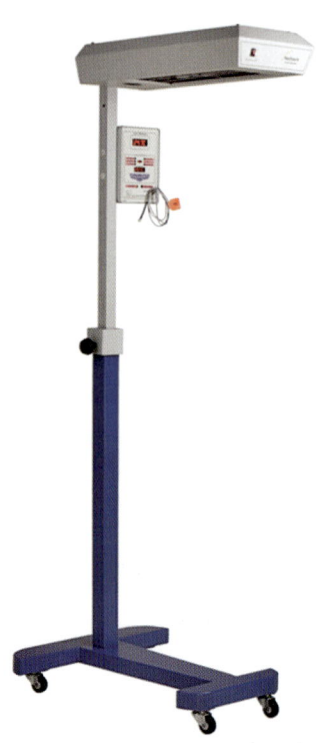

Fig. 4.23. Overhead radiant warmer

40% of heat loss is by radiation and 35% by convection. The warm wall will minimize the radiation loss and the warm air the convection loss. Once the child is cleaned and draped, the room temperature may be reduced to a comfortable level.

Overhead Radiant Warmer

These devices are useful at induction and cleaning when the baby is bare and again at the end after the drapes are removed. Prescribed distance from the body should be maintained to prevent burn injury (Fig. 4.23).

Warming Blankets

The blanket was used routinely in the past. They are either water circulating or electrical. As the heat loss due to conduction is <5%, its use has been decreased. It is often used in children less than 5 kg weight.[20]

Heated Humidifier in Circuit

Its role in preventing heat loss is not as good as believed. Its use is again limited to neonates and infants <5 kg.[21]

Forced Warm Air Devices

These are most effective devices to maintain body temperature (Fig. 4.24).[22,23] The disposable branded blankets are expensive. It has been observed that flowing the warm air under the drapes is good enough to maintain temperature (Fig. 4.25).[24] Sometimes two devices, one for upper part and other for the lower

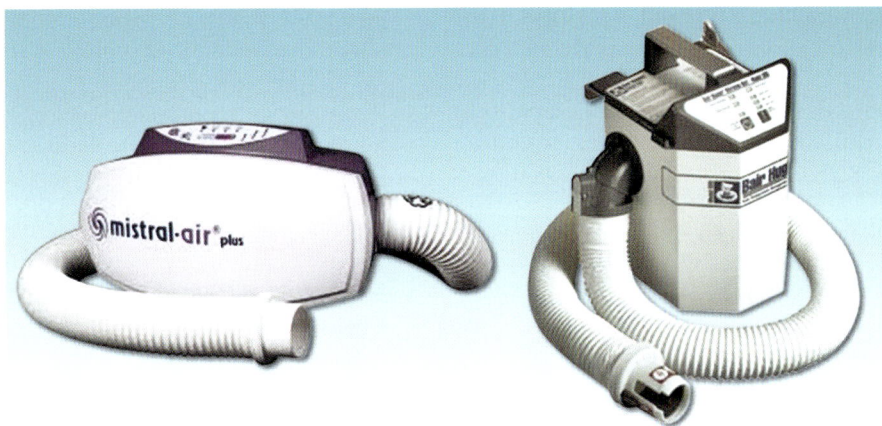

Fig. 4.24. Forced warm air devices

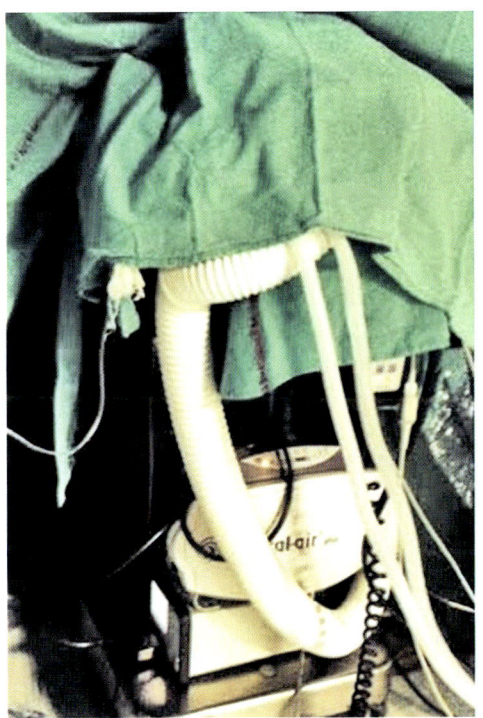

Fig. 4.25. Forced warm air device in use under the wraps

limb is used for children less accessible during surgery. It is important to see that the warm air does not directly reach the skin, the flow is diffused with a thick pad or something similar.

Fluid Warmers

Unless there is a large volume infusion/transfusion, these devices do not contribute much in preventing heat loss during maintenance therapy because the heat of the warmed fluid is lost along IV tubing between the warmer and child. However, the fluid warming devices, like hot line, warm IV line also are helpful.

Wrapping the child with cotton and pads prevents radiation and convective loss. It is a simple and cost-effective device. Covering the head is of importance as it has a large surface area

AIRWAY CART

Having a multi-drawer equipment cart especially for airway management is a necessity for patient safety. It should have masks, LMA, ET tubes of various sizes, airways, laryngoscopes, blades, suction catheters, bougies, tapes of all the sizes appropriate for different age group.

One can have a different cart for fibreoptic broncho-scope and video-laryngoscopes

In our country, it is important to have designated persons in charge of equipment who are responsible for cleaning, sterilization and maintenance of these life-saving equipment. Maintaining a logbook and record of these equipment go a long way in patient safety.

REFERENCES

1. Rendell-Baker L, Soucek DH. Newpaediatric face masks and anaesthetic equipment. Br Med J 1962;1:1690.
2. Osses H, Poblete M, Asenjo F. Laryngeal mask for difcult intubation in children. Paediatr Anaesth 1999;9:399–401.
3. O'Neill B, Templeton JJ, Caramico L, Schreiner MS. The laryngeal mask airway in pediatric patients: factors affecting ease of use during insertion and emergence. Anesth Analg 1994;78:659–662.

4. Koka BV, Jeon IS, Andre JM, MacKay I, Smith RM. Post intubation croup in children. Anesth Analg 1977;56: 501–505.

5. Khine HH, Corddry DH, Kettrick RG, et al. Comparison of cuffed anduncuffed endotracheal tubes in young children during general anesthesia. Anesthesiology 1997;86:627–631.

6. Weiss M, Dullenkopf A, Gysin C, et al. Shortcomings of cuffed paediatric tracheal tubes. Br J Anaesth 2004;92: 78–88.

7. Weiss M, Dullenkopf A, Gerber AC. Microcuff pediatric tracheal tube. A new tracheal tube with a high volume-low pressure cuff for children. Anaesthesist 2004;53: 73–79.

8. van den Berg AA, Mphanza T. Choice of tracheal tube size for children: nger size or age-related formula? Anaesthesia 1997;52:701–703.

9. Varghese E, Kundu R. Does the Miller blade truly provide a better laryngoscopic view and intubating conditions than the Macintosh blade in small children? Paediatr Anaesth 2014;24:825–829.

10. Jagannathan N, Sequera-Ramos L, Sohn L, Huang A, Sawardekar A, Wasson N, Miriyala A, De Oliveira GS. Randomized comparison of experts and trainees with nasal and oral fibreoptic intubation in children less than 2 year of age. Br J Anaesth 2015;114:290–296.

11. Holm-Knudsen R. The difcult pediatric airway: a review of new devices for indirect laryngoscopy in children younger than two years of age. Paediatr Anaesth 2011;21:98–103.

12. Ayre P. The T-piece technique. Br J Anaesth 1956;28:520–523.

13. Harrison GA. Ayer's T-piece: A review of its modications. Br J Anaesth 1964;36:115–120.

14. Berry Jr FA, Hughes-Davies DI. Methods of increasing the humidity and temperature of the inspired gases in the infant circle system. Anesthesiology 1972;37:456–462.

15. Lim B, Pawar D, Ng O. Pressure support ventilation vs spontaneous ventilation via ProSeal™ laryngeal mask airway in pediatric patients undergoing ambulatory surgery: a randomized controlled trial. Paediatr Anaesth 2012;22:360–364.

16. American Society of Anesthesiologists. Standards for basic anesthetic monitoring. Standards and Practice Parameters Committee (approved by the ASA House of Delegates on October 21, 1986, and last amended on October 20, 2010, with an effective date of July 1, 2011). Available at http://www.asahq.org/For.../ Standards-Guidelines-and-Statements.aspx (accessed October 16, 2012).

17. Coté CJ, Rolf N, Liu LM, et al. A single-blind study of combined pulseoximetry and capnography in children. Anesthesiology 1991;74:980–987.

18. Runciman WB, Webb RK, Barker L, Currie M. The Australian Incident Monitoring Study. The pulse oximeter: applications and limitations—an analysis of 2000 incident reports. Anaesth Intensive Care 1993;21:543–550.

19. Goldman JM, Petterson MT, Kopotic RJ, Barker SJ. Masimosignal extraction pulse oximetry. J Clin Monit Comput 2000;16:475–483.

20. Goudsouzian NG, Morris RH, Ryan JF. The effects of a warming blanket on the maintenance of body temperatures in anesthetized infants and children. Anesthesiology 1973;39:351–353.

21. Tausk HC, Miller R, Roberts RB. Maintenance of body temperature by heated humidication. Anesth Analg 1976;55:719–723.

22. Bräuer A, Quinte IM. Forced-air warming: technology, physical background and practical aspects. Curr Opin Anaesthesiol 2009;22:769–774.

23. Witt L, Dennhardt N, Eich C, Mader T, Fischer T, Bräuer A, Sümpelmann R. Prevention of intraoperative hypothermia in neonates and infants: results of a prospective multicenter observational study with a new forced-air warming system with increased warm air flow. Paediatr Anaesth 2013;23:469–474.

24. Kempen PM. Full body forced air warming: commercial blanket vs air delivery beneath bed sheets. Can J Anaesth 1996;43:1168–1174.

5

Fluid Management in Perioperative Period and Transfusion Therapy

Purnima Dhar, Chetan Mehra

- Preoperative fasting in children
- Amount of fluid required
- Composition of fluid required
- Colloids
- Postoperative fluid therapy
- Monitoring of fluid therapy
- Special concerns in neonate
- Transfusion of blood and blood products
- Complications of transfusion therapy

INTRODUCTION

Use of parenteral fluid therapy was first reported during the cholera epidemic in 1831 but was discarded afterwards because of reports of sepsis. The understanding of the composition of body fluids initiated by Claude Bernard along with the germ theory of disease by Joseph Lister paved the way for the modern knowledge of body fluids and their safe correction by means of oral and parenteral fluid therapy. Unfortunately, even now, failure to understand and appropriately treat fluid and electrolyte disturbances remains the leading cause of morbidity and mortality among children.

A lot of literature and recommendations have been published in recent years about perioperative fluid therapy and this account will try to address the various issues and the research as available currently.

PREOPERATIVE FASTING IN CHILDREN

The two most distressing things for parents of children undergoing surgery are preoperative fasting and postoperative pain. Various types of material empty from the stomach at different rates. Clear liquids and gastric secretions move rapidly out of the stomach; the 50% emptying time of water is approximately 12 minutes.[1] Glucose-containing fluids initially leave the stomach more slowly, but after 90 minutes the stomach is empty of clear liquids regardless of type.[2]

Gastric volume is a surrogate end point used in clinical studies because the incidence of aspiration is low. Although fasting to reduce the risk of aspiration during sedation or elective surgery makes intuitive sense, there is little evidence that this approach actually prevents aspiration. Most international anaesthesia societies (ASA, European Society of Anaesthesiology, Canadian Anesthesiologst's Society, Association of Anaesthetists in Great Britain and Ireland, etc.) have accepted the following recommendations for fasting before elective procedures are planned under general anaesthesia or deep sedation (Table 5.1).

Table 5.1	Preoperative fasting recommendations
Clear liquids	2 hours before induction
Breast milk	4 hours before induction
Non-human milk, infant formula, light meal	6 hours before induction
Fried or fatty food or meat	8 hours or more

Table 5.2	"4-2-1 Rule" for fluid requirement in children
Weight of child in kg	**Fluid required per hour**
Up to 10	4 ml/kg
10–20	40 ml + 2 ml/kg for weight above 10 kg
>20 kg	60 ml + 1 ml/kg for weight above 20 kg

Clear liquids include water, non-particulate fruit juice, such as apple juice, non-aerated clear drinks, clear coconut water. Infants and young children have a higher metabolic rate and a larger body surface area-to-weight ratio than adults and become dehydrated more easily than adults. Thus intake of clear liquids should be encouraged up until two hours prior to surgery for children who are considered to be at normal risk of aspiration/regurgitation during anaesthesia.[3]

AMOUNT OF FLUID REQUIRED

For the last half a century, we have been following the formula proposed by Holliday and Segar in 1957 for estimating the fluid requirement by children.[4] This formula was based on the fact that fluid requirement depended on the metabolic demand which varies with the age of the child. Using this formula, they proposed the 4-2-1 rule (Table 5.2).

This is the maintenance fluid requirement of an unanaesthetised resting child. A child undergoing surgery will have other losses, such as blood and other fluids that can vary from very little (1 ml/kg/hr) to large (15 ml/kg/hr) or very large.[5,6]

Correction of Preoperative Deficit

This has been a topic of debate lately. In 1975, Furman, et al. had proposed a fasting child is fluid deficient and the deficit should be calculated by the 4-2-1 formula. 50% of this should be administered in the first hour after induction and rest over next 2 hours. This fluid should be in addition to the intraoperative requirement as described later.[7] As most operations may not last for 3 hours or more, Berry simplified the calculation and advised a bolus to be administered after induction. As the requirement is more in smaller children, he proposed a bolus of 25 ml/kg for children 3 years and younger and 15 ml/kg for those 4 years and older, to be administered over the first hour after

induction.[8] This is convenient especially if the child is fasting for more than 6 hours and is the practice of the author. However, with the current libral fasting guidelines as described above, this correction may not be required, if the child is taking clear fluids until 2 hours before surgery or the child has been on parenteral fluids preoperatively. Studies in adults have shown that a normal vascular volume is maintained despite a prolonged fast.[9] No such data exists for children and so till such data becomes available it is recommended to correct the deficit unless the child has renal or cardiac issues.

Holliday, et al. revisited their original recommendations for surgical children and proposed a rather open-ended recommendation. For children admitted for surgery, they recommended that isotonic saline may be given as a measured expansion, 20–40 ml/kg followed by a "keep open" rate, modified as clinical events, during surgery and recovery, dictate.[10] It works out similar to the Berry's formula.

Intraoperative Fluid Requirements

If the child has been taking oral or parenteral fluids up to 2 hours preoperative, there is no need to do deficit correction. Deficit correction should be done, if the child has been fasting for long without intravenous fluids. During surgery, all children will require maintenance fluids for the period of surgery and replacement for ongoing losses, such as blood, plasma, ascetic or pleural fluids, evaporative losses from exposed tissues, etc. Both these should run concurrently unless otherwise indicated. The maintenance should be the same as calculated by 4-2-1 formula depending upon the weight of the child. The replacement fluid depends upon the degree of tissue trauma and the age of the child. The younger the child, the greater is the relative proportion of losses because of the large ECF volume in young infants compared with older children and adults.

Another concept complicating the intraoperative fluid therapy is that of "third space loss" proposed in the eighties. Third space loss refers to the sequestration of fluid to a non-functional extracellular space that is not in equilibrium with the vascular space.[11] Third space losses were reported to vary from 1 ml/kg/hr for minor surgical procedure to 15–20 ml/kg/hr for major procedures. Preterm babies with necrotizing enterocolitis may require up to 50 ml/kg/hr.[5,6] Adult literature has questioned

Table 5.3	Intraoperative fluid therapy (Maintenance to be calculated by 4-2-1 formula)
First hour	25 ml/kg for 3 yrs and younger 15 ml/kg for 4 yrs and older
Minor surgery with minimal trauma	Maintenance + Replacement 2 ml/kg/hr
Major surgery with moderate trauma	Maintenance + Replacement 4 ml/kg/hr
Major surgery with severe trauma	Maintenance + Replacement 6 ml/kg/hr
Replacement of blood loss	Crystalloid three times the loss, or colloid/ blood equal to the volume lost

the existence of third space[12] and there is evidence that crystalloid administration according to these calculations can lead to overloading resulting in deterioration of vascular barriers. The expansion of interstitial space contributes to postoperative complications, such as anastomotic leaks, cardiac failure, etc. No data exists for similar findings in children but this fact needs to be kept in mind while treating children as well.

So, as of now, we recommend the intraoperative fluid therapy as described by Berry (Table 5.3).[6,8]

In case of blood loss leading to hemodynamic disturbance, a bolus of 15–20 ml/kg of Ringer lactate solution administered over 15–20 min will re-establish cardiovascular stability. A second bolus of 15–20 ml/kg of crystalloid solution can be given, if there is no response to first bolus and the maximum allowable blood loss limit has not been crossed (*see later*). If there is continuing loss, administration of a colloid solution (albumin or synthetic colloid) to maintain intravascular osmotic pressure is indicated.[45] The formula of 3 : 1 rule, i.e. blood loss to be replaced with three times the volume with crystalloid, can also be used to correct hypovolaemia but it is not always possible to know the exact blood loss while the bleeding is going on. In addition, the point for starting colloids is related to assessment of losses. I, therefore, prefer to give two crystalloid boluses followed by colloid. Blood replacement is discussed separately.

COMPOSITION OF FLUID REQUIRED

Two main types of fluids are available for fluid therapy. The term 'crystalloids' is used to describe aqueous fluids that contain crystal-forming elements (electrolytes), which easily pass through vascular endothelial membrane barriers followed by water, leading to their equilibration between the intra-vascular and extracellular space. The examples are normal saline (0.9% sodium chloride), Ringer's lactate, Plasma-Lyte, Sterofundin, etc. The term 'colloids' refers to aqueous solutions that contain both large organic macromolecules and electrolytes. The large molecular size of the dissolved molecules limits their ability to cross the endothelial membrane. These molecules are retained within the intravascular space to a greater degree than pure crystalloids, owing to their higher oncotic pressure. The redistribution of water and electrolytes into the interstitial space results in smaller retained intravascular volume of the initial crystalloid infusion solution and development of oedema when compared to colloid solutions.[45] The examples of colloids are albumin (5%, 20%, 25%), hydroxyethyl starches (HES) and gelatins (Haemaccel, Gelofusin).

Isotonic vs Hypotonic Fluid

Holliday and Segar[4] had also described the electrolyte content of the intravenous fluid depending upon the daily requirements of sodium and potassium which were calculated to be 3 mEq/kg and 2 mEq/kg, respectively. The concentration of sodium in the infusion fluid for small babies worked out to be 0.18%, about 0.45% in older children and somewhere in between for smaller children. Both these solutions are hypotonic. The trauma of surgery leads to a state of increased ADH release, which exists intraoperatively and postoperatively. Increase in ADH leads to fluid retention and if combined with large volumes of hypotonic solutions can result in hyponatraemia with disastrous consequences, like seizures, brain damage and death.[14–17] Hence it is recommended to use iso-tonic saline, such as Ringer's lactate, or normal (0.9%) saline in the perioperative period. But despite con-vincing evidence, many anaesthesiologists continue to use hypotonic solutions intraoperatively.[18]

Hypochloraemic vs Hyperchloraemic Fluids

With more available clinical trial data, the debate behind fluid administration has expanded to include controversies surrounding particular solutions within the cryatalloid group. NS versus more balanced crystalloid solutions (Ringer's lactate, Plasma-Lyte,

Sterofundin, Normo Sol, etc.). Concerns have been raised about use of large volumes of normal saline as it leads to hyperchloraemia. Although clinical studies have not revealed adverse effects of hyperchloraemic acidosis on outcome,[18] it has now firmly been established that hyperchloraemic metabolic acidosis is a predictable consequence of saline-based, non-balanced intravenous fluid administration.[19] The hyperchloraemic acidosis was shown to be associated with reduced gastric mucosal perfusion on gastric tonometry.[20] Hyperchloraemia has been found to have profound effects on eicosanoid release in renal tissue, leading to vasoconstriction and a reduction of the glomerular filtration rate.[21] Therefore, although normal saline is safe in healthy children, in critically ill patients with other comorbidities, like renal disease, more physiological electrolyte solutions (e.g. Ringer's lactate solution) may be preferable, especially if boluses are being given.

COLLOIDS

The colloids available for clinical use can be divided into natural protein colloids (albumin) and synthetic colloids (hydroxyethyl starches [HESs], dextrans, and gelatins).

Albumin occurs naturally and is regarded as the colloid "gold standard." Albumin is derived from pooled human plasma. In India, albumin is available in concentrations of both 5% and 20%. An albumin 5% solution is osmotically equivalent to an equal volume of plasma, whereas a 20% solution is osmotically equivalent to 4 times its plasma volume. In other words, it draws water from the interstitium and expands the vascular compartment 4 times its volume. However, in subjects with increased intravascular permeability (e.g. critically ill, sepsis, trauma, and burn), the translocation of fluid from the interstitial compartment to the intravascular compartment may be decreased and colloids may actually leak into the interstitial space, thereby worsening oedema by pulling fluid from the intravascular compartment.[5] 20% albumin has limited role as a resuscitative fluid during surgery, as it needs to be given slowly, but can be used in the postoperative period.

There have been reservations about the use of synthetic colloids in children, especially HESs. HESs have been shown to increase the requirement for renal replacement therapy in adult ICU patients. However,

large retrospective analysis of data of children receiving HES for cardiac surgery has shown it to be as safe as albumin.[54] Moderate doses of HES (130/0.42/6:1) for perioperative plasma volume replacement seem to be safe even in neonates and small infants.[36]

Gelatins are polypeptides produced by the degradation of bovine collagen. Gelatins have a volume effect of 70 to 80%, are inexpensive, and have minimal effects on coagulation or renal function. Although safe to use in older infants and children, there is limited data to support the use of gelatin in neonates. Although a multicentre study done in preterm infants showed no adverse short-term outcomes related to gelatin use,[55] early volume expansion with gelatin in preterm infants has been found to marginally increase the risk of developing NEC.[56] Albumin was found to be better than gelatins in terms of survival in children suffering from malaria,[57] but was no better than other fluids in another meta-analysis of septic patients.[58]

So, except in septic children, both HES and gelatins are safe to use for routine replacement for blood loss in the operating room. However, in preterm and term neonates, presenting for major surgery, it may be safer to avoid the synthetic colloids and stick to 5% albumin, if colloids are needed.

When should one administer colloids? The choice of fluids is largely based on location, availability and cost. For example, in comparing the use of colloid to crystalloid for treating hypovolaemia, clinicians from the UK, China, and Australia rely primarily on colloid therapy (55 to 75% of time), whereas only 13% of clinicians in the US use colloid for treating hypovolaemia.[46,47] Within the colloids also, there is regional bias. Gelatins are not used in the United States, but fairly common in Europe and India. The cost of albumin is high, and it has a limited shelf-life, whereas starches and gelatins are cheaper and have a longer shelf-life.

Colloids should be used during surgery to replace blood loss and occasionally for replacement of large volume ascites drainage. There are enough studies in literature to favour crystalloids over colloids. Crystalloids (normal saline or Ringer's lactate) are first administered to treat absolute or relative blood volume deficits frequently observed during surgery in children. Their advantages include low cost, lack of effect on coagulation, no risk of anaphylactic reaction and no risk of transmission of infections but a higher incidence of pulmonary oedema and, weight gain and increased anion gap has been reported in patients receiving saline, in some studies.[48,49] However, this was not found by others.[50,51] A review by the WHO expert committee on the selection and use of colloids in paediatric trauma and burns patients concluded that "there is not sufficient evidence to recommend the inclusion of any colloid in the essential medicines list for children".[52] Studies on critically ill septic children from India have failed to show advantage of colloids over crystalloids[49] and in traumatic brain injury it may even be harmful.[53]

In our practice, in the operating room, blood loss is replaced with crystalloids first and colloids are given after the resuscitation with crystalloids has failed and blood is not immediately available or not indicated.

Perioperative Use of Dextrose

Hypoglycaemia and hyperglycaemia are both deleterious. Unrecognised and untreated hypoglycaemia (blood sugar <45 mg/dl) can cause serious neurological impairement.[22] However, the risk of preoperative hypoglycaemia has been demonstrated to be low in normal healthy infants and children (1–2%), despite prolonged fasting periods and almost always occurs when the child is fasted for more than 8 hrs.[23–26] Thus, it would appear that in the vast majority of patients, there is no need to administer glucose in the perioperative period nor is there a need to monitor blood glucose.[6]

Hyperglycaemia occurs in the perioperative period due to the hormonal response to surgical stress. Hyperglycaemia has also been recognised as detrimental for the nervous system.[27,28] Animal studies have shown that in the setting of an ischaemic or hypoxic event, due to the anaerobic metabolism of excess glucose causing an accumulation of lactate, a decrease in intracellular pH, and subsequently severely compromised cellular function and even cell death can result.[29–31] Hyperglycaemia also predisposes to wound infection and osmotic diuresis which can result in dehydration and electrolyte disturbance.

However, data are inadequate to eliminate glucose completely because the relevance of the animal data is not clear and the true incidence of hypoglycaemia is not known in different age group of fasted children. This issue is further complicated by the fact that different values are used to define hypoglycaemia, depending on the child's age.[32]

Therefore, it is recommended that intraoperative administration of glucose-free isotonic hydrating solutions should be the routine practice for most procedures in children over 4–5 years of age.[6] Neonates, malnourished children with poor glycogen stores, children on parenteral nutrition, those on glucose containing intravenous solutions preoperatively and children with endocrinopathies are prone to hypoglycaemia and should receive glucose infusion at a rate of 120–300 mg/kg/hr, which is sufficient to maintain an acceptable blood glucose level and prevent lipid mobilisation.[33] Therefore, 1% or 2% dextrose in Ringer's lactate is appropriate in infants and young children, but 5% dextrose solutions should be avoided.[34,35] It is recommended to monitor the blood sugar in children receiving glucose[36] as hyperglycaemia often sets in. It should be remembered that the glucose containing solutions should be used only for maintenance and given as a piggyback to replacement fluids. All replacement fluids and bolus fluids should be glucose free to avoid hyperglycaemia.

It is recommended to start glucose, if surgeries last for more than 3 hours. Children receiving regional anaesthesia along with general anaesthesia have lower blood sugars compared to those receiving general anaesthesia alone and this may be due to reduced stress response and they may be candidates for intraoperative glucose.[37,38]

It is important to remember that children, who are febrile or septic, will have increased fluid requirement.

POSTOPERATIVE FLUID THERAPY

1. When to start oral fluids
2. Volume of fluid to be administered
3. Composition of fluid to be administered

Unless contraindicated for surgical reasons, it is a general tendency to discontinue intravenous fluids and start oral fluids, as soon as the child is awake, especially for day care procedures. But studies have shown that delaying oral feeds up to 4–6 hrs post-op prevents PONV significantly.[39–41] In order to achieve this, 'superhydration' with up to 30 ml/kg/hr of fluid is also advocated during surgery especially for children highly prone to PONV, such as following squint surgery.[41] Superhydration has been shown to prevent PONV in adult daycare patients as well.

After major surgery, the increase in ADH continues in the immediate postoperative period and these children continue to be at risk of hyponatraemia in the postoperative period. Hence it is advocated to continue isotonic fluids in the postoperative period for 12 hours. It has been advised to reduce the volume to be infused to 2-1-0.5 formula for the first 12 hours post-op (2 ml/kg/hr for first 10 kg, 1 ml/kg/hr for next 10 kg and 0.5 ml/kg/hr above 20 kg) instead of 4-2-1 formula as they tend to retain fluid in this period. If oral feeds are not allowed after 12 hours, 4-2-1 formula should be followed and 0.45% saline with dextrose should be administered.[10,32] Others have recommended continuation of isotonic fluids with dextrose in the postoperative period unless the serum sodium is above 140 mmols/l in critically ill children after major surgery.[42,43] We continue to follow the 4-2-1 formula for maintenance fluids in the postoperative period (unless contraindicated due to medical reasons) with all replacements (nasogastric aspirate, all drains, wound soakage, etc.) replaced by isotonic fluid, colloid or blood products four to six hourly or earlier as the case may be. Modifications also need to be made in case the child is febrile or has sepsis.

MONITORING OF FLUID THERAPY

The main goal of intraoperative fluid therapy is to maintain tissue perfusion by optimizing intravascular volume status and stroke volume.

The patients undergoing surgery are at risk of underfilling (**hypovolaemia**) or overfilling (**hypervolaemia**). Hypovolaemia leads to vasoconstriction in the various vascular beds. Peripheral vasoconstriction may not be evident under anaesthesia but splanchnic vasoconstriction is an early response and is disproportionately higher than other vascular beds even under anaesthesia.[59] Within the splanchnic bed, the gut perfusion is affected before other organs. Hypervolaemia too, is quite common and weight gain of more than 10% from pre-op values has been shown to be associated with increased morbidity and mortality in adults.[60]

The main aim of monitoring a patient under anaesthesia and post-surgery is to maintain tissue perfusion. Clinical signs of impaired tissue perfusion, such as peripheral pulses, skin temperature and capillary refill, are a good guide but not entirely reliable and easy to check under anaesthesia especially in small babies although they may be very helpful post-op. Weight is a good monitor of fluid status post-surgery. Although ideally children should be weighed daily while on IV fluids, practically this is difficult in older children, or those who have undergone major surgery.

Therefore, routine monitors, such as heart rate, blood pressure, peripheral oxygen saturation, central venous pressure and urine output, are used to guide fluid therapy. Adult studies have shown that hypo- and hypervolaemic states are common despite all these monitors. Dynamic variables calculation, such as stroke volume variation, systolic pressure variation, pulse pressure variation derived from arterial or plethysmography waveform, may help. These monitors are not available for children yet and hence as of now, we cannot move away from protocol-based fluid therapy to goal-directed fluid therapy in children.

Serum lactate is a marker of tissue perfusion and has been used to measure the severity of shock in patients with sepsis. Lactate clearance has been used to monitor the response to therapy in hypovolaemic shock as well. Although not specifically studied in hypovolaemic shock, blood lactate may also be an indicator of severity of illness and lactate clearance a measure of response to fluid therapy. What sounds very exciting is the monitoring of microcirculation.[61]

Measures of tissue oxygenation, such as infrared oximetry and differences in sublingual PCO_2 and arterial PCO_2, are reported to detect subclinical hypoperfusion. Many other technologies are being investigated and newer monitors are in the pipeline.

SPECIAL CONCERNS IN NEONATES

The major concerns stem from three facts. Firstly, the newborns have a larger ECF volume, secondly, the renal system of newborns is immature and thirdly, they have low glycogen stores. During the first 48 hours, term babies make less urine, are volume expanded and hence require mainly 10% glucose at 60 ml/kg/day. Maintenance requirements for sodium, potassium, and chloride are approximately 1 to 2 mEq/kg/day. For infants receiving intravenous fluids, these electrolytes generally are not given during the first 24 hours after birth. Additional electrolyte losses beyond maintenance requirements should be replaced with isotonic fluid, plasma or albumin.

Preterm babies require more, up to 80–90 ml/kg/day in 1.5 kg baby due to larger surface area. Serum sodium can be an accurate marker of hydration in first two days of life, with hyponatraemia indicating fluid overload and hypernatraemia, dehydration. Fluid balance in sick surgical neonates should be meticulously monitored. Hypervolaemia in very low birth weight babies can prevent PDA closure and make them susceptible to nectrotising enterocolitis, in addition to causing intraventricular haemorrhage and bronchopulmonary dysplasia. Hidden fluid administration used to dilute antibiotics or analgesics should be taken into account, especially in neonatal anaesthesia where margin for error is miniscule.

Other points to remember are to always get rid of air bubbles in the intravenous administration set (risk of paradoxical air embolism via patent cardiac shunts) and warm the intravenous fluids whenever rapid infusions are being given.

TRANSFUSION OF BLOOD AND BLOOD PRODUCTS

Babies are born with foetal haemoglobin and premature infants have higher percentages of foetal haemoglobin (HbF) than their full-term counterparts (97% vs 70% of total haemoglobin) and decreased erythropoietin production which prevents them from responding to anaemia appropriately. HbF production diminishes during the first few months of life until only a trace is present at 6 months of age. HbF has lower oxygen unloading capacity at the tissue level. In the presence of congenital heart disease or lung disease, neonates may have, not only decreased unloading capacity at tissue level but a decreased ability to oxygenate the blood also. It is for these reasons that haemoglobin levels that are adequate for the older patient may be suboptimal in the younger infant or neonate and the threshold for transfusing RBCs to a neonate should be at a higher haemoglobin trigger than an older child or healthy adult. Maintaining higher haemoglobin levels will increase oxygen carrying capacity, and in the premature infant, may protect from post-anaesthetic apnoea of prematurity.[65]

The first step to managing blood loss in children is to know their normal haemoglobins (Table 5.4),[36,67] and the blood volumes (Table 5.5). Estimated circulating blood volume ranges from 84 ml/kg in infants at 1 to 6 months, to 71 ml/kg in adolescents.[68]

Table 5.4	Normal haemoglobin values for full-term and premature infants[36,67]	
	Full term (g/dl of blood)	Premature (g/dl of blood)
Birth	19.3	Slightly less than full term
0.5 months	16.6	15.4
1 month	13.9	11.6
Age at Hb nadir	9–12 weeks	6–10 weeks
Mean Hb at nadir	11.2	9.4
4 months	12.2	11.7
6 months	12.5	12.4

Table 5.5	Estimated blood volumes[36]
Age	Estimated blood volume (ml/kg)
Premature infant	90–100
Term infant 3 months	80–90
Children older than 3 months	70
Very obese children	65

A preoperative Hb level of ≥ 10 g/dl has been recommended for patients who will receive general anesthesia, because lower values are associated with an increase in perioperative complications.[70–72] Having said that, in a developing country like India, malnutrition is common and an Hb level less than 10 g/dl is very common and it is impractical to delay surgery in every case and minor surgeries are not postponed for this. Although there is no data, they tend to do fairly well. Neonates coming for surgery should have an Hb more than 12 g/dl. Older infant with no comorbidity can be accepted for surgery at a haemoglobin level more than 7 g/dl keeping in mind that this child will have practically zero allowable blood loss.

Transfusion Trigger and Maximum Allowable Blood Loss

The transfusion trigger will vary according to the age of the child and any associated cardiac or respiratory condition. Chronically anaemic children often tolerate haemoglobin (Hb) concentrations as low as 6 to 7 g/dl or a haematocrit (Hct) of 20%, because they are able to maintain adequate intravascular volume and tissue oxygenation by various physiological and biochemical adaptations.[69] On the other hand, patients with an acute loss of blood and hypovolaemia often require transfusion regardless of their level of Hb (Table 5.6).

Table 5.6	Approximate capillary Hb transfusion thresholds used fores 'restrictive' transfusion policies in studies evaluated by the Cochrane Review[73]	
Postnatal age	Respiratory support	No respiratory support
Week 1	115 g/l	100 g/l
Week 2	100 g/l	85 g/l
Week 3	85 g/l	75 g/l

It is important to calculate the patient's estimated blood volume (EBV) and the maximum allowable blood loss (MABL) for every case expected to bleed.

MABL = [(starting haematocrit – target haematocrit) ÷ starting haematocrit] × EBV

Blood loss less than the MABL should be replaced with balanced salt solution or a colloid. Crystalloid volume administered should be three times the loss and colloid volume should be equal to the blood loss. Albumin is the colloid of choice in neonates, but synthetic colloids can be used in older infants and children. Blood loss beyond MABL should be replaced with packed RBCs. RBC transfusion during surgery is also needed, if intraoperative blood loss is ≥15% of blood volume, regardless of the Hb or Hct level. Replacement for blood loss above the MABL(XBL) is made according to the following formula:

Volume of 100% RBCs blood to be transfused = XBL × desired haematocrit (30%)

As the approximate haematocrit in packed RBCs is 70%, the volume of packed RBCs in millilitres to be transfused will be = [XBL × desired haematocrit (suppose 30%)] ÷ 0.70. This can usually be simplified by transfusing approximately 0.5 ml packed RBCs for each millilitre of blood loss beyond the MABL; this will result in a slightly higher haematocrit than the target 30%, but since all of these calculations are estimates, the end result is usually close to the desired value.[73] The usual transfusion volume in children is 10 to 15 ml/kg; this volume is expected to raise the haemoglobin concentration by 2 to 3 g/dl.

It should be given over less than four hours. It should be remembered that the shelf-life of packed red cells after the bag is spiked is four hours.

Transfusion volumes and rates for children should be carefully calculated and prescribed in millilitre, not component units, to minimise dosing errors and reduce the risk of circulatory overload.[74]

Major Haemorrhage in Infants and Children

Massive transfusion in paediatric patients is usually defined as any one of the following:[77]

- Transfusion of more than 50% of total blood volume within three hours
- Transfusion of more than 100% of total blood volume in 24 hours
- Transfusion support to replace ongoing blood loss of more than 10% of total blood volume per minute.

There is limited research evidence to determine the clinical guidelines for the management of children with major haemorrhage. In general, principles developed in adult practice have been extrapolated to the care of children. Traditional 'massive transfusion' guidelines to reverse coagulopathy have been extrapolated from military practice and involve administration of packed RBCs, FFP and platelet concentrates in a 1:1:1 ratio. Where these transfusion ratios are employed, the ratio should be based on volume (ml), rather than 'units'. Once the patient has been stabilized by 'damage control resuscitation', transfusion is based on clinical signs and appropriate therapeutic targets which are: Hb 8 g/dl; fibrinogen >100 mg/dl; PT ratio <1.5; platelet count >75 × 10^3/mm^3.[74] There is a need for rapid coagulation testing in this situation. This is effectively managed by using a viscoelastic point-of-care device (ROTEM or thromboelastography). Hypothermia aggravates coagulopathy and should be prevented at all costs.

FFP transfusion should be with 15–20 ml/kg, if INR is more than 1.5. Acquired fibrinogen deficiency is a common finding and should be treated with cryoprecipitate. Fibrinogen level less than 150 mg/dl should be corrected with cryoprecipitate 5–10 ml/kg. One unit of cryoprecipitate per 10 kg body weight raises the plasma fibrinogen concentration by approximately 50 mg/dl in the absence of continued consumption or massive bleeding.

One random unit of platelets (obtained from 1 unit of whole blood) will raise the platelet count in an adult by 5,000–8,000/mm^3. In children, 0.1–0.2 units/kg will increase the platelet count by 30–50,000/mm^3 [78] that works out to about one such unit for 10 kg.

Based on current literature, routine use of recombinant factor VIIa is not supported,[75] however, it is widely used off-label as a 'last ditch' therapy for patients with major haemorrhage.

Based on the CRASH-2 study in adults, the Royal College of Paediatrics and Child Health now recommends the use of tranexamic acid in children after major trauma in a dose of 15 mg/kg (maximum 1,000 mg) infused intravenously over 10 minutes followed by 2 mg/kg/h (maximum 125 mg/h) until bleeding is controlled.[74]

Ultimately, it is the well-rehearsed local protocols, good communication with the blood bank, the laboratory, the housekeeping staff and involvement of staff with paediatric expertise that lead to successful outcomes.

COMPLICATIONS OF TRANSFUSION THERAPY

Although most of the complications associated with paediatric blood transfusions are similar to those encountered in adults, the rate is much higher. The rate of transfusion reaction in children reported in United States, is approximately 1%,[80] but a Brazilian study reported an overall incidence of 3.8%.[81] Main complications reported are overtransfusion, metabolic complications and transfusion reactions.

Overtransfusion is the most common complication. Metabolic complications also occur more readily and with a greater frequency in children (e.g. hypocalcaemia, hyperkalaemia and hypothermia).[66] Transfusion reactions are not so common these days. The product most frequently involved in transfusion reactions, is platelet concentrate (50.9%).[81] Transfusion reactions consist mostly of the allergic type, which are generally mild. Furthermore, children aged 1 to 2 years are more susceptible to febrile non-haeamolytic reaction, while those older than 2 years are more prone to allergic reactions.[81]

More serious transfusion reactions are haemolysis (early and delayed), transfusion-related acute lung injury (TRALI) and transfusion-associated graft versus host disease (TA-GVHD).

Transfusion-related acute lung injury (TRALI) is an important cause of transfusion-related mortality, and should be suspected, if a patient develops dyspnoea, pulmonary oedema, hypotension, and fever within six hours of a transfusion.

SUMMARY

1. Children can safely be allowed clear fluids 2 hours before surgery without increasing the risk of aspiration.
2. Food should normally be withheld for 6 hours prior to surgery in children aged 6months or older.
3. In children under 6 months of age, it is probably safe to allow a breast milk feedup to 4 hours before surgery.
4. Dehydration without signs of hypovolaemia should be corrected slowly.
5. Hypovolaemia should be corrected rapidly to maintain cardiac output and organ perfusion.
6. In the child, a fall in blood pressure is a late sign of hypovolaemia.
7. Maintenance fluid requirements should be calculated using the formula of Holliday and Segar Body weight Daily fluid requirement
   - 0–10 kg 4 ml/kg/hr
   - 10–20 kg 40 ml/hr + 2 ml/kg/hr above 10 kg
   - >20 kg 60 ml/hr + 1 ml/kg/hr above 20 kg
8. A fluid management plan for any child should address 3 key issues:
   - Any fluid deficit which is present
   - Maintenance fluid requirements
   - Any losses due to surgery, e.g. blood loss, 3rd space losses
9. During surgery, all of these requirements should be managed by giving isotonic fluid in all children over 1 month of age.
10. The majority of children over 1 month of age will maintain a normal blood sugar, if given non-dextrose containing fluid during surgery.
11. Children at risk of hypoglycaemia, if non-dextrose containing fluid is given, are those on parenteral nutrition or a dextrose containing solution prior to theatre, children of low body weight (<3rd centile) or having surgery of more than 3 hours duration and children having extensive regional anaesthesia. These children at risk should be given dextrose-containing solutions or have their blood glucose monitored during surgery.
12. Blood loss during surgery should be replaced initially with crystalloid or colloid, and then with blood once the haematocrit has fallen to 25%.

Children with cyanotic congenital heart disease and neonates may need a higher haematocrit to maintain oxygenation.

13. Fluid therapy should be monitored by daily electrolyte estimation, use of a fluid input/output chart and daily weighing, if feasible.

14. Acute dilutional hyponatraemia is a medical emergency and should be managed in PICU.

REFERENCES

1. Hunt JN. Some properties of an alimentary osmoreceptor mechanism. J Physiol 1956;132–267.

2. Nygren J, Thorell A, Jacobsson H, et al. Preoperative gastric emptying. Effects of anxiety and oral carbohydrate administration. Ann Surg 1995;222–728.

3. Brady M, Kinn S, O'Rourke K, et al. Preoperative fasting for preventing perioperative complications in children. Cochrane Database Syst Rev 2005;CD005285.

4. Holliday MA, Segar WE. The maintenance need for water in par-enteral fluid therapy. Pediatrics 1957;19:823–832.

5. Bailey AG, McNaull PP, Jooste E, Tuchman JB. Perioperative crystalloid and colloid fluid management in children: Where are we and how did we get here? Anesth Analg 2010;110:375–390.

6. Murat I, Dubois M. Perioperative fluid therapy in pediatrics. Paediatric Anaesth 2008;18:363–373.

7. Furman E, Roman DG, Lemmer LA, Jairabet J, Jasinska M, Laver MB. Specific therapy in water, electrolyte and blood volume replacement during pediatric surgery. Anesthesiology 1975;42:187–193.

8. Berry F. Practical aspects of fluid and electrolyte therapy. In: Berry F, (Ed). Anesthetic Management of Difficult and Routine Pediatric Patients. New York: Churchill Livingstone, 1986; p.107–135.

9. Jacob M, Chappell D, Conzen P, Finsterer U, Rehm M. Blood volume is normal after preoperative overnight fasting. Acta Anaesthesiol Scand 2008;552:522–529.

10. Holliday MA, Ray PE, Friedman AL. Fluid therapy for children: facts, fashions and questions. Archives Dis Child 2007;92(6):546–550.

11. Shires T, William J, Brown F. Acute change in extracellular fluids associated with major surgical procedure. Ann Surg 1961;154(5):803–810.

12. Chappell D, Jacob M, Hofmann-Kiefer K, Conzen P, Rehm M. A rational approach to perioperative fluid management. Anesthesiology 2008;109:723–740.

13. Montañana PA, Modesto iAlapont V, Ocón AP, López PO, LópezPrats JL, Toledo Parreño JD. The use of isotonic fluid as maintenance therapy prevents iatrogenic hyponatremia in pediatrics: a randomized, controlled open study. Pediatr Crit Care Med 2008;9:589-597.

14. Halberthal M, Halperin ML, Bohn D. Lesson of the week: Acute hyponatraemia in children admitted to hospital: retrospective analysis of factors contributing to its development and resolution. Br Med J 2001;322:780–782.

15. Arieff AL. Postoperative hyponatraemic encephalopathy following elective surgery in children. Paediatr Anaesth 1998;8:1–4.

16. Moritz ML, Ayus JC. Hospital-acquired hyponatremia: why are there still deaths? Pediatrics 2004;113:1395–1396.

17. Paut O, Remond C, Lagier P, et al. Severe hyponatremic encephalopathy after pediatric surgery: report of seven cases and recommendations for management and prevention. Ann Fr Anesth Reanim 2000;19:467–473.

18. Gunnerson KJ, Saul M, He S, Kellum JA. Lactate versus non-lactate metabolic acidosis: a retrospective outcome evaluation of critically ill patients. Crit Care 2006;10:R22.

19. Prough DS, Bidani A. Hyperchloremic metabolic acidosis is a predictable consequence of intraoperative infusion of 0.9% saline. Anesthesiology 1999;90:1247–1249.

20. Wilkes NJ, Woolf R, Mutch M, Mallett SV, Peachey T, Stephens R, Mythen MG. The effects of balanced versus saline-based hetastarch and crystalloid solutions on acid-base and electrolyte status and gastric mucosal perfusion in elderly surgical patients. Anesth Analg 2001;93: 811–816.

21. Bullivant EMA, Wilcox CS, Welch WJ. Intrarenal vaso-constriction during hyperchloremia: role of thromboxane. Am J Physiol 1989;256:152–157.

22. Burns CM, Rutherford MA, Boardman JP, Cowan FM. Pattern of cerebral injury and neurodevelopmental outcomes after symptomatic neonatal hypoglycemia. Pediatrics 2008;122:65–74.

23. Aun CS, Panesar NS. Paediatric glucose homeostasis during anaesthesia. Br J Anaesth 1990;64:413–418.

24. Jensen BH, Wernberg M, Andersen M. Preoperative starvation and blood glucose concentrations in children undergoing inpatient and outpatient anaesthesia. Br J Anaesth 1982;54:1071–1074.

25. Nilsson K, Larsson LE, Andreasson S, et al. Blood-glucose concentrations during anaesthesia in children. Effects of starvation and perioperative fluid therapy. Br J Anaesth 1984;56:375–379.

26. Welborn LG, McGill WA, Hannallah RS, et al. Perioperative blood glucose concentrations in pediatric outpatients. Anesthesiology 1986;65:543–547.

27. Sieber FE, Smith DS, Traystman RJ, et al. Glucose: a reevaluation of its intraoperative use. Anesthesiology 1987;67:72–81.

28. Leelanukrom R, Cunliffe M. Intraoperative fluid and glucose management in children. Paediatr Anaesth 2000; 10:353–359.

29. Nakakimura K, Fleischer JE, Drummond JC, et al. Glucose administration before cardiac arrest worsens neurologic outcome in cats. Anesthesiology 1990;72:1005–1011.

30. Drummond JC, Moore SS. The influence of dextrose administration on neurologic outcome after temporary spinal cord ischemia in the rabbit. Anesthesiology 1989; 70:64–70.

31. Steward DJ, Da Silva CA, Flegel T. Elevated blood glucose levels may increase the danger of neurological deficit following profoundly hypothermic cardiac arrest [letter]. Anesthesiology 1988;68:653.

32. Cote CJ, Pediatric anesthesia. In: Miller RD (Ed). Miller's Anesthesia, 8th edn, Elsevier Saunder's 2015; p. 2757–2798.

33. Nishina K, Mikawa K, Maekawa N, Asano M, Obara H. Effects of exogenous intravenous glucose on plasma glucose and lipid homeostasis in anesthetized infants. Anesthesiology 1995;83:258–63.

34. Dubois M, Gouyet L, Murat I. Lactated Ringer with 1% dextrose: an appropriate solution for peri-operative fluid therapy in children. Paediatr Anaesth 1992;2:99–104.

35. Hongnat J, Murat I, Saint-Maurice C. Evaluation of current paediatric guidelines for fluid therapy using two different dextrose hydrating solutions. Paediatr Anaesth 1991;1: 95–10

36. Arya VK. Basics of fluid and blood transfusion therapy in paediatric surgical patients. Indian Journal of Anaesthesia 2012;56(5):454–462.

37. Nakamura T, TakasakiM. Metabolic and endocrine responses to surgery during caudal analgesia in children. Can J Anaesth 1991;38(8):969–973.

38. Gouyet I, Dubois MC, Murat I, Saint-Maurice C. Comparison of two anesthesia techniques on perioperative insulin response to IV glucose infusion in children. Acta Anaesthesiol Scand 1993;37(1):12–16.

39. Kearney R, Mack C, Entwistle L. Withholding oral fluids from children undergoing day surgery reduces vomiting. Paediatr Anaesth 1998;8:331–336.

40. Schreiner MS, Nicolson SC. Pediatric ambulatory anesthesia: NPO–before or after surgery? J Clin Anesth 1995;7:589–596.

41. Goodarzi M, Matar MM, Shafa M, et al. A prospective randomized blinded study of the effect of intravenous fluid therapy on postoperative nausea and vomiting in children undergoing strabismus surgery. Pediatr Anesth 2006;16:49–53.

42. Moritz ML, Ayus JC. Prevention of hospital-acquired hyponatremia: a case for using isotonic saline. Pediatrics 2003;111:227–230.

43. Duke T, Molyneux EM. Intravenous fluids for seriously ill children: time to reconsider. Lancet 2003;362:1320–1323.

44. Hahn RG. Volume kinetics for fluid infusion. Anesthesiology 2010;113:470–481.

45. Lira A, Pinsky M. Choices in fluid type and volume during resuscitation: impact on patient outcomes. Ann Intensive Care 2014;4:38.

46. Singer M. Management of fluid balance: a European perspective. Curr Opin Anesthesiol 2012;25:96–101.

47. Finfer S, Liu B, Taylor C, Bellomo R, Billot L, Cook D, et al. Resuscitation fluid use in critically ill adults: an international cross-sectional study in 391 intensive care units. Crit Care 2010;14:R185.

48. Rackow EC, Falk JL, Fein IA, Siegel JS, Packman MI, Haupt MT, et al. Fluid resuscitation in circulatory shock: a comparison of the cardiorespiratory effects of albumin, hetastarch, and saline solutions in patients with hypovolemic and septic shock. Crit Care Med 1983;11:839–850.

49. Sumpelmann R, Schurholz T, Marx G, et al. Haemodynamic, acid-base and electrolyte changes during plasma replacement with hydroxyethyl starch or crystalloid solution in young pigs. Paediatr Anaesth 2000;10:173–179.

50. Upadhyay M, Singhi S, Murlidharan J, Kaur N, Majumdar S. Randomized evaluation of fluid resuscitation with crystalloid (saline) and colloid (polymer from degraded gelatin in saline) in pdiatric septic shock. Indian Pediatr 2005 Mar;42(3):223–231.

51. Choi P, Yip G, Quinonez LG, Cook DJ. Crystalloids vs colloids in fluid resuscitation: A systematic review. Crit Care Med 1999;27:200–210.

52. Huwer, C. "Are colloid solutions essential for the treatment of pediatric trauma or burn patients?" Review for the Expert Committee on the Selection and Use of Essential Medicines, WHO, Geneva, Switzerland November 2012.

53. Myburgh J, Cooper DJ, Finfer S, Bellomo R, Norton R, Bishop N, et al. SAFE Study Investigators; Australian and New Zealand Intensive Care Society Clinical Trials Group; Australian Red Cross Blood Service; George Institute for International Health. Saline or albumin for fluid resuscitation in patients with traumatic brain injury. N Engl J Med 2007;357:874–884.

54. Van der Linden P, Dumoulin M, Lerberghe C, Torres CS, et al. Efficacy and safety of 6% hydroxyethyl starch 130/0.4, for perioperative volume replacement in children undergoing cardiac surgery. Crit Care 2015;19(1):87.

55. The Northern Neonatal Nursing Initiative [NNNI] Trial Group. A randomized trial comparing the effect of prophylactic intravenous fresh frozen plasma, gelatin or glucose on early mortality and morbidity in preterm babies. Eur J Pediatr 1996;155:580–588.

56. Osborn DA, Evans N. Early volume expansion for prevention of morbidity and mortality in very preterm infants. Cochrane Database Syst Rev 2004;(2):CD002055. Review.

57. Akech S, Gwer S, Idro R, Fegan G, Eziefula AC, et al. (2006) Volume expansion with albumin compared to gelofusine in children with severe malaria: results of a controlled trial. PLoS Clin Trials1:e21.

58. Libing Jiang, Shouyin Jiang, Mao Zhang, Zhongjun Zheng, Yuefeng Ma, James D. Chalmers, (Eds). Albumin versus Other Fluids for Fluid Resuscitation in Patients with Sepsis: a Meta-Analysis. PLoS One 2014;9(12): e114666.

59. Chieveley-Williams S, Hamilton-Davies C. The role of the gut in major surgical postoperative morbidity. Int Anesthesiol Clin 1999;37:81.

60. Lowell JA, Schifferdecker C, Driscoll DF, et al. Postoperative fluid overload: not a benign problem. Crit Care Med 1990;18:728.

61. Knotzer H, Hasibeder WR. Microcirculatory function monitoring at the bedside—a view from the intensive care. Physiol Meas 2007;28:R65.

62. Fergusson DA, Hébert P, Hogan DL, et al. Effect of fresh red blood cell transfusions on clinical outcomes in premature, very low-birth-weight infants: the ARIPI randomized trial. JAMA 2012;308:1443.

63. Lacroix J, Hébert PC, Hutchison JS, et al. Transfusion strategies for patients in pediatric intensive care units. N Engl J Med 2007;356:1609.

64. Rouette J, Trottier H, Ducruet T, et al. Red blood cell transfusion threshold in postsurgical pediatric intensive care patients: a randomized clinical trial. Ann Surg 2010; 251:421.

65. Coté CJ, Zaslavsky A, Downes JJ, Kurth CD, Welborn LG, Warner LO, et al. Postoperative apnea in former preterm infants after inguinal herniorrhaphy. A combined analysis. Anesthesiology 1995;82:809–22.

66. Barcelona SL, Thompson AA, Cote CJ. Intraoperative pediatric blood transfusion therapy: A review of common issues. Part I: Hematologic and physiologic differences from adults; metabolic and infectious risks. Paediatr Anaesth 2005;15:716–26.

67. Brown MS. Physiologic anemia of infancy: Normal red-cell values and physiology of neonatal erythropoiesis. In: Stockman JA III, Pochedly C, (Eds). Developmental and Neonatal Hematology. New York: Raven Press 1988; pp. 249–274.

68. Riley AA, Arakawa Y, Worley S, et al. Circulating blood volumes: a review of measurement techniques and a meta-analysis in children. ASAIO J 2010;56:260.

69. Homi J, Reynolds J, Skinner A, et al. General anaesthesia in sickle-cell disease. Br Med J 1979;1:1599.

70. Carson JL, Duff A, Berlin JA, et al. Perioperative blood transfusion and postoperative mortality. JAMA 1998; 279:199.

71. Carson JL, Noveck H, Berlin JA, Gould SA. Mortality and morbidity in patients with very low postoperative Hb levels who decline blood transfusion. Transfusion 2002; 42:812.

72. Roseff SD, Luban NL, Manno CS. Guidelines for assessing appropriateness of pediatric transfusion. Transfusion 2002;42:1398.

73. Barcelona SL, Thompson AA, Cote CJ. Intraoperative pediatric blood transfusion therapy: a review of common issues. Part II: Transfusion therapy, special considerations, and reduction of allogenic blood transfusions. Paediatr Anaesth 2005;15:814–830.

74. Effective transfusion in pediatric practice. Section 10 in Transfusion Handbook. 5th edn. Jan 2014. Joint United Kingdom (UK) Blood Transfusion and Tissue Transplantation Services Professional Advisory.

75. Haas T, Mauch J, Weiss M, Schmugge M. Management of dilutional coagulopathy during pediatric major surgery. Transfus Med Hemother 2012;39:114–119.

76. Transfusion management of major haemorrhage. Section 7.3 in Transfusion Handbook. 5th edn. Jan 2014. Joint United Kingdom (UK) Blood Transfusion and Tissue Transplantation Services Professional Advisory.

77. Diab YA, Wong EC, Luban N. Massive transfusion in children and neonates. Br J Haematol 2013;161(1):15–26.

78. Arya RC, Wander G, Gupta P. Blood component therapy: Which, when and how much. J Anaesthesiol Clin Pharmacol 2011;27(2):278–84.

79. Floss AM, Strauss RG, Goeken N, Knox L. Multiple transfusions fail to provoke antibodies against blood cell antigens in human infants. Transfusion 1986;26:419–22.

80. Slonim AD, Joseph JG, Turene WM, Sharangpani A, Luban NL. Blood transfusions in children: a multi-institutional analysis of practices and complications. Transfusion 48(2008);pp.73–80.

81. Anna KKV Pedrosa, Francisco JM Pinto, Luiza DB Lins, Grace M Deus. Blood transfusion reactions in children: Associated factors. Jornal de Pediatria (Versãoem Português), Vol.89, Issue 4, July–August 2013;pp 400–406 (English Translation).

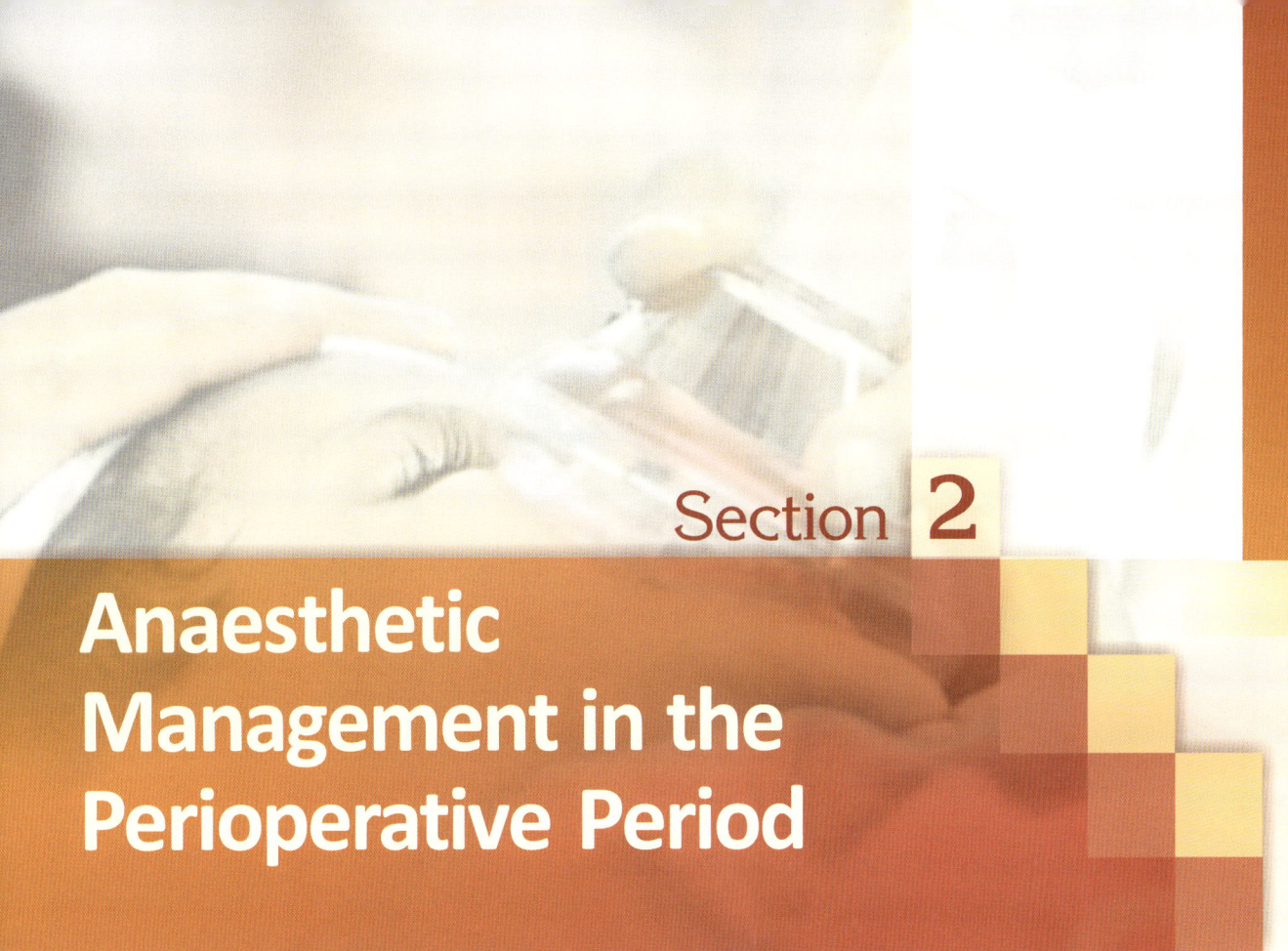

Section 2

Anaesthetic Management in the Perioperative Period

ANAESTHESIA IN SPECIAL SITUATIONS

6

Preoperative Evaluation of Paediatric Patients

Purnima Dhar, Rajeshwari Subramaniam, Renu Sinha, Hemkumar Pushparajan

- Timing and content of preoperative visit
- Value of preoperative laboratory testing
- Psychological effects of hospitalization and surgery
- Approaches to psychological preparation
- Pharmacological preparation (premedication)
- Special Situations
  - Ex-preterm infant
  - Child with upper respiratory tract infection
  - Child with a cardiac murmur
  - Preoperative evaluation of syndromic child

INTRODUCTION

The basis for any successful anaesthetic is the preoperative evaluation of the patient and accordingly the preparation for the conduct of anaesthesia. The outcome of any anaesthetic is determined by how well prepared the anaesthesiologist is, to handle that particular patient and that particular surgery. Anaesthesia-related mortality amongst healthy children undergoing surgery is rare. An incidence of 0.98 per 10000 anaesthetics was reported and all were attributable to pre-existing medical problems mainly in newborns.[1]

Anaesthesia-related mortality is higher in children with heart disease and in particular those with pulmonary hypertension.[2]

Therefore, the goals of preoperative evaluation would include:

- To obtain baseline information about patients' current physical status by thorough clinical examinations and appropriate investigations.
- Detection of comorbid conditions and optimization of these if any, e.g. URI, anaemia.
- Assessment of risk and obtaining informed consent from parent/guardian/child as appropriate.
- Allaying anxiety of child/parent by effective communication and premedication wherever applicable.

Should the child be evaluated in the preanaesthetic clinic or after hospitalization for surgery? Preanaesthetic clinics are now the norm because of the large number of surgeries being done as day care procedures. In addition, it gives an opportunity to the patient to look at anaesthesiologist as a physician and not as a technician. Even in the developed world, 35–40% of patients coming for surgery do not consider anaesthesiologists as physicians.[3] The numbers in third world countries would be much higher. The preanaesthesia clinic helps to an extent in creating an awareness about the speciality. The preoperative visit is as important to the anaesthetist as the process of diagnosis is for the surgeon.

TIMING AND CONTENT OF PREOPERATIVE VISIT

It has been long established that personal preoperative communication with patients can result in both physiologic and psychological improvements in patient care and a good preanaesthetic communication with patients the evening before surgery was even shown to result in less postoperative opioid use and earlier discharge.[2] But nowadays, with the growing pressure on hospital beds and economics of healthcare, the preoperative visit by the anaesthesiologist rarely takes place the evening before and it is also possible that the team doing the preoperative evaluation may not be involved in administering anaesthesia.

Therefore, preoperative programmes must adopt several strategies to ensure that anaesthesia providers in the operating room will be satisfied with the quality of outpatient preoperative assessment. There should be consensus within the department for determining the criteria for cancelling or postponing the surgery for medical reasons. There should also be a standardization of the documentation of preanaesthetic assessment in the clinic so that nothing is missed. Some anaesthetic groups have initiated work on consensus-based documentation standards for all preanaesthesia assessments.[4] The American Society of Anaesthesiologists (ASA) published specific standards for the conduct of preoperative anaesthesia evaluation.[5]

The patients should have an anaesthetic assessment whenever the child is scheduled for surgery. It may be in the preanaesthetic clinic or in the hospital after admission. A child seen in the preanaesthetic clinic can be called directly on the day of surgery, if found fit. The parents can be instructed to inform telephonically in case the child develops a respiratory or any other illness so that they can be advised to come to the hospital or not. In third world countries where the literacy levels and communication means are low, it becomes challenging because such delays can mean considerable financial loss to poor parents who work as daily wagers.

If a child is not an appropriate candidate for outpatient surgery, such as a child with OSA, and needs to be admitted overnight we should not allow patients, insurance companies, or surgeons make us change our practice for convenience or cost reduction. "We need to do what is right for our children, even if it means a poor bundle fee and less money in our own pocket."[6]

During the Preoperative Visit

- The anaesthesiologist evaluates the medical condition of the child.

- The problems related to the surgical procedure.
- History of past experience with anaesthesia, general medical history, antenatal and neonatal history in case of infants (prematurity and gestational age) and allergies if any.
- Medication history particularly corticosteroids, cardiorespiratory medications (inhalers, ophthalmic drugs), anticonvulsants, and chemotherapy. It is useful to know which chemotherapeutic drug the child has been on. Look for pulmonary (bleomycin), cardiac (adriamycin) or renal (cisplatin) side effects.[11]
- History of familial anaesthesia-related conditions, such as malignant hyperthermia, pseudocholinesterase deficiency, muscular dystrophy, sickle cell disease, thallasaemia, etc. Pseudocholinesterase deficiency is prevalent in Vysya community of India.[11]
- General physical examination and systemic examination including airway examination and examination of the spine and local site, if planning for regional anaesthesia.
- The psychological makeup of the child and family. The anxiety felt by the parents is always transmitted to the child and hence reassurance of the parents is critical. An explanation about the induction methods and control of postoperative pain is appropriate at this time.

All this can take time and in a study of patient-centred communication during a model preanaesthesia visit (including opening and closing interview; and gaining patient's perspective) took about 17.4 vs 14.5 minutes depending on standardized patient type.[7] This may be difficult to achieve in a busy preanaesthetic clinic. Therefore, means to improve efficiency and at the same time not to miss any important information needs to be ensured. Many centres in the West use nurses to do the preliminary screening. A trained nurse can pickup problem case and refer them to the anaesthetist. This is not the practise in our country but can be tried.

Finally, risk assessment and its documentation needs to be done as per the ASA classification. The fact that infants, especially neonates, and children undergoing procedures at remote locations are more at risk, is not included in this classification and that is a drawback.

ASSESSMENT OF AIRWAY

Aim of airway assessment preoperatively is to identify a difficult airway so that plan can be made for managing problems that may occur during spontaneous ventilation, bag mask ventilation, laryngoscopy or intubation (The management of difficult airway is discussed separately).

Paediatric airway has been described as being different from adults. These differences, most evident in children less than two to three years of age, include, a large occiput which affects positioning. A large tongue and small mouth that may make laryngoscopy difficult, larynx may be harder to locate with the laryngoscope because it is higher and more anterior than in an adult and the epiglottis is relatively large, U-shaped, floppy and difficult to control. Having said that, a large, prospective, multicentre observational study of paediatric emergency department intubations was conducted and found to be associated with a high success rate and a low rate of serious adverse events. The authors concluded that paediatric intubation as practised in academic emergency departments, with most initial attempts by emergency and paediatric residents and fellows under attending physician supervision, is safe and highly successful.[8] That is a reason that even big centres may be unprepared with equipment and gadgets to manage difficult airway in children of different age groups.

Unlike adults, no fixed classifications exist which would help in determination of patients at risk of difficult bag mask ventilation or intubation. The following points will help in anticipating a difficult airway. The LEMON approach described for adults can be used used for children as well.[9]

1. L: Look
   a. Misshapen head as in craniosynostosis, hydrocephalus
   b. Facial asymmetry as in syndromes with craniofacial abnormalities
   c. Masses in the neck. Congenital masses, such as cystic hygroma, teratomas, etc.
2. E: Evaluate
   a. Mouth opening. Microstomia may be a feature of Freeman-Sheldon syndrome and other syndromes. The mouth opening should be at least two patient's finger width.
   b. Mandibular hypoplasia (receding jaw) as a part of common syndromes, such as Robin sequence

and Treacher Collins' syndrome, leads to difficulty in intubation. Thyromental distance should be three patient's finger breadths and distance between the mandible and thyroid cartilage should be width of two patient's fingers.
   c. Large and protruding tongue (mucopolysaccharidosis, Down's syndrome, etc.) is an indicator of obstructed airway under sedation and anaesthesia can lead to airway obstruction.
3. M: Mallampati score
   Assigning a Mallampati score may be difficult in young children. It may be possible to see the inside of the mouth in a crying child or by offering a candy. For the obtunded, supine patient, a crude assessment can be made using a tongue blade.
4. O: Obstruction
   Signs of airway obstruction, such as stridor, drooling, muffled voice, indicate a difficult bag mask ventilation and intubation.
5. N: Neck mobility
   Limited neck mobility (as occurs with Klippel-Feil syndrome) may interfere with intubation. Cervical spine instability (which can occur with Down syndrome and the mucopolysaccharidoses) will require care during positioning.

VALUE OF PREOPERATIVE LABORATORY TESTING

The aim of performing preoperative laboratory tests includes identifying unpredictable situations that may complicate the anaesthesia and surgery. We are moving from "test everything" to "test selective". It is not only the cost that is incurred but indiscriminate testing has been found to lead to further tests and unnecessary stress in case of borderline results that are clinically irrelevant. There is broad consensus that routine blood testing is not indicated in children with negative history or examination; with this action superfluous stress for the child can be avoided and costs can be saved without compromising safety and quality. Testing should be based on findings of history and physical examination, if a clinical examination warrants it.[10–12]

Having said that routine testing is still necessary in our country, where malnutrition and parasitic infections are common especially amongst the lower socioeconomic group. It may not alter the anaesthesia plan but will identify malnutrition and hence start treatment. It is particularly indicated in infants below

6 months with physiological anaemia and exprematures who are prone to iatrogenic anaemia from repeated investigations and resultant apnoea risk.[13]

PSYCHOLOGICAL EFFECTS OF HOSPITALIZATION AND SURGERY

Induction of anaesthesia may be the most stressful procedure a child experiences during his hospitalization. Psychological and behavioural changes can be observed in three different aspects; preoperative anxiety, emergence delirium and postoperative behavioural changes.[14]

The causes of preoperative anxiety can be categorised into two categories, child-related and operating room-related. The child-related causes are, age less than 5 years, developmental maturity, lack of social adaptability, previous medical experience, patient and parental anxiety, lower educated parents. And operating room-related causes are number of people in the induction room, level of noise, and intensity of lights.[15] In one study, post-hospitalization behaviour changes were demonstrated by 52% of children on day 1 and 22% on day 7; and were associated with: a previous traumatic healthcare experience, male sex, and distress during induction of anaesthesia.[16] Children with more anxiety had more pain, required more analgesia, had more emergence delirium, sleeping problems and more delayed oral intake.[17] Although immediate negative behavioural responses develop in a relatively large number of young children following surgery, the magnitude of these changes is limited, and long-term maladaptive behavioural responses develop in only a small minority.[14]

Children who have had previous surgeries, long hospital or ICU stays may suffer lasting psychological effects. They require more effort to establish rapport, but it is definitely worth the time and energy spent.[13]

APPROACHES TO PSYCHOLOGICAL PREPARATION

Suggested approaches to a fearful child:
- In an older child who can verbalize his/her concerns, reassurance, establishing a rapport and explaining the induction technique can often overcome this problem.
- In a younger child, allaying anxiety in the parent (transmitted anxiety) and a suitable premedication goes a long way in dealing with the situation.

Psychological assurance is needed in neonates and infants less than 6 months in the form of gentle handling. They are comfortable with anybody who handles them gently since communication is more by touch than verbal.[13]

Infants more than 6 months resent separation from parents and it is advisable to either have the parent hold the child or sedate the child. Without this individualized attention, infants and toddlers 6 months to 5 years, may develop post-hospitalization regressive behaviour, fear of separation, clinging to mother in presence of strangers, screaming on entering a closed room, poor sleeping, feeding, nightmares, bedwetting, loss of toilet training, etc.[13]

Children older than 4–6 years from a cosmopolitan upbringing are easier to communicate with. Our children from rural areas or reclusive or small families with limited interaction with people may be shy and overawed. They need an honest, reassuring explanation of the premedication and induction, etc. It is best to liken the sedation and anaesthesia to their normal routine, like sleeping at night and waking up next morning.[13]

PHARMACOLOGICAL PREPARATION (PREMEDICATION)

A good premedication is the presence of the parent till the child goes to sleep and a number of non-pharmacological methods of distracting a child have worked well in reducing the anxiety in a child and the parents. These include toys, stories, videos, etc. However, pharmacological premedication with midazolam provided better reduction in anxiety.[18] Oral midazolam was found to be more effective than either parental presence or no intervention for managing a child's and parent's anxiety during the preoperative period in other studies as well.[19] Premedication is not normally necessary for the average 6-month-old infant but is warranted for a 10 to 12-month-old who is afraid and oral route is the most preferred and provides effective and reliable sedation in children, the only drawback being splitting out or vomiting following administration.

Midazolam

Midazolam is accepted as the most preferred drug for achieving the goals of premedication in children weighing less than 20 kg. The benefits are faster onset of action and lesser side effects. It can be given orally 20–30 minutes prior to induction. Oral dose is 0.5 mg/kg body weight.

Clonidine

This alpha 2 agonist is emerging as a popular alternative due to its sedative, analgesic, antiemetic and calming effects. It also causes a decrease in salivation. It is said to reduce emergence agitation associated with inhalation agents, such as sevoflurane. Dosage is 4 µg/kg, to be given 60–90 min prior to induction of anaesthesia. Peak effect can take a long time to come (60–90 min) which can be a challenge in a busy surgical setup.[20]

Dexmedetomidine

It is a more selective alpha 2 agonist. Tasteless and odourless, it has both sedative and analgesic, properties. Causes minimal respiratory depression[21] and prevents emergence delirium.[22] Bradycardia, hypotension and hypertension can occur based on the age of the child. The main disadvantage for premedication is the 45–60 minutes needed for clinical effect. Intranasal dexmedetomidine 2 µg/kg causes sedation in 30 min. It was shown to be better than midazolam in one study and worse in another. Hence, more studies are needed.[15]

Ketamine

Ketamine can be used by intramuscular, intravenous, oral or nasal route. IM ketamine is useful for an out of control, combative child. Increased secretions, psychomimetic side effects and PONV are some disadvantages. 2–7 mg/kg IM produces adequate sedation in 3–5 min. Oral ketamine in a dose of 5–6 mg has onset in 10 min. This dose is often mixed with midazolam. 0.3–0.5 mg/kg to prevent psychomimetic effects.[23]

Anticholinergics

Atropine and glycopyrolate are not used in routine practice any more. They may be given in special circumstances, such as before airway surgery to reduce secretions. Atropine is indicated before squint surgery and bronchoscopy to prevent vagal response. Some people continue to use it in the very young child to prevent bradycardia at induction although the

authors do not recommend it. Dose of oral atropine is 0.02 mg/kg 30 min prior to induction. Animal studies have reported hypertension, if atropine is used with dexmedetomidine.

Fasting

It has now been well established that in the absence of obstruction or pylorospasm, the gastric emptying time for clear liquids is not more than 2 hours and there is no advantage in withholding fluids for longer. Breast milk takes longer to leave the stomach, and should be withheld 4 hours prior to induction. Formula feed and solids should be given 6 hours prior to surgery. Details are discussed in Chapter 5 on fluid therapy.

SPECIAL SITUATIONS

Ex-premature Child

A baby born before 37 weeks is called preterm and these babies who were born preterm are increasingly coming for hernia repair and ophthalmic surgeries. Those born very preterm have usually been through a long stay in the nursery and suffered some degree of bronchopulmonary dysplasia as well. The course of stay in nursery should be ascertained from the records. The main postoperative risk in these babies is postoperative apnoea which is defined as apnoea lasting more than 15 seconds or less than 15 seconds but associated with bradycardia (HR<80/min).[24] The main risk factors for this are:

- Post-conceptional age (PCA)
- Gestational age (GA)
- Haemoglobin levels

Apnoea is likely to occur up to 60 weeks PCA[25] although it is more common in PCA less than 46 weeks.[26] Gestational age is an independent factor too. Lesser the gestational age the higher the chances of apnoea for a similar post-conceptional age.[24] Anaemia (haematocrit <30% or Hb <10 gm/dl) was found to be an important predisposing factor for postoperative apnoea by Welborn et al[27] and this risk is not altered by the PCA. An anaemic preterm baby is at risk of apnoea irrespective of the PCA. An absence of preoperative apnoeic spells and normal haemoglobin does not eliminate the chance of apnoea in the postoperative period completely. Apnoea has been shown to occur with newer inhalational agents and sedatives, like ketamine, midazolam. The risk is lesser when regional anaesthesia is used without sedation but not eliminated completely.[28,29] High dose caffeine (10 mg/kg) has been found to be effective[30] but lasts only 6 hours and first episode of apnoea can occur even 12 hours post-op.[31] Therefore, all preterm babies less than 60 weeks PCA should not be operated on a daycare basis and should be in a monitored facility post-op. Elective surgery should be postponed till 60 weeks PCA. Anaemia should be corrected by blood transfusion, if surgery is relatively urgent, such as an obstructed hernia.

Child with Upper Respiratory Tract Infection

The dilemma and debate of whether to go ahead, or postpone anaesthesia and surgery in a child presenting with features of an ongoing/recent upper respiratory tract infection (URTI), still continues. School children and preschoolers experience 3–9 (on an average, 7) episodes per year of URTI.

Till recently, and even amongst some contemporary paediatric anaesthesiologists, it was/is common practice to postpone elective surgery till the child becomes asymptomatic. This was due to a presumed risk of increase in adverse outcomes compounded by fear of litigation. However, accumulating clinical data suggests that only certain children are at risk of these adverse outcomes, which can be anticipated and treated. Further, postponement causes economic as well as emotional impact on the family. Better understanding of how URTI impacts the intra- and post-operative period and identification of risk factors has led to a more 'permissive' and liberal approach. The final decision often rests on the comfort and confidence level of the individual anaesthesiologist in managing potential complications of URTI.

One of the earliest series to report adverse respiratory events in children with URTI presenting for surgery was by McGill, Covener and Epstein, in 1979. This series of 11 children undergoing a variety of surgical procedures had complications ranging from desaturation to atelectasis.[32] Careful history and physical examination with a chest X-ray and postponement of elective surgery was recommended. De Soto reported that children aged 1–4 years with signs and symptoms of URTI/history of URTI were at increased risk of developing transient post-operative hypoxaemia.[33] A retrospective review of 3,585 cases in 1987 consisting of asymptomatic, currently symptomatic children and those with history of recent infection found adverse effects only in children with history of recent infection.[34] In another study involving children undergoing myringotomy (without intubation), it was demonstrated that there was no increased morbidity in children with mild URTI receiving anaesthesia.[35] However, yet another study involving 93 infants and 295 children with URTI receiving anaesthesia, most of whom were intubated, observed 'critical' incidents (incidents that could result in morbidity or mortality) in a significantly high number of children with URTI (71% vs 26% in infants; 30% vs 12% in children).[36] An editorial in 1991 attempted to explain these conflicting findings; it was postulated that the obviously 'symptomatic' children probably had symptoms of a chronic nature (allergic, mild nasopharyngitis) whereas the children recovering from 'recent' URTI had actually had a viral infection with predilection for super added bacterial infection and airway hyper-reactivity, which explained the increased occurrence of adverse events.[37] In a subsequent study, it was determined that children with a preoperative URTI (n=1283) were 2–7 times more likely to experience respiratory-related adverse events during intra- and post-operative periods and that endotracheal intubation increased risk of respiratory complications 11-fold. This study concluded that administration of general anaesthesia (GA) to children was a serious matter with children requiring careful observation through the perioperative period.[38] A series by Schreiner et al (1996) reported that children with active upper respiratory infection were twice as likely to have laryngospasm. The other factors increasing predilection of laryngospasm were younger age, airway surgery and **supervision by a less experienced anaesthesiologist**.[39]

A survey of 2051 children by Parnis et al presenting for surgery, attempted to determine the variables which would predict adverse events.[40] Of these children, nearly 23% had symptoms of URTI, and nearly 50% had history of URTI in the last 6 weeks. The findings which strongly correlated with development of an adverse event were:

1. Airway management: ETT>LMA>Facemask
2. Parent states child has a cold
3. Child snores
4. History of passive smoking (parent smoker)

5. Airway surgery
6. Induction agent: Thiopental > Halothane > Sevoflurane > Propofol
7. Child producing sputum
8. Child has nasal congestion

These findings were confirmed in a study which prospectively evaluated 1078 children aged 1 month to 18 years appearing for surgery.[41] It was found that the incidence of breath holding, desaturation and other adverse events were significantly higher in children with active/recent URTI, although events like laryngospasm and bronchospasm were distributed evenly. This study added the following risk factors to Parnis' list:

1. Use of ETT in children <5 years
2. History of bronchospastic disease
3. Prematurity (<37 weeks)
4. Surgery on the airway

In another study by Tait and Malviya, children with congenital heart disease and URTI presenting for corrective/palliative procedures were found to have a significantly increased incidence of respiratory events, bacterial infection and ICU stay, although there was no impact on the overall outcome.[42]

Pathophysiological Effects of URTI

Nearly 30–40% respiratory infections in children are caused by rhinovirus species with significant contribution from coronavirus, RSV, parainfluenza and influenza. Symptoms may be the prodromal features of more ominous conditions, like croup (laryngotracheobronchitis), epiglottitis, influenza, herpes simplex pneumonia and streptococcal sore throat.

Although mainly present in the upper airway, URTI has the potential of affecting lung parenchyma. Oedema, debris from epithelial shedding in small airways and alveoli, combined with decreased physical clearance results in decreased FEV_1, FVC and VC and a seven-fold increase in bronchial reactivity and receptors. Asthma is present in up to 20–25% children. In the upper airway, viral URTI results in inflammation, increased secretions and oedema of the nasal mucosa and the throat. These children are prone to nasal obstruction and an irritable throat and airway predisposing to coughing, bronchospasm and desaturation.

Effects of URTI

a. Systemic effects of infection: Pyrexia, malaise, lethargy, myalgia and toxemia may result, depending on the severity and the virulence of the infection. URTI may be the prodrome of severe exanthematous infection like, measles and varicella.
b. Bronchoconstriction due to hyper-reactivity is a major reason of morbidity and has been shown to be vagally mediated. Thus physical (endotracheal tube) or chemical (inhalational agent) stimuli can result in bronchoconstriction. This can be partly blocked by atropine. Influenza and parainfluenza cause low/dysfunctional M_2 receptor[43] activity by two methods. (These receptors in the airway contain sialic acid which binds released acetylcholine, preventing bronchospasm.)
   - Viral neuraminidases directly depress activity of M_2 receptors
   - Viral infections decrease airway neural endopeptidase activity, facilitating tachykinin activity, which leads to bronchoconstriction.
c. Viral infections increase the volume and consistency of secretions, promoting atelectasis.
d. Rarely, death has been reported.[44,45] The child in one of the reports was subsequently found to have undiagnosed viral myocarditis.

Effect of URTI on Anaesthesia

1. Obstruction of nasal airway during induction and recovery
2. Laryngospasm, stridor during induction and recovery
3. Bronchospasm
4. Coughing, breath holding
5. Desaturation.[46]

Preoperative Assessment

A detailed history is mandatory. This should be aimed to determine the severity of the infection. Presence of fever >38°C, productive cough, loss of appetite, wheezing and lethargy are indicative of more than a mild infection. Parent's report on the child's condition is a sensitive measure of illness. Parents should be questioned on the activity levels, dyspnoea, rib retractions and productive cough. Parents are attuned to their child's condition and usually provide an accurate picture of the situation. Smoking by any or both of the parents should be documented. History of snoring, mouth breathing are important in that they have a bearing on mask ventilation, postoperative airway obstruction and its management.

Physical examination should be focused and detailed. Children may not co-operate to open their mouths and crying may interfere with auscultation, and appropriate efforts should be made to cover these aspects. Fever should be documented. Respiratory rate, enlarged and inflamed tonsils, nasal discharge, crusting and congestion should be documented. Every effort should be made to rule out more ominous conditions, like laryngotracheobronchitis, pneumonia and epiglottitis. Finally, the lungs should be auscultated, and presence/absence of breath sounds, rhonchi and crepitations documented.

If the child presents for emergency surgery, a well-documented history of URTI alerts the anaesthesiologist to the potential for complications, and to plan an appropriate anaesthetic technique.

Laboratory Testing

Laboratory tests are neither cost-effective, nor practical in the scenario of URTI. Nasopharyngeal swabs/aspirates have limited sensitivity for viral infections. The total leucocyte count (TLC) may not always be high. Chest X-rays have limited utility except before cardiac surgery; they may be done if there is a suspicion of lower respiratory infection. Generally chest X-ray findings lag behind the child's symptoms.

Explanation to Parents

When the child is obviously ill, it is not difficult to convince all concerned about postponement; if the child is playful and active, with a clear 'runny' nose, scheduled for a minor procedure not requiring intubation, it is not a difficult decision to proceed. It is the child with in-between symptoms where the decision is difficult. A clear and correct explanation to parents on the type and severity of complications to expect goes a long way in not only allaying anxiety, but to obtain an informed and 'participatory' consent. Parents should be given the option of postponement, but also told that it is beneficial only if the wait is for more than 4–6 weeks. They should be told that the likelihood of adverse events, like breath holding or fall in oxygen saturation, is higher, if the child is premature, or if one of the parents is a smoker. At all points, however, parents should be reassured that the child will get the best possible care and appropriate and suitable anaesthetic technique.[47]

A note should be placed in the case record that these possibilities have been discussed with the surgeon and the parents, and that everyone has agreed to proceed. Tait and Malviya[17] have proposed a useful algorithm for managing a child with URTI (Fig. 6.1).[48]

Conclusions

Children with mild URTI may be safely anaesthetized without significant morbidity. Technology to foresee and treat complications (monitoring, muscle relaxants, LMA, etc.) is available. However, unknown myocarditis can still occur.

Elective surgery should be ideally postponed for at least 4 weeks, if children have more 'serious' symptoms: mucopurulent secretions, fever >38°C, lethargy and signs of pulmonary involvement. The child should be placed on appropriate antibiotics.

Children presenting for antegrade or retrograde oesophageal dilatation (generally consequent to corrosive-induced oesophageal stricture and surgery) form a unique group in that they invariably have signs and symptoms of lower respiratory infection resulting from repeated aspiration due to their inability to swallow food and saliva. Timely dilatation is necessary to reduce aspiration. These children, therefore, are not refused the minor anaesthetic with endotracheal intubation.

A guide to which children with URTI may need postponement of their surgery has been suggested by Bhatia (Table 6.1).[49]

Table 6.1	Guide to schedule/cancel elective surgery[49]	
Schedule	**Cancel**
▪ Clear runny nose	▪ Child < 1 year
▪ Dry cough	▪ Purulent nasal discharge
▪ Minor surgery	▪ Productive cough
	▪ Wheezing/crepitations on auscultation
	▪ Systemic features of being unwell, i.e. fever >38°C, malaise, headache, feeding problems
	▪ Parental confirmation of child being unwell

(Also consider patient comorbidities, type or urgency of surgery, and experience of anaesthetist.)

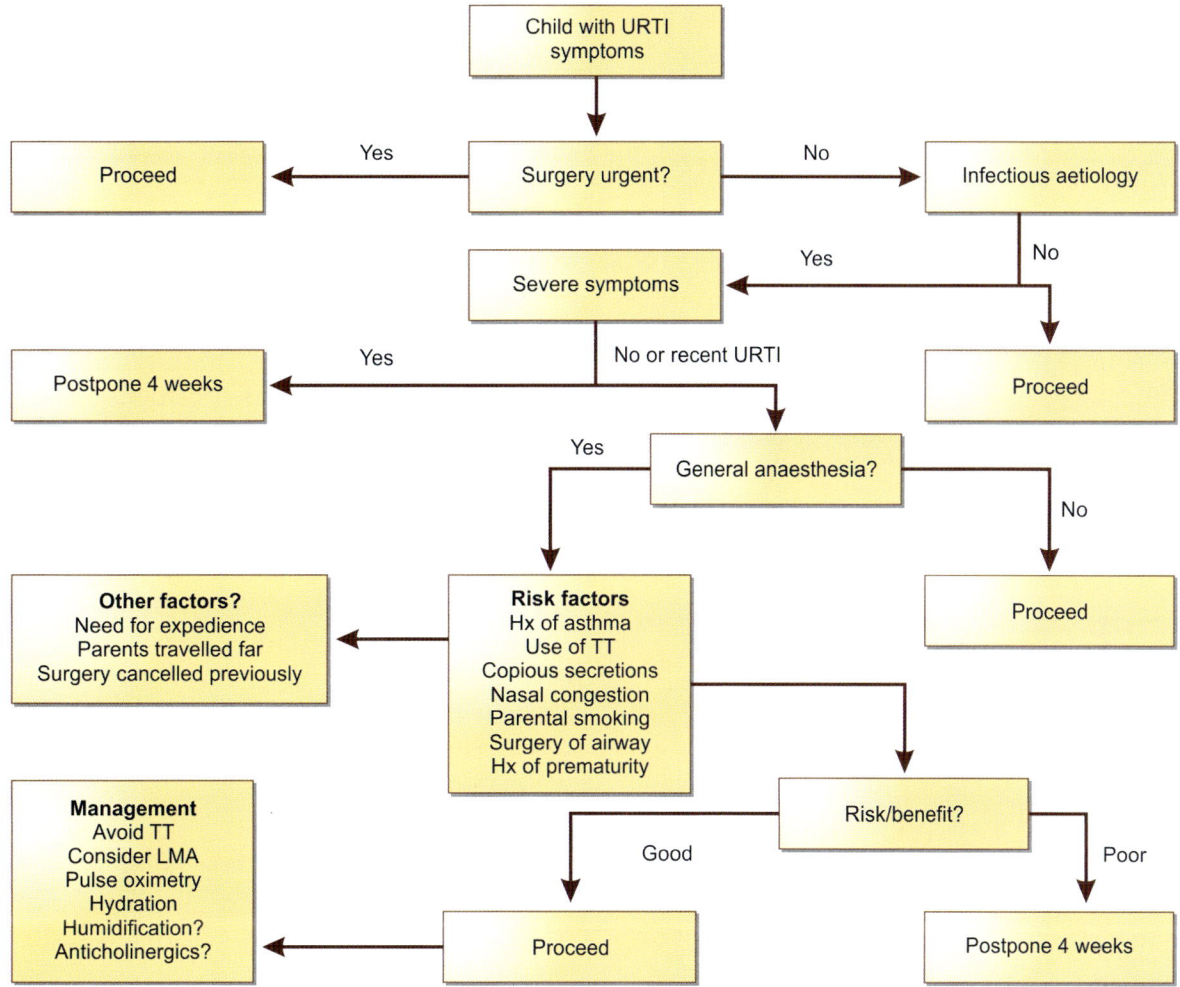

Fig. 6.1. Algorithm for managing child with URTI

CHILD WITH A CARDIAC MURMUR

Many children have a murmur noticed during the preoperative evaluation, by the anaesthesiologist. Murmurs are a common finding in healthy infants, children and adolescents. The prevalence of innocent murmurs in childhood may be as high as 75–90%, but the incidence of significant CHD is 1%. Amongst newborns, approximately 1% are diagnosed with a murmur; in this age, there is on an average, more than 50% (31–86%) chance of structural heart disease. The important point is that a murmur may be the only manifestation of life-threatening cardiac disease at any age (hypertrophic obstructive cardiomyopathy, aortic stenosis), and it is, therefore, important to ensure accurate diagnosis before the child is scheduled for surgery. Further, anaesthetic techniques, if not selected appropriately, can alter the balance between SVR and PVR and result in avoidable morbidity. CHD can increase mortality after non-cardiac surgery by a factor of 2.

Preoperative Evaluation[50]

History. Factors that increase likelihood of cardiac disease are:

1. Family history of sudden cardiac death
2. Family history of CHD
3. *In utero* exposure to medication (SSRI, Li, valproate)/alcohol
4. Maternal diabetes mellitus

5. Maternal infection
6. Genetic disorders

Syndromes associated with congenital heart disease (CHD):[51]

1. CHARGE (Coloboma, Heart defects, Atresia of the choanae, Retardation, Genital/urinary defects, Ear defects)
2. VATER (Vertebral, Anorectal, Tracheal and Esophageal fistula, Radial anomalies)
3. Di-George syndrome
4. Down
5. Turner syndrome
6. Kawasaki disease

Common presenting features in infants and toddlers are:

1. Recurrent chest infections
2. Cyanosis at rest or on crying
3. Sweating, grunting
4. Squatting
5. Feeding difficulties
6. Failure to thrive

Older children may present with different symptoms:

1. Dyspnoea
2. Nausea–vomiting
3. Fatigue
4. Cough
5. Rarely, chest pain or syncope.

Age-appropriate exercise tolerance should be ascertained. In neonates and infants, the best features in favour are difficulties and sweating during feeding; in older children, capability to participate in team sports should be assessed.

Children with HOCM/critical AS may be asymptomatic except for a murmur; ECG will reveal LVH and LAD.

Physical Examination

The appearance of the child, activity level, colour and respiratory efforts should be noted. All four extremities should be examined for cyanosis, peripheral pulses and capillary refill (should be less than 3 seconds). Characteristics of pulse should include rate, rhythm, volume, character and presence, if any, of radiofemoral delay. The neck should be inspected for prominent vessels and pulsations, and palpated for thrills/bruits. The JVP is rarely increased in children. The chest should be examined for sternal abnormalities, abnormal pulsations, displacement of the apex beat and any thrill/s.

A focused examination of the respiratory and cardiovascular systems and the abdomen should be performed. Congenital anomalies are present with CHD in nearly 25% patients.

Auscultation of the heart sounds should be carried out in the standing, supine position and during a Valsalva manoeuvre. Small children can be asked to push their abdomen against the anaesthesiologist's hand (Fig. 6.2).

It is an essential and useful skill for paediatric anaesthesiologists to be able to differentiate between innocent and pathological murmurs.

Murmurs are described by their location, quality, intensity and pitch.

The intensity is graded on a scale of 6 as follows:

I. Barely audible
II. Faint, but heard
III. Heard easily, loud
IV. Heard over a wide area, no thrill
V. Heard over a wide area, with palpable thrill
VI. Heard with stethoscope off the chest

The murmur of HOCM tends to decrease in intensity with leg elevation/squatting.

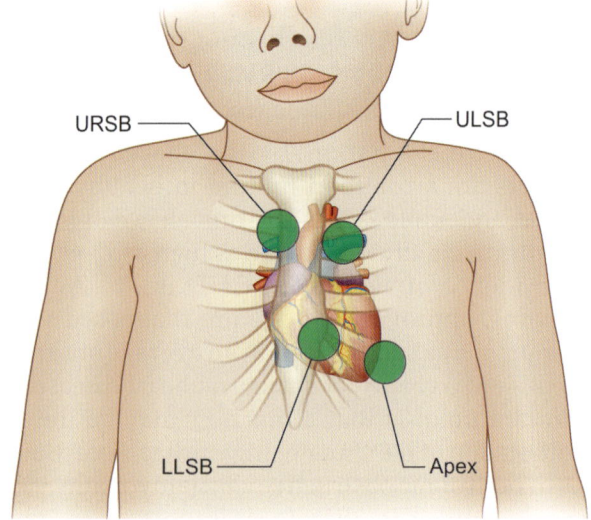

Fig. 6.2. Auscultatory points

Table 6.2	The 'Seven Ss' of innocent murmur

- **S**ensitive (changes with child's position or with respiration)
- **S**hort duration (not holosystolic)
- **S**ingle (no associated clicks or gallops)
- **S**mall (murmur limited to a small area and non-radiating)
- **S**oft (low amplitude)
- **S**weet (not harsh sounding)
- **S**ystolic (occurs during and is limited to systole)

'Red flags' for pathological murmurs:

1. Holosystolic
2. Harsh quality
3. Maximum intensity at left upper sternal border
4. Systolic click
5. Diastolic murmurs
6. Increasing intensity on standing

On the other hand, innocent murmurs have seven qualities (Table 6.2).

The other diagnostic criteria for innocent murmurs are:

1. No other physical finding except murmur
2. Child is asymptomatic
3. No findings in maternal/family history increasing risk of cardiac disease
4. Increase in intensity when supine
5. Features specific to the innocent murmur present

However, it must be remembered that these criteria are NOT applicable for infants <1 year. These children have a high rate of asymptomatic structural heart disease.

The lungs should be auscultated for crackles (crepitations, signaling pulmonary congestion) and wheezing (pulmonary oedema). The abdomen should be palpated for the liver (situs, enlargement).

Table 6.3 gives a brief description of innocent murmurs.

Investigations

Chest X-ray (CXR) and ECG are rarely useful in assessment of murmurs. In asymptomatic murmurs

Table 6.3	Brief description of innocent murmurs	
Lesion/murmur	**Features**	**Description and explanation**
1. Peripheral pulmonary stenosis	Seen in very young. Common in clavicular area, L > R Disappears by 6 months	■ Branch PA given off at sharp angle ■ Blood flow audible due to acceleration ■ With growth vessels increase in size, angulation reduced
2. Basal ESM	Preschool, school Near pulmonic area High-pitched, blowing To be differentiated from AS/PS	■ Caused by eddies created in blood ejected from RV during systole ■ Disturbance of stationary blood above pulmonary valve
3. Still's murmur (Fig. 6.3)	Late pre-school Musical, vibratory Left middle/lower sternal border Intensity increases in supine position	■ Resonation of blood in LVOT and aorta ■ Smaller aorta with higher peak velocities
4. Venous hum	School age Continuous, through systole and diastole Low-pitched Increases with inspiration	■ Due to blood draining down collapsed cervical veins into dilated intrathoracic veins ■ Vein walls flutter ⟶ hum ■ Absent when supine—differentiated from PDA
5. Supraclavicular bruit	Majority of children 40% young adults Increased velocity of LV ejection	■ Proximal subclavian artery ■ Delayed after I sound ■ Maximum intensity in neck ■ Brief duration ■ Differentiates from AS, PS

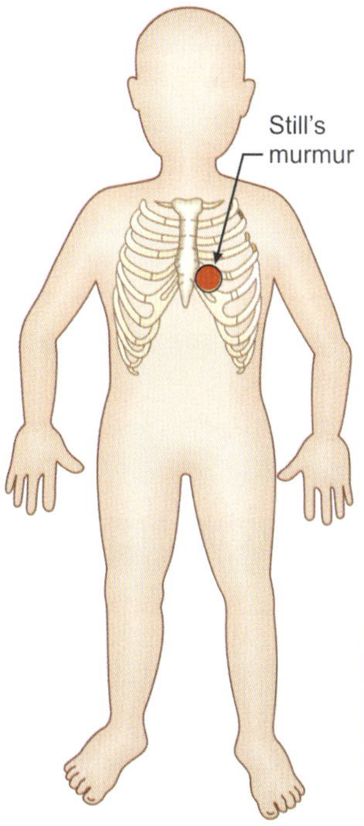

Still's murmur

Fig. 6.3. Still's murmur

in newborns, CXR does not assist clinical diagnosis or influence management. Similarly, addition of ECG to clinical assessment does not improve sensitivity or specificity of detecting structural heart lesion. However, CXR in symptomatic newborns with structural heart disease are usually diagnostic, with specific features. These X-rays will often reveal an abnormal cardiac silhouette, pulmonary plethora or oligemia.

ECG in structural heart disease may reveal abnormal rate, rhythm or evidence of atrial/ventricular hypertrophy. Voltage criteria for children differ from adults as follows:

RVH: R in V1   >1.75 mV (<5 years), or

                   >1.25 mV (5–12 years), or upright T

LVH: R in V5 or V6 >4 mV

Recommendations[52,53]

1. Active children >1 year of age, with innocent murmur, who do not have any features in history or examination to suggest structural heart disease, with normal ECG can proceed with surgery. They may get investigated later. If there is a doubt about the nature of the murmur, echocardiography should be done.
2. Children with corrected CHD (ASD/VSD repair, PDA ligation) can be anaesthetized in non-specific centres.
3. Complex conditions/single ventricle circulation need to be managed in specialized centres with paediatric ICU facilities.
4. Children on cardiac medications, those with prolonged QT interval, or residual cardiac disease should not be offered the option of outpatient surgery.

A useful algorithm is given in Table 6.4 and Figure 6.4 .

PREOPERATIVE EVALUATION OF SYNDROMIC CHILD

During preoperative evaluation, it is not uncommon to have a child with known or unknown syndromic association. These children may have abnormal facies due to craniofacial involvement and may be diagnosed during preanaesthetic assessment. The syndromes commonly encountered are the Down, Goldenhar, Marfan, Apert and Pierre-Robin sequence. Comprehensive descriptions of syndromes with their systemic involvement can be easily accessed in standard text books or Internet.

A detailed history and careful examination is mandatory in these children, along with relevant investigations to rule out other systemic association. If surgery is elective, these children can be referred to genetic clinics for detailed evaluation and confirmation of genetic diagnosis.

Records of the previous hospital visits and admission are very informative relating to difficulties in endotracheal intubation, vascular cannulation, abnormal drug responses and postoperative complications/care provided.

If the child is visually/mentally challenged or deaf/mute, parents become the main source of information and also for calming/reassuring the child.

History

Birth history. Prematurity, birth weight, history of cyanosis, apnoea, respiratory distress, need for intubation and mechanical ventilation, duration of neonatal intensive care stay should be documented.

Respiratory system. History of repeated chest infections, sore throat/tonsillitis, detection of cardiac murmur, asthma/allergies requiring hospitalization should be enquired and documented. Presence of snoring, apnoeic spells (obstructive sleep apnoea), tachypnoea should be noted. Many children with large

Table 6.4	Conclusion and recommendations for investigations	
Clinical recommendation		**Evidence rating**
▪ Structural heart disease is more likely when the murmur is holosystolic, diastolic, grade 3 or higher associated with a systolic click; when it increases in intensity with standing; or when it has a harsh quality.		C
▪ Chest radiography and electrocardiography rarely assist in the diagnosis of heart murmurs in children		B
▪ Family physicians should order echocardiography or consider referral to a paediatric cardiologist for newborns with a heart murmur, even if the child is asymptomatic, because of the higher prevalence of structural heart lesions in this population		B

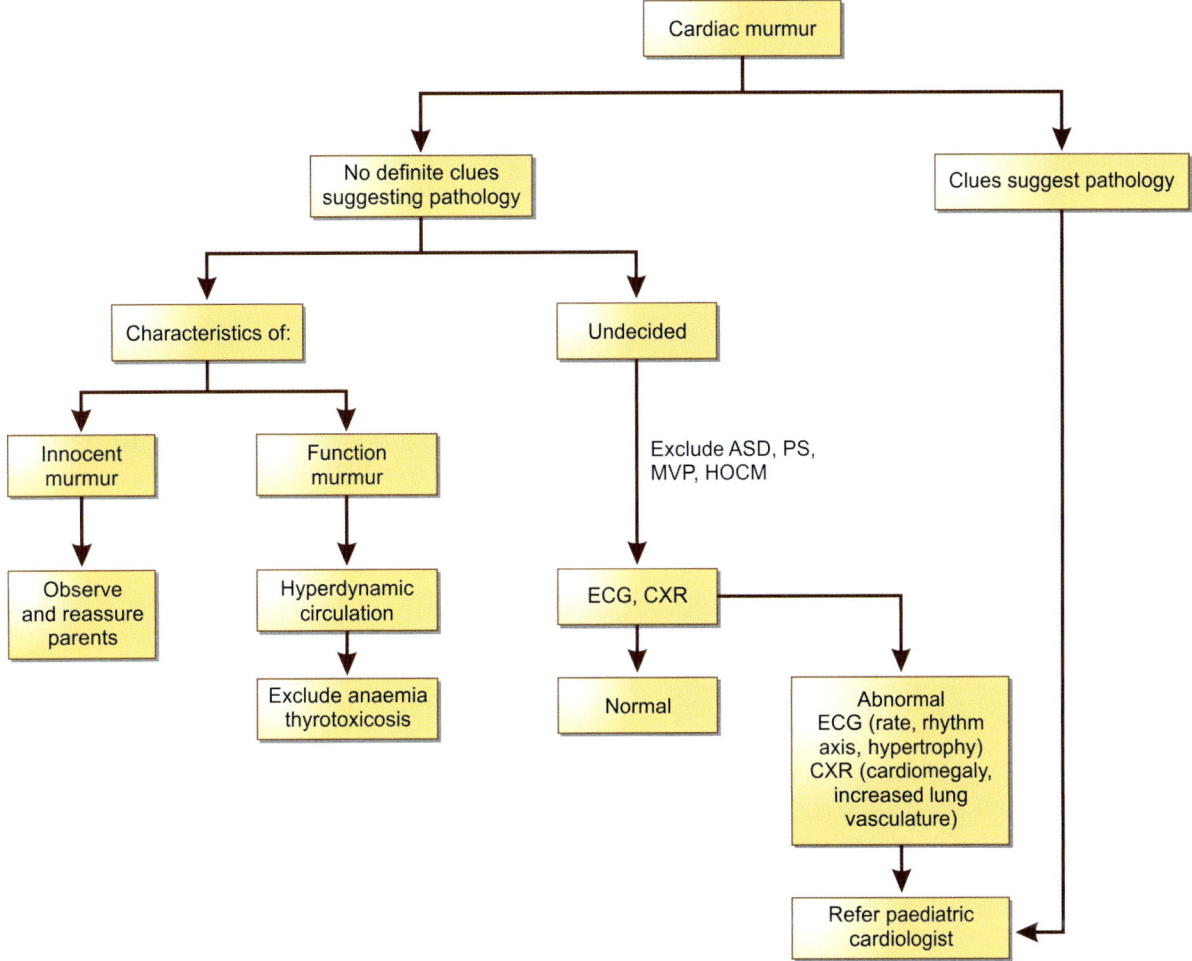

Fig. 6.4. Algorithm for management of children with cardiac murmur (Adapted from Chye QS, Ling WM. In: Assessment of cardiac murmurs in children, The National University Hospital, Bulletin. 5, September 1998)

tongue or nasal obstruction are mouth breathers. They keep their mouth open with slight protrusion of the tongue. The child's preferred position during sleep is important to note: sleeping in prone position in children with large tongue or tonsillar hypertrophy is common to avoid airway obstruction. These children have a high risk of airway obstruction after extubation in supine position.

Cardiovascular system. Feeding difficulty, choking or cyanosis during feeding, prolonged apnoea with cyanosis during crying should be noted.

Nervous system. Parents should be asked for details of inability to sit or walk unsupported, gait, school performance and types of activity. History of seizures, abnormal movement, hearing ability, vision, speech should be taken.

Endocrine system. Lethargy (due to hypothyroidism), overactive, diabetes, tetany.

Renal system. History of repeated urinary tract infections, pedal oedema, facial puffiness should be asked.

Gastrointestinal system. History of reflux, repeated vomiting should be taken.

Drug history. Some children may be on regular medication (antiepileptic, diuretics, steroid, digoxin) due to systemic involvement. Plasma levels and their side effects should be seen.

Examination

General examination. The child's posture, communication, intelligence, growth retardation, weight (less or more for age) and height should be observed .

Craniofacial. Abnormal shape of head, cranio-synostosis, microcephaly, hydrocephalus, proptosis, receding hairline or hair till nape of neck, eye abnormalities ranging from microophthalmos to buphthalmos, cataract and presence of ear tags may be pointers for syndromes.

Airway examination. Reduction or difficulty in mouth opening, Mallampati scores >2, reduced neck movements, abnormal dentition, large tongue size, nasal patency, deviated nasal septum, turbinate hypertrophy, tonsillar hypertrophy, cleft lip and cleft palate, microsomia/macrosomia may point to airway difficulties. Profile view of the face gives a better idea of micrognathia, retrognathia, pointed chin and maxillary abnormalities.

Cardiorespiratory system. Chest abnormalities (pectus excavatum), intercostal and suprasternal retraction, paradoxical respiration, respiratory rate, abnormal breath sounds, heart rate, rhythm, murmur or abnormal heart sounds should be looked for.

Nervous system. The child's ability to walk with or without support, motor skill according to age, mental retardation, IQ level, comprehensive speech, hand eye coordination, myopathy, hypotonia should be noted.

Musculoskeletal system. Joint involvement is present in some of the syndromes. This has implications in positioning the child. Down syndrome associated with instability of the atlanto-occipital and atlantoaxial joints warrants special investigations.[54]

Skin involvement. Children with thick and dry skin have difficult intravenous line like in Down syndrome. Since a significant proportion of these children are mentally challenged, they may not be co-operative for insertion of intravenous cannulae even after application of topical anaesthetic cream.

Investigations

Haematological investigations also depend on the type of syndrome, i.e. thyroid function test in Down syndrome, renal function test in Apert syndrome,[55] serum calcium levels, blood sugar, etc. Other investigations will also depend on type of syndrome and their associated system involvement, i.e. ECG and echocardiography. X-rays of chest, cervical spine, head and neck, airway (AP, lateral views) may be done, if indicated. Advanced evaluation, like computerized tomogram (CT) or MRI of chest/brain, would be done in many children to plan surgical procedures as well. EMG, EEG and muscle biopsy will be indicated in children with myopathy for diagnostic and prognostic considerations. Fibreoptic laryngoscopy may be required to rule out laryngeal web and other laryngeal abnormalities associated with Fraser syndrome.

Table 6.5	Common syndromes and their anaesthetic significance[56–59]		
S.No	Name of syndrome	Findings with anesthetic significance	Investigations required
1.	Down syndrome	Macroglossia, subglottic stenosis, atlantoaxial instability, ASD, VSD, TOF, GERD, sleep apnoea, LRTI	X-ray cervical spine Echocardiogram
2.	Treacher Collins syndrome	Macroglossia, limited mouth opening, mandibular hypoplasia, adenotonsillar hypertrophy	Repeated airway assessments
3.	Apert syndrome	Midface hypoplasia, tracheal stenosis, fused cervical vertebrae, G6PD deficiency, difficult IV access, cardiac defects, polycystic kidneys	Radiology of cervical spine, renal function, airway assessment
4.	Sturge-Weber syndrome	Hemangiomas in skin, airway, CNS; seizure disorders	Airway evaluation ICP, seizure prophylaxis
5.	Glycogen storage disorders: Hurler syndrome	Kyphosis, macroglossia, short neck, raised ICP, restrictive lung disease, asthma, OSA	Airway evaluation ABGs
6.	Laurence-Moon-Biedl syndrome	Obesity, short neck, CHD, difficult venous access	Airway, EKG, echocardiogram
7.	Muscular dystrophies	Hyperkalaemia to succinylcholine, malignant hyperthermia, poor recovery from neuromuscular blockade, ventilator dependency	Muscle biopsy, PFTs, MH prophylaxis/preparedness

Although rare in themselves, a few of the syndromes are more commonly encountered in paediatric anaesthetic practice due to their association with lesions requiring surgical correction. They are outlined in Table 6.5.

CONCLUSION

The key to successful and safe anaesthesia is proper clinical evaluation and accordingly being prepared for any eventuality.

Preoperative anxiety has far more serious effects than generally perceived and all efforts should be made to allay it. Pharmacological and non-pharmacological methods should all be used to effect it.

Parental anxiety is transmitted to the child and hence their counselling is equally if not more important. Prolonged fasting is one of the major parental concerns and can be easily addressed by the new liberal guidelines. More than anything else a paediatric anaesthesiologist has to be compassionate and flexible so as to help a child through a very difficult period in his or her life.

REFERENCES

1. van der Griend BF, Lister NA, McKenzie IM, Martin N, Ragg PG, Sheppard SJ, Davidson AJ. Postoperative mortality in children after 101,885 anesthetics at a tertiary pediatric hospital. Anesth Analg 2011;112(6):1440–1447.

2. Egbert LD, Battit GE, Welch CE, Bartlett MK. Reduction of postoperative pain by encouragement and instruction of patients. N Engl J Med 1964;270:825–827.

3. Klafta JM, Roizen MF. Current understanding of patients' attitudes toward and preparation for anesthesia: A review. Anesth Analg 1996; 83:1314–1321.

4. Ahmadian L, Cornet R, Kalkman C, et al. Development of a national core dataset for preoperative assessment, Methods Inf Med 2009;48:155–161.

5. Apfelbaum JL, Connis RT, NIckinovich DG, et al. Practice advisory (for preanesthesia evaluation: an updated report by the American Society of Anesthesiologists Task Force on Preanesthesia Evaluation, Anesthesiology 2012;116: 522–538.

6. Cote CJ. "Risk, error, outcome, and prevention in pediatric anesthesia: so many issues, lots of good solutions, but where do we find the resources?" Paediatr Anaesth 2011;21(7):713–715.

7. Sagarin MJ, Chiang V, Sakles JC, Barton ED, Wolfe RE, Vissers RJ, Walls RM. National Emergency Airway Registry (NEAR) investigators. Rapid sequence intubation for pediatric emergency airway management. Pediatr Emerg Care 2002;18(6):417.

8. Walls RM, Luten RC, Murphy MF, Schneider RE (Eds). Manual of Emergency Airway Management. Philadelphia: Lippincott Williams & Wilkins, 2000.

9. Zollo RA, Lurie SJ, Epstein R, Ward DS. Patterns of communication during the preanesthesia visit. Anesthesiology 2009;111(5):971–997.

10. Munro J, Booth A, Nicholl J. Routine Preoperative Testing: A Systematic Review of the Evidence, Health Technology Assessment 1997;1(12):I–IV;1–62.

11. Meneghini L, Zadra N, Zanette G, Baiocchi M, Giusti F. The usefulness of routine preoperative laboratory tests for one-day surgery in healthy children. Paediatr Anaesth 1998;8(1):11–15.

12. García-Miguel FJ, Serrano-Aguilar PG, López-Bastida J. Preoperative assessment. Lancet 2003;362(9397): 1749–1757.

13. Vas L. Preanaesthetic evaluation and premedication in paediatrics. Ind J Anaesth 2004;48(5):347–354.

14. Kain ZN, Mayes LC, O'Connor TZ, Cicchetti DV. Preoperative anxiety in children. Predictors and outcomes. Arch Pediatr Adolesc Med 1996;150(12):1238–1245.

15. Williams ES, Watch MF. Evaluation and preparation of pediatric patient for surgery. World Clin Anesth Crit Care Pain 2014;2(2):177–190.

16. Beringer RM, Segar P, Pearson A, Greamspet M, Kilpatrick N. Observational study of perioperative behavior changes in children having teeth extracted undergeneral anesthesia. Paediatr Anaesth 2014;24(5): 499–504.

17. Kain ZN, Mayes LC, Caldwell-Andrews AA, Karas DE, McClain BC. Preoperative anxiety, postoperative pain, and behavioural recovery in young children undergoing surgery. Pediatrics 2006;118:651–658.

18. Patal A, Scheble T, Davidson M, Tran MC, Schoenberg C, DelphinE, et al. distraction with a hand held video game reduces preoperative anxiety. Paedtr Anaesth 2006;16: 1019–1027.

19. Kain ZN, Mayes LC, Wang SM, Caramico LA, Hofstadter MB. Parental presence during induction of anesthesia versus sedative premedication: which intervention is more effective? Anesthesiology 1998;89(5): 1147–1156.

20. Bergendahl H, Lönnqvist PA, Eksborg S Clonidine. An alternative to benzodiazepines for premedication in children. Curr Opin Anaesthesiol 2005;18:608–613.

21. Mason KP, Lerman J. Review article: Dexmedetomidine in children: current knowledge and future applications. Anesth Analg 2011;113:1129–1142.

22. Phan H, Nahata MC. Clinical uses of dexmedetomidine in pediatric patients. Paediatr Drugs 2008;10:49–69.

23. Warner DL, et al. Ketamine plus midazolam, a most useful premedicant in children. Paediatr Anaesth 1995;5:293.

24. Coté CJ, Zaslavsky A, Downes JJ, Kurth CD, Welborn LG, Warner LO, Malviya SV. Postoperative apnoea in former preterm infants after herniorraphy. A combined analysis. Anesthesiology 1995;82:809.

25. Kurth CD, Spitzer AR, Broennle AM, Downes JJ. Postoperative apnoea in preterm infants. Anesthesiology 1987;66:483.

26. Malviya S, Swartz J, LermanJ. Are all preterm infants less than 60 weeks postconceptual age at risk for post-anaestheticapnoea? Anesthesiology 1993;78:1076.

27. Welborn LG, Hannallah RS, Luban NL, Fink R, Rüttimann Ueli. Anaemia and postoperative apnoea in former preterm infants. Anesthesiology 1991;74:1003.

28. Welborn LG, Rice LJ, Hannallah RS, Broadman LM, Ruttimann UE, Fink R. Postoperative apnoea in former preterm infants; a prospective comparison of spinal and general anaesthesia. Anesthesiology 1990;72:838.

29. Krane EJ, Haberkern CM, Jacobson LE. Postoperative apnoea , bradycardia and oxygen desaturation in former preterm infants. Prospective comparison of spinal and general anaesthesia. Anesth Analg 1995;80:7.

30. Welborn LG, Hannallah RS, Fink R, Ruttimann UE, Hicks JM. Highdose caffeine suppresses postoperative apnoea in former preterm infants. Anesthesiology 1989; 71:347.

31. Coté CJ, Zaslavsky A, Downes JJ, et al. Postoperative apnea in former preterm infants after inguinal herniorrhaphy. A combined analysis. Anesthesiology 1995;82: 809–822.

32. McGill WA, Coveler LA, Epstein BS. Subacute upper respiratory infection in small children. Anesth Analg 1979; 58:331–333.

33. DeSoto H, Patel RI, Soliman IE, Hannallah RS. Changes in oxygen saturation following general anesthesia in children with respiratory infection signs and symptoms undergoing otolaryngological procedures. Anesthesiology 1988;68:276–279.

34. Tait AR, Knight PR. The effects of general anesthesia on upper respiratory tract infections in children. Anesthesiology 1987;67:930–935.

35. Tait AR, Knight PR. Intraoperative respiratory complications in patients with upper respiratory tract infections. Can J Anaesth 1987;34:300–303.

36. Liu LMP, Ryan JF, Cote CF, Goudsouzian NG. Influence of upper respiratory infections on critical incidents during anesthesia. Ninth World Congress of Anesthesiologists 1988;2:A786.

37. Cohen MM, Cameron CB. Should you cancel the operation when a child has an upper respiratory tract infection? Anesth Analg 1991;72:282–288.

38. JacobyDB, Hirshman CA. General anesthesia in patients with viral respiratory infections: an unsound sleep? Anesthesiology 1991;74:969–972.

39. Schreiner MS, O'Hara I, Markakis DA, Politis GD. Do children who experience laryngospasm have an increased risk of upper respiratory tract infection? Anesthesiology 1996;85:475–480.

40. Parnis SJ, Barker DS, Van der Walt JH. Clinical predictors of anestheticcomplicationsin children with upper respiratory tract infections. Paediatr Anaesth 2001;11:29–40.

41. Tait AR, Malviya S, Voepel-Lewis T, et al. Risk factors for perioperative adverse respiratory events in children with upper respiratory tract infections. Anesthesiology 2001; 95:299–306.

42. Malviya S, Voepel-Lewis T, Siewert M, et al. Risk factors for adverse post operative outcomes in children presenting for cardiac surgery with upper respiratory tract infections. Anesthesiology 2003;98:628–632.

43. Maria de Andrade Castro J, Resende RR, Mirotti L, et al. Role of M2 selected for minimal or maximal acute inflammatory response. Bio Med Research International Volume 2013:12.

44. Jones A. Anaesthetic death of a child with a cold. Anaesthesia 1993;48:171.

45. Bloch EC. Anaesthetic death of a child with a cold. Anaesthesia 1993;48:171.

46. Kinouchi K, Tanigami H, Tashiro C, et al. Duration of apnea in anesthetized infants and children required for desaturation of hemoglobin to 95%; the influence of upper respiratory infection. Anesthesiology 1992;77:1105–1107.

47. Cote CJ. The upper respiratory infection (URI) dilemma: fear of complication or litigation? Anesthesiology 2001; 95:283–285.

48. Tait AR, Malviya S. Anesthesia for the child with an upper respiratory infection: still a dilemma? Anesth Analg 2005; 100:59–65.

49. Bhatia N, Barber N. Dilemmas in the pre operative evaluation of children. Cont Edu Anaesth Crit Care Pain (CEACCP) 2011;11:214–218.

50. Frank EJ, Jacobe KM. Evaluation and management of heart murmurs in children. Am Fam Physician 2011;84(7): 793–800.

51. Bhatia N, Barber N. Dilemmas in the pre operative evaluation of children. Cont Edu Anaesth Crit Care and Pain 2011;11:214–218.

52. White CM, Peyton JM. Anaesthetic management of children with congenital heart disease for non-cardiac surgery. Cont Edu Anaesth Crit Care Pain (CEACCP) 2012;12:17–22.

53. Chye QS, Ling WM. NUS Bulletin 5, September 1998.

54. Hata T, Todd MM. Cervical spine considerations when anesthetizing patients with Down's syndrome. Anesthesiology 2005;102:680–685.

55. Gupta N, Rath GP, Bala R, et al. Anesthetic management in children with Hurler's syndrome undergoing emergency ventriculoperitoneal surgery. Saudi J Anaesth 2012; 6:178–180.

56. Gandhi M, Iyer H, Sehmbi H, Datir K. Anaesthetic management of a patient with Sturge-Weber syndrome undergoing oophorectomy. Indian J Anaesth 2009;53: 64–67.

57. Dhulkhed VK, Shetti AN, Dhulkhed PV. Anaesthetic management of a patient with Laurence Moon Biedl syndrome undergoing ostiumprimum atrial septal defect closure. Anesth Essays Res 2013;7(2): 276–278.

58. Boku A, Hanamoto H, Kudo C, Morimoto Y, et al. Airway Management for Treacher Collins Syndrome with Limited Mouth Opening. Open Journal of Anesthesiology 2013;3: 90–92.

59. Patel K, Chavan D, Sawant P. Anesthesia management in a patient of Apert syndrome. Anesthesia: Essays and Researches 2013;7:133–135.

7

Difficult Paediatric Airway

Aparna Sinha, AK Sethi

- **Assessment of airway in a child**
- **Acquired causes of difficult airway in children**
- **Anticipated difficult airway and anaesthesia plan**
- **Preparing the child**
- **Unanticipated difficult airway**
- **Laryngospasm**

INTRODUCTION

Identification of difficult airway is the corner stone of anaesthetic practice, and the single most important step in preventing failure!! No manoeuvre is 100% reliable but failure to evaluate the airway to predict difficulty is the single most important reason to encounter failure. Problems may even occur in the experienced and extensively trained hands during paediatric airway management. Surveys and literature continue to demonstrate that respiratory complications are the second most common cause for perioperative cardiac arrest in children and remain a major cause of morbidity and mortality, that is largely preventable.

Most children have airway that can be easily handled and managed in experienced hands. However, in inexperienced hands, even a straight forward airway may become difficult! Caution needs to be exercised in 'occasional paediatric anaesthesiologists'.

The goal of preoperative assessment and airway examination in paediatric patients should be to be able to identify the patients in whom the airway may become challenging or difficult.[1] Respiratory complications due to inappropriately managed airway continue to remain second most common cause of morbidity and mortality in this age group.[1-3]

The limited body reserves and higher demand of infants and children make them very prone to desaturation much earlier than in adults. It may become impossible to resuscitate the child, if oxygenation and ventilation cannot be restored immediately. Hence, airway management remains the most significant component of perioperative management in paediatric patients (Box 7.1).

> **Box 7.1: Child's difficult airway differs from that of adult**
>
> - Difficult to gain child's cooperation
> - Handling miniature equipment needs training/additional care
> - Prone to hypoxaemia
> - Needs experienced anaesthesiologist

ASSESSMENT OF AIRWAY IN A CHILD

A thorough assessment of airway should be mandatory in every, apparently normal looking, child prior to an anaesthesia to rule out and identify any indicators of difficult airway. Careful history and pre-procedure or preoperative physical examination is

Table 7.1	Conditions known to be associated with difficult airway in children
Conditions that improve with age	**Conditions that worsen with age**
■ Pierre Robin syndrome	■ Treacher Collins
■ Goldenhar syndrome	■ Apert-Pfeifer
■ Cleft palate	■ Glycogen storage disorders
	■ Bechwith-Weidmann
	■ Arthrogryposis
	■ Freeman-Sheldon

likely to reveal several facts, which can be complimented by investigations, if required.

Coming to discuss difficult paediatric airway (Table 7.1), it is usually associated with dysmorphic features and poor visualization of larynx with direct laryngoscopy (Figs 7.1 to 7.5).

There have been no standardized screening tests applicable to children and the suggested tools for the adults cannot be extrapolated to children particularly neonates and infants. However, a systematic and thorough preoperative screening can identify many potential difficult airways. An important question to ask oneself during preoperative visit is whether ventilation by facemask is likely to be difficult.

History

History should have emphasis on:

■ Upper respiratory tract infection
■ Any respiratory problems—such as snoring with or without apnoeic episodes during sleep, mouth breathing, noisy breathing, change of voice, recurrent croup.
■ Any previous surgery on head and neck or face
■ Previous anaesthetic events
■ Any difficulty in feeding

Examination of a child should commence from the nares and proceed down the airway. Such as choanal

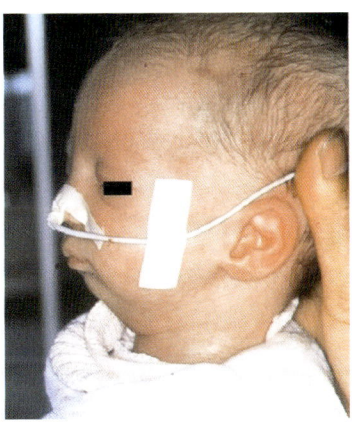

Fig. 7.1. Pierre-Robin syndrome

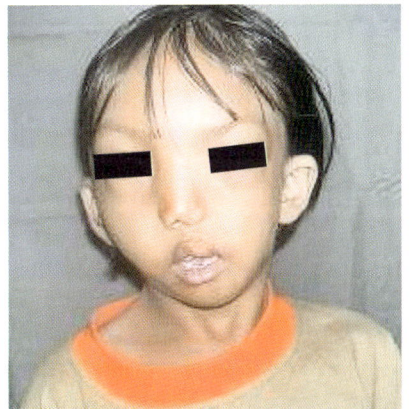

Fig. 7.2. Goldenhar syndrome

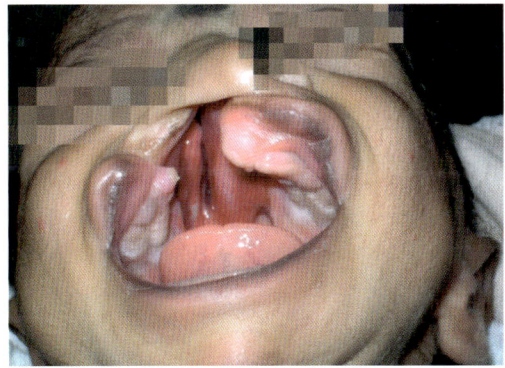

Fig. 7.3. Cleft palate

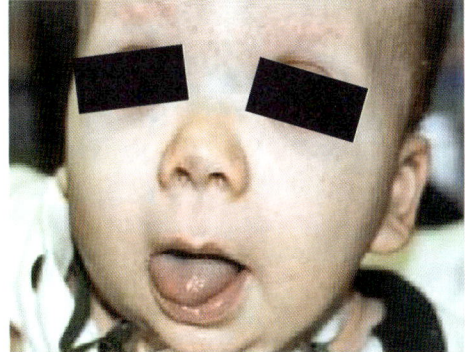

Fig. 7.4. Bechwith-Weidmann syndrome

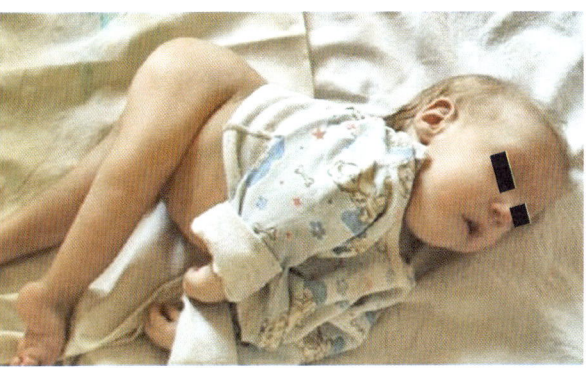

Fig. 7.5. Arthrogryposis

stenosis in the newborn can occur as an isolated finding and be life-threatening.

There can be association with craniofacial anomalies, such as Apert and Crouzon syndromes. Nasal patency of the nasal airway be carried out.

Physical Examination

Airway examination must assess (Table 7.2):

- Mouth opening
- Presence of loose or protruding teeth
- Size of the tongue
- Presence of other soft tissue mass, such as cystic hygroma/cysts/Ludwig's angina in the mouth
- Mandibular size
- Neck mobility/presence of swelling around the head and neck (meningocoele/cystic hygroma)
- Temporomandibular joint movement

General physical examination should focus on the facial symmetry, neck symmetry, adequacy of mouth opening, mentohyoid distance, thyromental distance, and adequacy of neck flexion and extension. Presence of receding jaw, micrognathia or reduced thyromental distance (less than 3 fingers of patient) should immediately alert the anaesthesiologist of the possibility of anterior larynx and hence a difficult direct laryngoscopy.

The physical features suggestive of a difficult airway have been summarized in Table 7.2.

Wherever possible, the Mallampati and Cormach and Lehane should be recorded for future reference. Though there are no standard values thyromental and horizontal, mandibular lengths do not exist for the paediatric patients. Mandibular space assessment is used to predict difficult airways in older children only. Clinical evaluation should also be carried out from the side to assess for micrognathia.

In general age less than 1 year, Mallampati III or IV, BMI > 35 kg/m^2, patient posted for ENT surgery, cardiac or maxillofacial surgery has higher possibility of a difficult airway.[4,5]

Some external features have been shown to be associated with difficult airway management (Tables 7.1 and 7.2). A special note should be made of these features, e.g. any abnormality of external ear, i.e. microtia. So, in children presenting for ear reconstruction extra caution should be exercised. Incidence of difficult airway (Cormach and Lehane III/IV) is significantly higher in bilateral microtia when compared to unilateral microtia.[4]

The rising prevalence of obesity has brought into focus the obese and morbidly obese children who may represent a unique group of children. Due to high prevalence of obstructive sleep apnoea in these children a high degree of suspicion needs to be maintained. Airway management and securing the airway may be very challenging due to reduced safe apnoea time.[5] BMI, thyromental distance and neck circumference are useful predictors of difficult airway in these patients.[6-11]

Other phenotypic features associated with difficult airway in children are seen with various congenital anomalies and genetic syndromes, like Pierre-Robin sequence, Goldenhar syndrome and Treacher Collins syndrome.[1] Various syndromes and their impact on airway management have been nicely reviewed by Butler et al.[8]

Table 7.2 Features suggestive of difficult paediatric airway	
Mouth opening	With mouth fully open < two finger breadth (patient's) and Mallampati 3 or 4
Palate	Narrow and high arched
Teeth	Long teeth or malaligned allow less space for the laryngoscope and the tube
Jaw protrusion/upper lip bite test	Indicator of mask ventilation
Small submandibular space/thyromental distance	Less than 3 fingers of patient
Length of neck	Short neck
Size of neck	Fat deposition around neck
	Limits the extension and makes identification of landmarks difficult
Neck movement	Neck extension and side to side movement

One or the above mentioned features have been combined into scoring systems from time to time and may be clinically beneficial.[12,13]

While making airway assessment, one should include assessment of:

- Any associated signs of respiratory distress
- Baseline pulse oximetry
- Presence of cyanosis
- Any stridor? Inspiratory/expiratory

ACQUIRED CAUSES OF DIFFICULT AIRWAY IN CHILDREN

Acute obstruction: Infection (epiglottitis, retropharyngeal abscess)

- Foreign body aspiration
- Trauma
- Poor mouth opening or mobility of jaw, neck
  - Temporomandibular joint disease, e.g, infection
  - Spinal fusion
  - Burns contractures
  - Measles stomatitis.

Chronic obstruction:

- Tonsillar hypertrophy
- Glottic web
  - Haemangioma
  - Subglottic stenosis

The anticipated DA: Whenever there is a history suggestive of a difficult airway in a previous anaesthetic or there are features suggestive of a potential difficult airway (Box 7.2), a risk-benefit analysis must be performed. A clear plan of action with respect to securing the airway and extubation should be in place. Plan B and C should also be formulated. To completely eliminate the possibility CICV scenario, in patients with poorly defined neck landmarks, ultrasound can be used to mark out the location of cricothyroid membrane using ultrasound machine and provision of surgical airway should be ensured well in time.[15,16]

ANTICIPATED DIFFICULT AIRWAY AND ANAESTHESIA PLAN

When there is past history suggestive of potential difficult airway (difficult mask ventilation or difficult endotracheal intubation), risk benefit analysis must

---

Box 7.2: Points to ponder before decision-making

- Ensure whether the surgery is emergency or elective
- Any further evaluation required to substantiate a difficult airway
- Any intervention required to improve patients general condition and bring up the oxygen reserves
- Is awake intubation planned? Define the type of anaesthesia/sedation.
- What premedication/antisialogogues/nasal decongestants need to be administered
- How to maintain a quiet spontaneously breathing patient
- How is the intubation planned: nasal/oral
- Delineate the desired equipment
- Define plan B and C
  - In case of failure will the patient be awakened?
  - Will an alternative device be used?
- Assess if an ENT surgeon/anaesthesiologist proficient in tracheostomy will be required in operation theater

---

be done. Run through a department protocol to ascertain some pertinent issues.

1. Ascertain whether the procedure/surgery is an emergency.
2. Any intervention is required prior planned procedure/surgery to further optimise the present clinical condition.
3. Is the child adequately fasting?
4. Does the child require any further evaluation to ascertain the degree of difficulty?
5. Ascertain the present level of sensorium.
6. Decide the anaesthesia plan.
7. Does positioning need to be further optimised/modified?
8. Can the airway be optimised before anaesthesia or sedation?
9. Ascertain the level of consciousness of the child while securing the airway: awake, sedated or anaesthetized?
10. Can spontaneous ventilation be maintained during sedation or anaesthesia?
11. Route of endotracheal intubation: oral versus nasal?
12. Additional airway devices required.
13. What are plans B and C? Awaken the patient vs advanced airway procedures?

14. Is an ENT surgeon required at time of anaesthetic induction?
15. Need for sternotomy or extracorporeal membrane oxygenation.

Preparing the Child

Ensure fasting strictly prior to elective surgery. A variety of premedication drugs are available:

- EMLA/Prilox cream prior intravenous cannulation
- Midazolam—0.5 mg/kg PO or intranasal, max dose 20 mg
- Contraindicated in sleep disorders
- Glycopyrrolate (0.008 mg/kg IV)

If EMLA is applied in time, intravenous access can be initiated in the ward itself and premedication and necessary nebulization, etc. administered. This would in all probability give a quiet and fully optimised patient.

In older kids, if awake intubation is planned sedation and dexmedetomidine infusion can be initiated well in time.

The plan for anaesthesia will vary from patient to patient, the situation and experience of the care provider. Every effort should be made to maintain spontaneous respiration initially and to provide incremental dose of the anaesthetic. In anticipated difficult mask ventilation, the induction of anaesthesia should be considered carefully—in children with Apert's syndrome or adenotonsillar hypertrophy, breathing spontaneously on a facemask often leads to obstruction, but intubation is not usually a problem, so it is suggested to proceed with intravenous induction rather than inhalational induction. Conversely, children with Hunter or Hurler's syndrome have a difficult mask airway and difficult intubation—a careful inhalational induction is preferred.

It is preferred to use inhalational induction in children with a difficult airway. The child's ventilation can be gradually assisted with increasing depth of anaesthesia. Muscle relaxant can be administered only when mask ventilation has been ensured. Inhalational induction may be associated with airway obstruction, which can be resolved by careful repositioning, opening the mouth, gentle application of jaw thrust, the use of CPAP.

Introduction of dexmedetomidine into anaesthetic practice has brought new promises especially to

> **Box 7.3: Guiding principles for difficult paediatric airway**
>
> - Limit the number of attempts
> - Maintain and teach proficient paediatric mask airway skills
> - Involve experienced paediatric anaesthesiologist
> - Ask for help early
> - Maintain oxygenation at all times
> - Keep Plan B and C ready

patients with burn contracture of neck, etc. where sedation can be produced with no risk of apnoea or respiratory depression.

The supraglottic devices can be used as rescue to maintain ventilation and oxygenation during inhalational anaesthesia or as a conduit for intubation using a fibreoptic scope. It can also be used in a *cannot intubate/cannot ventilate* situation (Box 7.3).

Child Requiring Fibreoptic Bronchoscopy (FOB)

Before considering a patient for FOB through nasal route, it is important to rule out any nasal anomaly, and procure a detailed history making a special note of features suggestive of nasal patency, mouth breathing and snoring, etc.

Nasal mucosa can be prepped with decongestant, endotracheal tube can be warmed to soften it and secretions can be reduced using antisialogogues.

While performing FOB in a child caution has to be exercised all the time to have a spontaneously breathing quiet child. Either administering slow incremental concentrations of sevoflurane in oxygen or resorting to intravenous techniques can achieve this. One or more of the agents, like propofol, dexmedetomidine, midazolam, fentanyl and ketamine can be used. Lately dexmedetomidine has given very encouraging results.

Availability of oxygen supply and resuscitative means must be ensured before administering any of these agents. Only anaesthesiologist very well versed with the technique should attempt the procedure.[14–16]

Maintenance of spontaneous ventilation continuous oxygenation, provision of bag-mask ventilation when required and use of alternative techniques. It is suggested to prefer using familiar devices and techniques rather than unfamiliar newer techniques, which might be reportedly better (Boxes 7.4 to 7.6; Fig. 7.6).

Box 7.4: Tips for successful FOB in children

- Maintain spontaneous ventilation
- Lubricate the scope well
- Nasal trumpet with 15 mm adapter in contralateral nostril for oxygenation
- Consider antisialogogues
- Experienced help

Box 7.5: Factors affecting decision-making

- Whether procedure is an emergency
- Long-standing condition vs acute onset
- Pulmonary vs airway problem
- Experience of the anaesthesiologist

Box 7.6: Limitations of paediatric FOB

- The endotracheal tube needs to be longer
- The fibrescopes are much smaller have either a flexible tip or suction at a time
- The scope occupies almost the entire tube so continuous oxygenation is difficult
- Scope is too floppy to stay in midline
- Nasal intubation allows very small tubes so very high airway resistance
- Takes longer to secure the airway

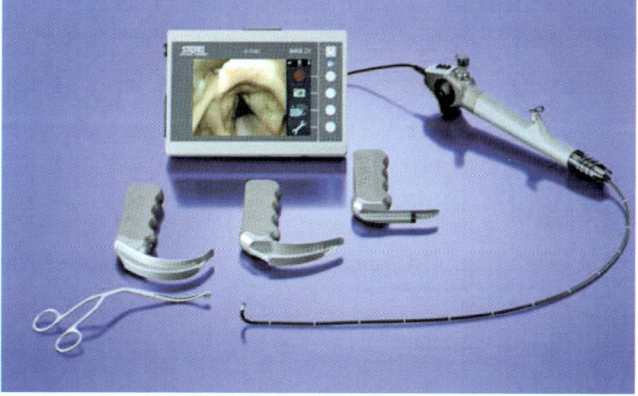

Fig. 7.6. Optical stylet

Device Options and Techniques

- **Indirect laryngoscopy**: C-MAC (Karl Storz, Tuttlingen, Germany), Glidescope® (Verathon Inc, Bothwell, WA).
- **Endotracheal intubation** using the fibreoptic bronchoscope LMA to facilitate endotracheal intubation (awake intubation or under general anaesthesia or sedation).
- **Supraglottic device**: Intubating LMA or endotracheal intubation through the LMA using fibreoptic guidance.
- **Optical stylet**: Similar to the rigid bronchoscope. It is loaded with a tracheal tube, and advanced using a video screen into the trachea. (Bonfils, Karl Storz, Tuttlingen, Germany) .

UNANTICIPATED DIFFICULT AIRWAY

Every anaesthesiologist must have an algorithm to guide through an unanticipated difficult airway or CICV (cannot intubate cannot ventilate) scenario. This anaesthetic catastrophe has poorer outcome in younger children. The time available to establish a surgical airway is much shorter in paediatric patients when compared to adults. The importance of a thorough preoperative assessment to rule out any possibility of CICV cannot be over emphasized. Familiarity with the guidelines and algorithms and to have basic equipment and rescue devices available in the operation theatre should be mandatory prior to taking up any paediatric patient under anaesthesia. The ultimate aim in case of CICV should be to maintain oxygenation and prevent trauma.

The immediate rescue measure in such a situation should be to call for help, readjust the mask, reassess the head and neck position, attempt four-hand and six-hand ventilation, consider the possibility of repeating direct laryngoscopy, changing the laryngoscope or its blade size and use of supraglottic device. In case of failure to rescue using a supraglottic device, use of indirect laryngoscopy or video-laryngoscopy should be attempted prior to a surgical airway. If a rigid bronchoscope is handy, it may be attempted to by placing the tracheal tube over it. These alternatives are preferred over an emergency surgical airway as the latter has very poor outcomes in neonates and small children.

Clinicians must familiarize themselves with the new generation devices, like GlideScope and C-MAC in elective and non-emergency situations, as these can be made available within 60 seconds in most situations.

Conscious decision should be taken to awaken the patient, avoid repeated futile attempts at laryngoscopy to prevent 'cannot intubate but can ventilate' scenario to a CICV situation.[17–21]

In case of failure to re-establish ventilation, one must follow the adult guidelines and consider cricothyroidotomy, though jet ventilation should be avoided in small children. Jet ventilation is known to endanger subcutaneous emphysema, tension mediastinum, and air-embolism and tension pneumothorax.[21–23]

However, in situations of persistent failure, the decision of a surgical access to the airway should not be delayed. The entire exercise should wind up in a few minutes. In children especially neonates and smaller children, the time available for rescue measures is extremely limited and the surgical airway interventions are very challenging.

LARYNGOSPASM

This is a very frequently encountered problem in perianaesthesia period, which occurs due to obtundation of laryngeal reflexes. Under normal course, this reflex is meant to prevent aspiration by causing glottic closure. However, during induction/emergence or otherwise this may become sustained thereby making ventilation and oxygenation difficult. This can be precipitated by light plane of anaesthesia, turbulent airflow, secretions, suctioning in a child with hyper-reactive airway.[23–25] It can present as stridor, where the spasm is partial, associated with desaturation and inability to maintain exchange and ventilation. With increasing severity of spasm, the breath sounds diminish or become absent and paradoxical movement of chest and abdomen can be perceived. This is associated with hypoxaemia, bradycardia and can be life-threatening.

Airway manoeuvres are helpful to maintain a clear and patent airway in mild cases.

Administration of FiO_2 1.0, increasing depth of anaesthesia and maintaining CPAP are the most initial manoeuvres.[26]

Subhypnotic dose of 0.5–1 mg/kg of propofol is suggested. In more severe cases, a prompt call for help and immediate and definitive pharmacologic interventions to prevent irreversible complications.

While awaiting help trial of CPAP is along with definitive pharmacological interventions. Failure to re-establish ventilation warrants the administration of a full dose of neuromuscular blocking agent and

potent intravenous anaesthetic agent (2–3 mg/kg of propofol).[27–29]

Principles to guide difficult paediatric airway: Proficiency in mask ventilation should be acquired. Practitioners in poorly equipped centres should refer the elective surgery and with anticipated difficult airway to centres with expertise and infrastructure.

One must ask for help after first failed intubation attempt and limit the number of attempts at intubation with the same technique and device. Must master alternative techniques too!!

SUMMARY

To summarise, features of a normal paediatric airway, the knowledge of conditions leading to difficult mask ventilation as well as equipment essential for management taking a difficult paediatric airway include the important consideration for successful management of difficult airway in a child (Boxes 7.7 to 7.9; Fig. 7.7).

Box 7.7: Features of the normal paediatric airway

- Large occiput
- Large tongue relative to oral space
- Cephalad position of the larynx
- Floppy, omega-shaped epiglottis
- Angled vocal cords
- Redundant soft tissue/ adenotonsillar
- Hypertrophy

Box 7.8: The difficult mask ventilation in a child

- **Anatomical:**
  - Maxillofacial anomaly
  - Any mass in oropharynx
  - Adenotonsillar hypertrophy
- **Macroglossia**
  - Hurler's/Hunter's syndrome (mucopolysaccharidoses) (Fig. 7.8)
  - Beckwith-Wiedemann syndrome
  - Down's syndrome (Fig. 7.9)
- **Functional:**
  - Laryngospasm
  - Inadequate depth of anaesthesia
  - Bronchospasm
  - Thoracic rigidity
  - Overinflated stomach

Box 7.9: Essential equipment for managing DA

- Nasal airways: various sizes
- Oral airways: various sizes
- Stylets/intubating guides (Fig. 7.10)
- Tube exchangers/gum elastic bougies
- Endotracheal tubes: Conventional armored/uncuffed/cuffed
- Laryngoscope blades: Curved/straight/hybrid
- Laryngoscope handles: Regular/short
- Laryngeal mask airways: Classic, intubating and ProSeal, etc. (Fig. 7.11)
- Face masks
- Combitubes
- Lung isolation devices: Bronchial blockers/double lumen tubes
- Surgical airway access kits
- Accessory equipment: EtCO$_2$/ambu bag, suction catheters/ Magills
- Fibreoptic bronchoscope
- Indirect laryngoscopes

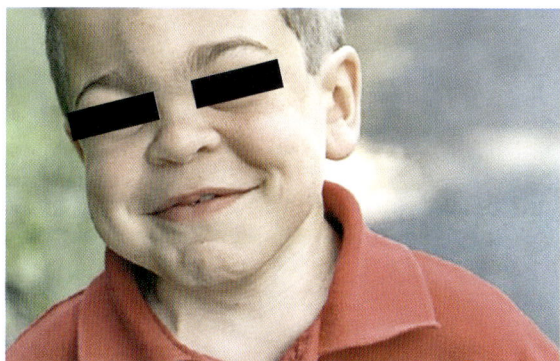

Fig. 7.8. Hurler's mucopolysaccharidoses

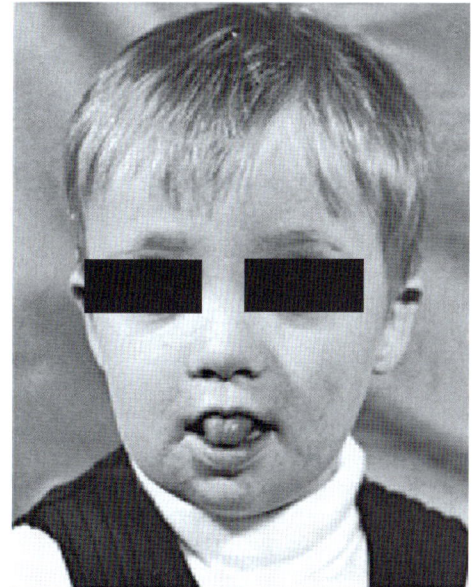

Fig. 7.9. Trisomy 21

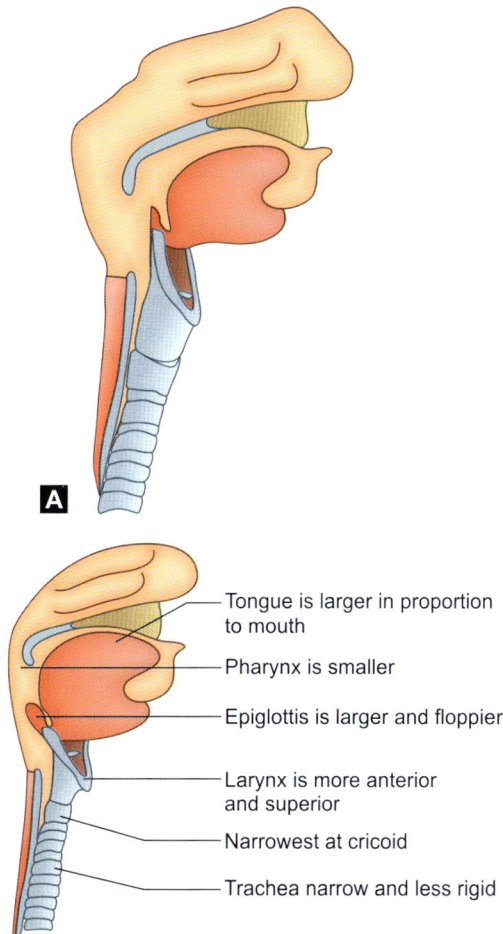

Tongue is larger in proportion to mouth

Pharynx is smaller

Epiglottis is larger and floppier

Larynx is more anterior and superior

Narrowest at cricoid

Trachea narrow and less rigid

Fig. 7.7. (A) Adult upper airways and (B) Children upper airway

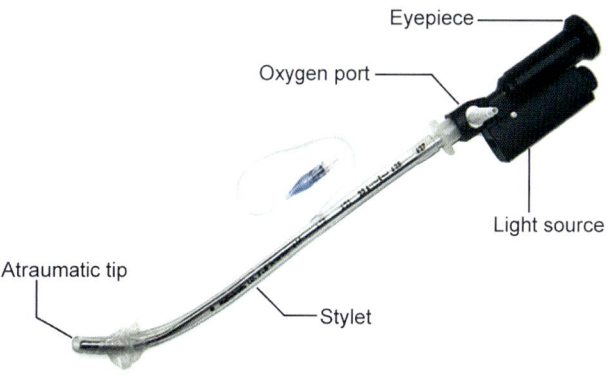

Eyepiece

Oxygen port

Light source

Atraumatic tip

Stylet

Fig. 7.10. Stylets/intubating guides

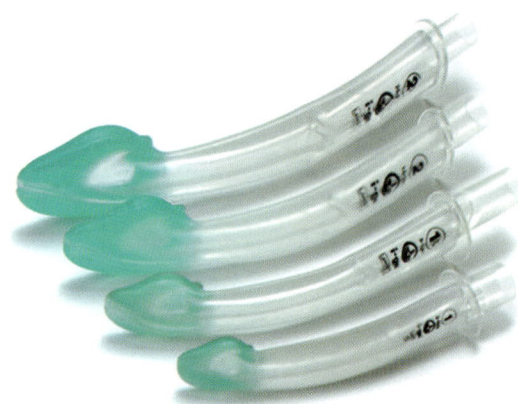

Fig. 7.11. Supraglottic airway device—i-gel

REFERENCES

1. Heinrich S, Birkholz T, Irouschek A, Ackermann A, Schmidt J. Incidences and predictors of difficult laryngoscopy in adult patients undergoing general anaesthesia: a single-center analysis of 102,305 cases. J Anesth 2013; 27:815–821.

2. Bhananker SM, Ramamoorthy C, Geiduschek JM, Posner KL, Domino KB, Haberkern CM, et al. Anesthesia-related cardiac arrest in children: update from the paediatric perioperative cardiac arrest registry. Anesth Analg 2007; 105:344–350.

3. Jimenez N, Posner KL, Cheney FW, Caplan RA, Lee LA, Domino KB. An update on paediatric anesthesia liability: a closed claims analysis. Anesth Analg 2007;104:147–153.

4. Uezono S, Holzman RS, Goto T, Nakata Y, Nagata S, Morita S. Prediction of difficult airway in school-aged patients with microtia. Paediatr Anaesth 2001;11:409–413.

5. Jense HG, Dubin SA, Siverstein PI, et al. Effect of obesity on safeduration of apnea in anesthetized humans. Anesth Analg 1991;72:89–93.

6. Butler MG, Hayes BG, Hathaway MM, Begleiter ML. Specific genetic diseases at risk for sedation/anesthesia complications. Anesth Analg 2000;91:837–855.

7. Magalhães E, Oliveira MF, Sousa Govêia C, Araújo Ladeira LC, Lagares J. Use of simple clinical predictors on preoperative diagnosis of difficult endotracheal intubation in obese patients. Rev Bras Anestesiol 2013; 63:262–266.

8. Kim WH, Ahn HJ, Lee CJ, Shin BS, Ko JS, Choi SJ, Ryu SA. Neck circumference to thyromental distance ratio: a new predictor of difficult intubation in obese patients. Br J Anaesth 2011;106:743–748.

9. Wilson ME, Spiegelhalter D, Robertson JA, Lesser P. Predicting difficult intubation. Br J Anaesth 1988;61: 211–216.

10. Shiga T, Wajima Z. Predicting difficult intubation in apparently normal patients: a meta-analysis of bedside screening test performance: Anesthesiology 2005;103: 429–437.

11. Bryant J, Krishna SG, Tobias JD. The difficult airway in pediatrics. Advan Anesth 2013;31:31–60.

12. Shiga T, Wajima Z. Predicting difficult intubation in apparently normal patients: a meta-analysis of bedside screening test performance: Anesthesiology 2005;103: 429–437.

13. Bryant J, Krishna SG, Tobias JD. The difficult airway in pediatrics. Advan Anesth 2013;31:31–60.

14. Pott LM, Murray WB. Review of video laryngoscopy and rigid fiberoptic laryngoscopy. Curr Opin Anaesthesiol 2008;21:750–758.

15. Chou HC, Tseng WP, Wang CH, et al. Tracheal rapid ultrasound exam (TRUE) for confirming endotracheal tube placement during emergency intubation. Resuscitation 2011;82:1279–1284.

16. Elliott DSJ, Baker PA, Scott MR, et al. Accuracy of surface landmark identification for cannula cricothyroidotomy. Anaesthesia 2010;65:889–894.

17. Schramm C, Knop J. Role of ultrasound compared to age-related formulas for uncuffed endotracheal intubation in a pediatric population. Pediatr Anesth 2012;22:781–786.

18. Kristensen MS. Ultrasonography in the management of the airway. Acta Anesthesiol Scand 2011;55:1155–1157.

19. Curtis RP. Persistent "can't intubate, can't oxygenate" crisis despite reversal of rocuronium with sugammadex: the importance of timing. Anaesth Intensive Care 2012; 40:722–723.

20. Ezri T, Evron S. Sugammadex and the cannot intubate/cannot ventilate scenario in patients with predicted difficult airway. Br J Anaesth 2012;109:459–461.

21. Tait AR, Malviya S, Voepel-Lewis T, Munro HM, Seiwert M, Pandit UA. Risk factors for perioperative adverse respiratory events in children with upper respiratory tract infections. Anesthesiology 2001;95:299–306.

22. Curtis RP. Persistent "can't intubate, can't oxygenate" crisis despite reversal of rocuronium with sugammadex: the importance of timing. Anaesth Intensive Care 2012; 40:722–723.

23. Ezri T, Evron S. Sugammadex and the cannot intubate/cannot ventilate scenario in patients with predicted difficult airway. Br J Anaesth 2012;109:459–461.

24. Batra YK, Ivanova M, Ali SS, et al. The efficacy of a subhypnotic dose of propofol in preventing laryngospasm following tonsillectomy and adenoidectomy in children. Paediatr Anaesth 2005;15:1094–1097.

25. Al-Alami AA, Zestos MM, Baraka AS. Pediatric laryngospasm: prevention and treatment. Curr Opin Anaesthesiol 2009;22:388–395.

26. Walker RM, Sutton RS. What port in a storm? Use of suxamethonium without intravenous access for severe laryngospasm. Anaesthesia 2007;62:757–759.

27. Hannallah RS, Oh TH, McGill WA, et al. Changes in heart rate and rhythm after intramuscular succinylcholine with or without atropine in anesthetized children. Anesthesiology 1986;65:1329–1332.

28. Tobias JD, Nichols D. Intraosseous succinylcholine for orotracheal intubation. Pediatr Emerg Care 1990;6:108–109.

29. Difficult Airway Society. Guidelines for management of the unanticipated difficult intubation. Anaesthesia 2004;59:675–694.

8

General Anaesthesia Considerations in Paediatric Patient

Rajeshwari Subramaniam, Renu Sinha

- **Preparation of operation room**
- **Techniques of IV cannulation**
- **Monitoring**
- **Induction of anaesthesia**
  - **Inhalation induction**
- **Securing the airway in the child**
  - **Mask ventilation and endotracheal intubation**
- **Positioning**

PREPARATION OF OPERATION ROOM (OR)

Careful OR preparation is an integral part of good and safe anaesthesia practice. Apart from routine check of the anaesthesia workstation, an efficient working wall suction and spare oxygen supply, the following aspects need to be addressed when dealing with paediatric patients:

1. **Ambient temperature:** OR needs to be warmed for all paediatric patients, especially neonates and infants. Forced-air warming blankets, heat convectors, warming gel pads are all appropriate. Very effective radiant warmers are now available which should be in place for neonates, preterm babies and small infants. Cling wrap, Saran wrap and/or plastic sheets, cotton and gamgee padding should be kept ready for preterm babies who rapidly lose body heat when exposed. All skin prepping fluids should be warmed.

2. **IV fluids:** Fluid appropriate for the child's age should be prepared and warmed. Fluids tend to lose their warmth when being infused slowly, so should ideally be warmed by systems, like Hotline® (Smiths Medical), especially where large-volume infusion and/or transfusion is planned. Warmed fluids may have bubbles which should be shaken and brought to the surface.

   IV fluid dispensing equipment appropriate for the child's age should be set up, e.g. paediatric burette sets for infants and toddlers, and infusion pumps for neonates and preterm babies. Special care should be taken to meticulously de-air all IV tubing.

3. **Airway equipment:** In spite of various formulae available to calculate appropriate endotracheal tube size in children, there is wide variability in the size depending on the physical build of the child. Further, it is not rare for congenital airway malformations, e.g. tracheal stenosis, to be diagnosed for the first time during anaesthesia. Facemasks appropriate in shape and size for the facial contour (e.g. Rendell-Baker-Soucek for the neonate) should be readied (Fig. 8.2C). Endotracheal tubes one size larger and smaller should be kept ready, with ready access to tubes of other sizes. Airway rescue devices (oropharyngeal, nasopharyngeal and laryngeal mask airways, paediatric video-laryngoscopes) are now part of standard equipment in busy paediatric facilities. Paediatric airway stylets and bougies should be available and accessible.

   A number of rolls of varying sizes, along with 'doughnuts' or head rings to support the head should be at hand during induction of anaesthesia and positioning the baby.

4. **Drug preparation:** If all the drug from the parent ampoule is drawn up in a single 5 ml or 10 ml syringe (e.g. 50 mg atracurium) not only is dosing difficult (e.g. in an infant weighing 6 kg), but wastage very high since the syringe will be discarded with unused drug at the end of the list. Although anaesthetic drug usage per patient in the paediatric OR is significantly lower than ORs with adult patients, attention needs to be paid to drug preparation in order not only to reduce wastage, but to have life-saving drugs drawn up and ready for use. It is a good idea to prepare 'master' syringes with all the contents of an ampoule drawn up, and use small-volume syringes with suitable dose and dilution for each small baby. Further, atropine, ephedrine and suxamethonium can be prepared in one set of syringes and kept readily available in the nurses' bay in between 2 shared ORs. These are the drugs that are maximally wasted in ORs.

TECHNIQUE OF IV CANNULATION

A large part of safe paediatric anaesthetic management relates to secure IV access. In general, veins in pre-school children and adolescents are easy to cannulate as their caliber is satisfactory. In chubby or obese infants, veins may be completely invisible. Secondly, in small babies pressure in the veins is so low that there is no back flash into the cannula. The experienced operator can tackle these situations successfully, and it is a part of learning to watch the art of good venous cannulation. Since the majority of children fear needles, IV cannulation is best attempted when the child is asleep. This facilitates holding the wrist firmly and 'tapping' the vein rendering it prominent (Fig. 8.1A), and reduces chances of the child wriggling its wrist, thereby dislodging the cannula. Veins can be felt as fluid-filled structures under the skin. For neonates, the appropriate way to make a vein prominent is to retract the skin over the wrist away with a single finger (Fig. 8.1B). A few gadgets are available which claim to make IV cannulation easy in

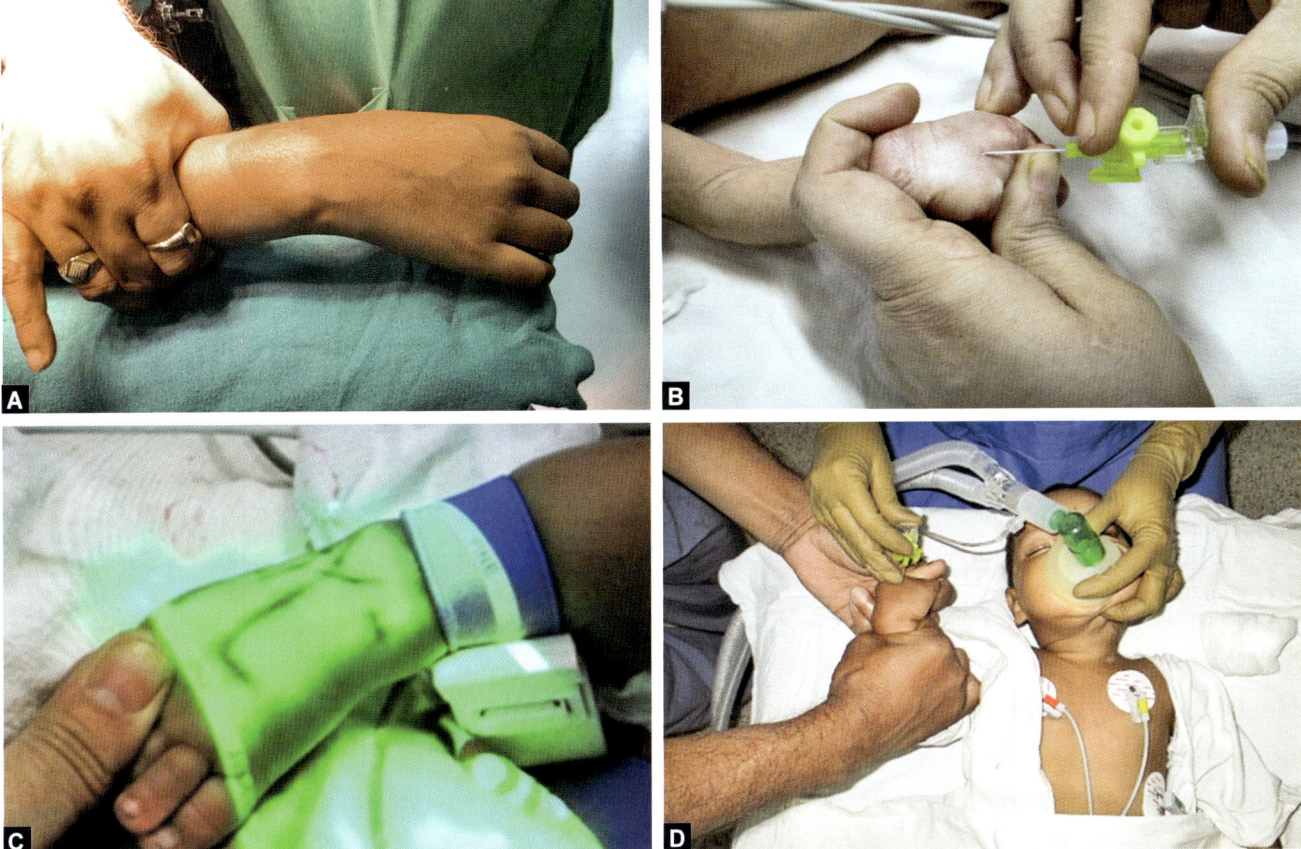

Fig. 8.1A to D. (A) IV cannulation, (B) IV cannulation in neonate, (C) The 'Vein-viewer', (D) Cannulation while holding mask

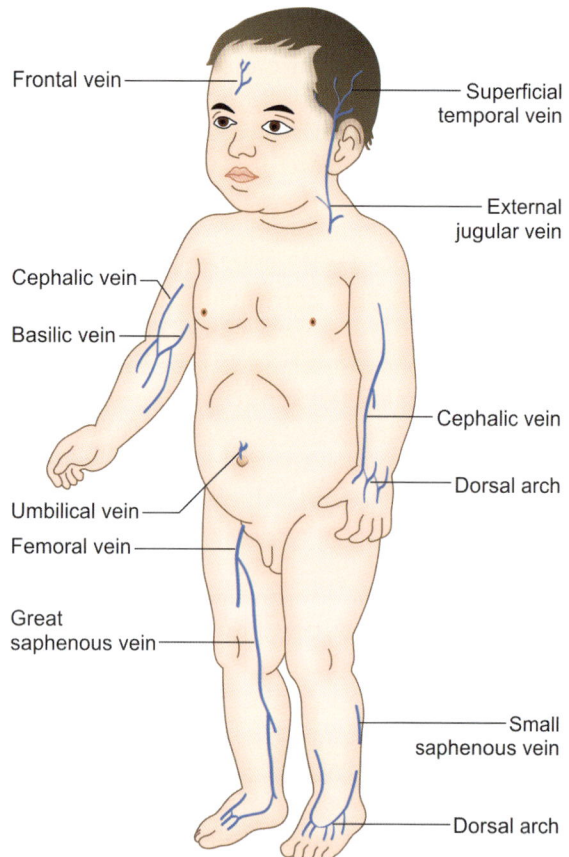

Frontal vein

Superficial
temporal vein

External
jugular vein

Cephalic vein

Basilic vein

Cephalic vein

Dorsal arch

Umbilical vein

Femoral vein

Great
saphenous vein

Small
saphenous vein

Dorsal arch

Fig. 8.1E. Suitable sites for IV access

the paediatric patient (Fig. 8.1C and 8.1E). Over time the skilled paediatric anaesthesiologist can perform IV cannulation with a single hand while holding the mask (Fig. 8.1D).

MONITORING

As is mandatory for any anaesthetic, ASA guidelines are applicable to paediatric anaesthesia as well. Mandatory monitoring includes pulse oximetry, ECG, non-invasive blood pressure (NIBP), and end-tidal CO_2 in intubated patients. Temperature monitoring is very important in small babies and is recommended in all children except those undergoing very brief peripheral procedures.

Pulse oximeter probes come in a variety of models to suit varying sizes of fingers. Adult size probes can be used on the great toe of smaller children. Pulse oximetry is a safe, non-invasive, inexpensive, and reasonably sensitive test that will detect many cases of critical CHD in neonates. Swenson et al recommend

that abnormal pulse oximetry readings persisting for more than 2 hours in newborns, or accompanied by physical findings, warrant an echocardiogram. Conventional pulse oximetry in newborns suffers from artifacts due to motion. Movement by the newborn results in irregular movement of venous blood which sends a confounding signal to the pulse oximeter sensor. The resulting trace, depending on the magnitude of movement, may be larger than the SpO_2 trace, but does not represent the true value. Further, when noise or motion artefact is introduced both into red and infrared channels, the ratio is driven towards unity, which is translated into an SpO_2 value $\infty 82\%$ which can set off the lower limit alarm. Inaccurate SpO_2 values may add up to >50% of the trace. Recently, Masimo has introduced the 'signal extraction' technology which identifies and verifies the energy produced by the arterial pulse, thereby eliminating other sources of interference.

When should pulse oximetry be measured in the upper and lower limbs simultaneously?

Simultaneous, or immediate sequential monitoring of SpO_2 in the right upper and right lower limb has been recommended to screen newborns for critical congenital heart disease (CCHD). A reading of <90% in either probe, persistent values between 90 and 94% in either limb or a difference of >3% between upper and lower limbs increases the likelihood of detection of CCHD.

Pulse oximeters, being non-invasive, can, and should be applied before induction.

Automated non-invasive blood pressure monitoring is useful in all children and correlates well with volume loss.

Temperature monitoring may be carried out through oesophageal or nasopharyngeal routes. If available or indicated, bladder or tympanic temperatures may be used. Cutaneous probes may not reflect actual core temperature, especially in low-perfusion states.

Invasive pressure monitoring has now become feasible even in small neonates with the availability of appropriately-sized arterial and central venous cannulae. It is important for the full-time paediatric anaesthesiologist to become adept at these skills, as they provide valuable inputs in patient management during prolonged and major surgery, or in the child with trauma.

INDUCTION OF ANAESTHESIA

As far as paediatric patients are concerned, induction of anaesthesia can be a terrifying or a calm and pleasant experience, and is heavily influenced by adequate planning and judgment on the part of the anaesthesiologist. During preoperative evaluation, the older child can be asked to exercise his/her choice of induction technique—whether by inhalational or intravenous route.

Inhalational Induction

For older children, inhalational induction can be likened to blowing a balloon during the preoperative visit. Many anaesthesiologists carry a small reservoir bag and facemask to familiarize the child with what to expect in the OR. In the OR, after attaching the pulse oximeter probe and ECG, the circuit is primed with sevoflurane or halothane, and the child is encouraged to place the facemask on his/her face and reminded to breathe deeply. Single-breath induction can also be taught to the child. Younger (pre-school) children usually are unable to fully comprehend and cooperate with inhalational induction. Larger masks are sometimes useful to engage the whole face and distract the child (Fig. 8.2A).

Toddlers and pre-school children are usually comfortable in their parents' arms, and a parent may accompany the child into the OR. The parent, however, should be explained that they would be required to leave as soon as the child loses consciousness, and reassured that he/she will be safe. In case a child is sleeping when brought into the OR, 'steal induction' can be carried out; 70% N_2O is blown over the child's face, and the facemask gently brought into contact with the face. When the child does not respond to facemask placement, halothane/sevoflurane is introduced and the concentration gradually stepped up, and all monitoring devices are applied.

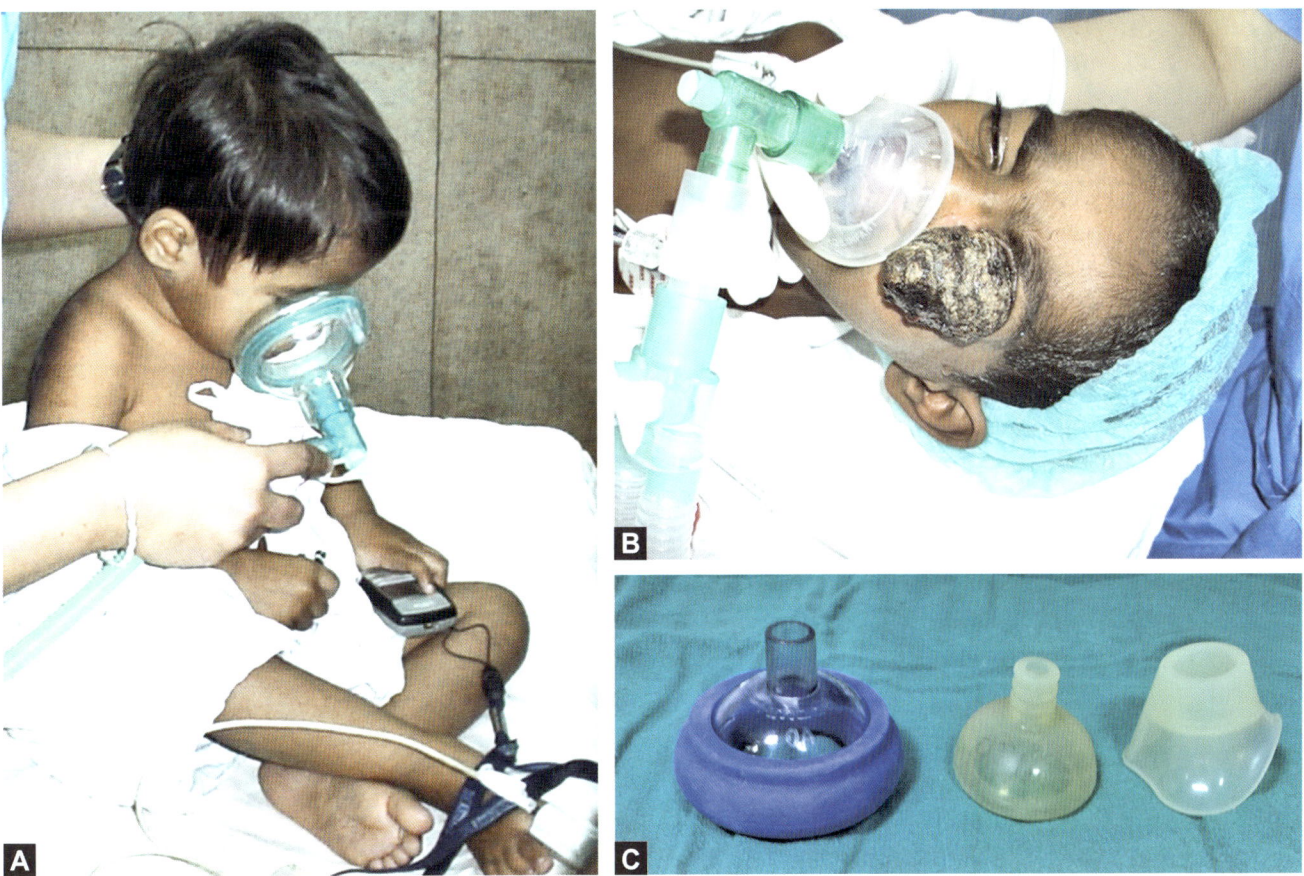

Fig. 8.2A to C. (A and B) Inhalation induction; (C) Facemask used for inhalation induction

If the child has an indwelling IV cannula, the pulse oximeter is applied, and induction can be made straightforward and pleasant with a narcotic and intravenous induction. The dose of propofol in children is higher (2–4 mg/kg) compared to adults. Thiopentone is a good choice for neonates and infants, specially when a functional IV cannula is in place.

AIRWAY MANAGEMENT

There are basic anatomical and physiological differences between the airway of a child and adult. The approach to management of the airway in a child, therefore, differs significantly from that of an adult. Different paediatric age groups need different approaches for securing a definitive airway. A wide variety of techniques and devices are presently available to secure the airway in children.

Mask Ventilation and Endotracheal Intubation

After induction of anaesthesia and loss of consciousness, the majority of smaller children (toddlers, infants and neonates) need airway assistance prior to placement of a definitive airway. A correct selection of mask size is vital not only to prevent leaks on a normal facial structure, or, if there is a lesion, like proptosis, to prevent injury to the eye (Fig. 8.2B).

Mask holding especially for small babies is an art and needs to be practiced so that optimal ventilation can be achieved without air trapping in the lungs (which can occur, if expiration is incomplete, as with a tongue partially obstructing the airway) or gastric distension. It is important not to pull up the mandible with pressure on the soft submandibular space, as it forces the tongue on the palate, thereby closing off the oropharyngeal airway. The mask needs to be delicately held with the thumb and forefinger, with the ring finger providing the required seal from the chin end and the small finger supporting the mandible (Fig. 8.3A). It is also important to check that the mask is not pinching the nostril shut (Figs 8.3B and C).

POSITIONING

A pillow under the head is not needed in neonates and smaller children due to the prominent occiput. The infant's head is large with respect to the body size, and the chin tends to flex on the neck (vide infra). This situation is corrected by placing a small rolled towel below the baby's shoulders and neck, which raises the chest, prevents neck flexion and stabilizes the head. In neonates and infants, the shoulder roll not only provides stability to the head, but also aids in neck extension (Fig. 8.3A).

Intubation can be done with direct laryngoscopy, indirect laryngoscopy, rigid or flexible bronchoscopy.

Laryngoscopy

Both Miller and Macintosh blades have been used for intubation depending on operator choice and the airway anatomy. The Miller blade is inserted in the center of the mouth so that the tongue is pressed and displaced into the floor of the mouth by the blade. The tip of the Miller blade is placed on the posterior (ventral) surface of epiglottis to lift it for glottic exposure in neonates and smaller infants, whose epiglottis is large, U-shaped and floppy. The Macintosh blade is inserted from the right angle of the mouth and moved towards the center, displacing the tongue towards the left side to provide an intraoral space similar to adult laryngoscopy. The tip of the Macintosh blade is inserted in the glossoepiglottic fold and the epiglottis lifted indirectly.

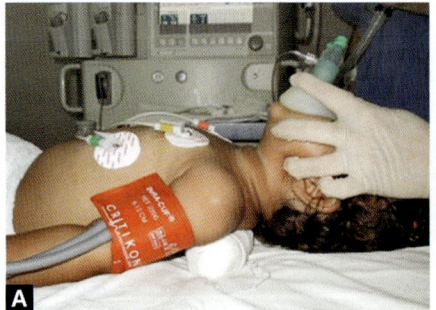 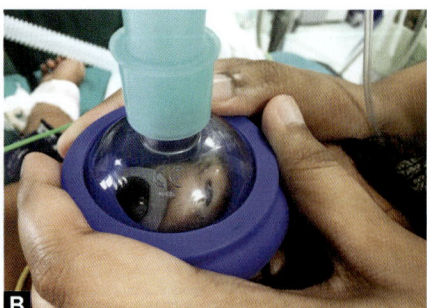 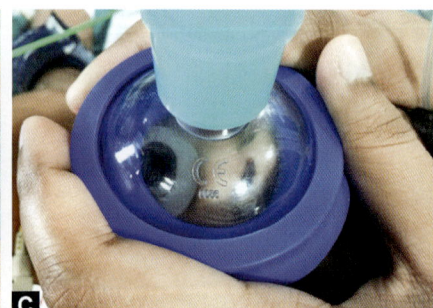

Fig. 8.3A to C. Procedure of inhalation induction

During laryngoscopy in neonates and smaller infants, the little finger of the left hand can be used to press the cricoid for better visualization of the glottis. (Fig. 8.4A).

The endotracheal tube (ETT) is inserted through the C-shape space provided in the Miller blade and from the right angle of the mouth with the Macintosh blade. Stretching the angle of the mouth on the right side by an assistant during ETT insertion provides better space (Fig. 8.4B).

Recently different video-laryngoscopes (Glide-Scope, C-MAC, TruView) have been used for intu-bation (Figs 8.5A to C). They provide a magnified glottic view in the monitor and passage of the ETT can be seen in the monitor. Since video-laryngoscopes have different types of blades, the technique of laryngoscopy and insertion of ETT varies with each device. Training with video-laryngoscopes is necessary even for experienced anaesthesiologists as it has been observed that intubation is difficult even with best glottic view. Hand-eye coordination is needed as the magnified view provided results in a small movement of ETT perceived as a major movement on the monitor.

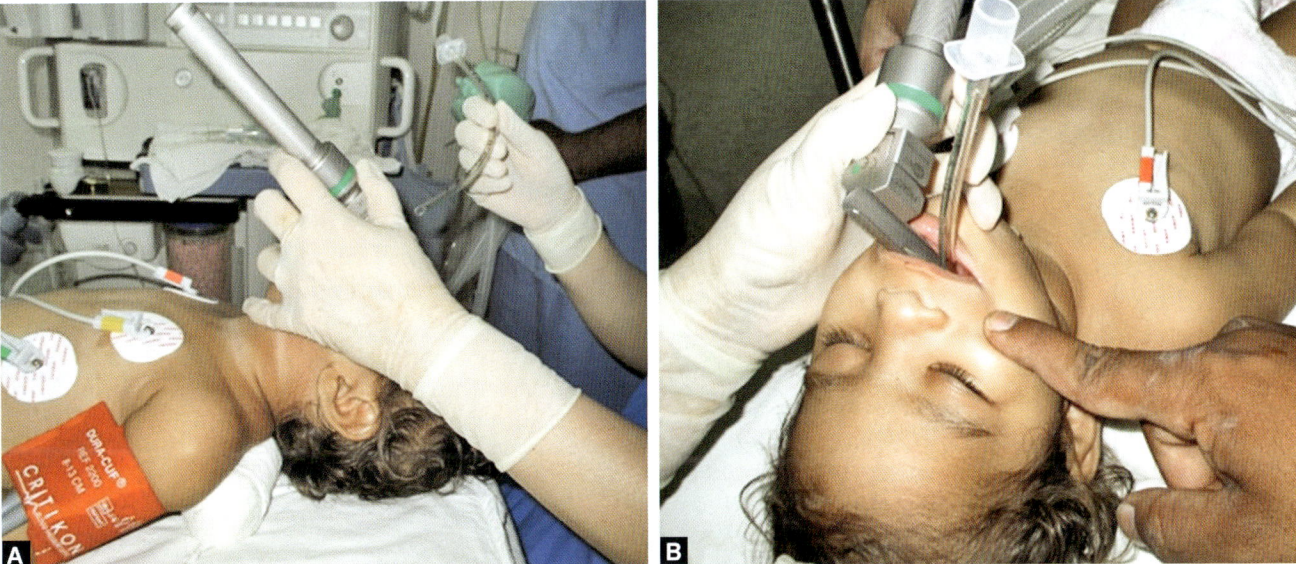

Fig. 8.4A and B. Positioning for laryngoscopy and intubation

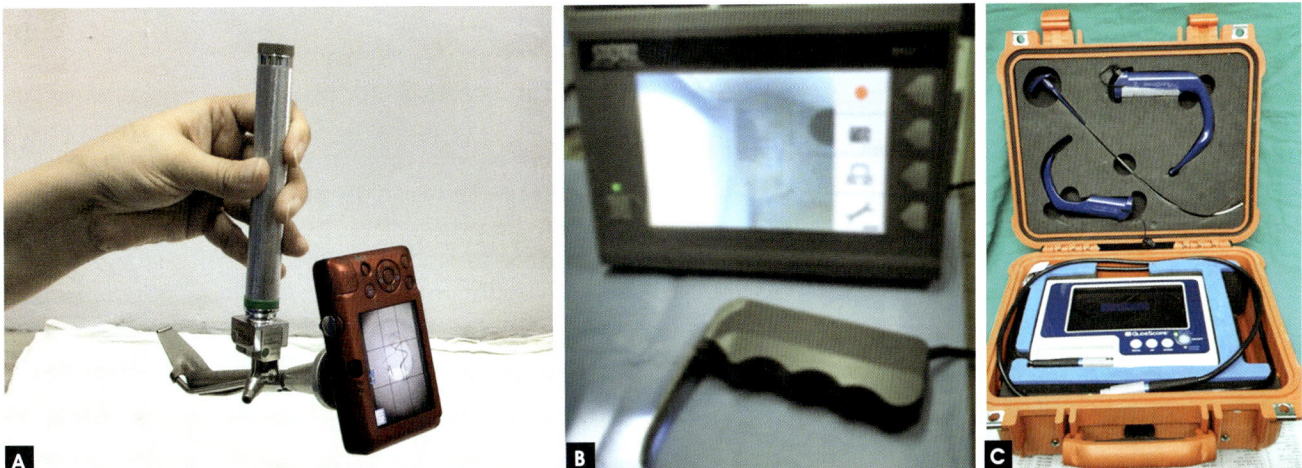

Fig. 8.5A to C. Videolaryngoscopes: (A) Truview, (B) C-MAC, (C) GlideScope

It is important that the tip of the video-laryngoscope should be placed under direct vision behind the tongue to prevent inadvertent injury of oropharyngeal and perilaryngeal structures.

Supraglottic Airways

Apart from endotracheal tube, supraglottic airways (SGAs) are also an effective means of securing the paediatric airway. Various types of SGAs are available, e.g. prototypes of laryngeal mask airway (LMA): Classic, Proseal, Flexible, Ambu ; the Air-Q Intubating Laryngeal Airway (ILA), Laryngeal Tube, Cobra perilaryngeal airway, i-gel, Streamlined Liner of Pharyngeal Airway (SLIPA), etc. (Fig. 8.6).

A number of studies comparing SGAs showed that the choice of airway device should depend on various factors, like age of the child, type of surgery, duration of surgery and the experience of the anaesthesiologist. Some of these devices have a channel (gastric drain;) (Proseal, i-gel), others (Air-Q ILA and Ambu Aura) are specially designed for endotracheal intubation. SGAs with gastric drain are better for children with gastric reflux or when the surgery is planned in lateral or prone position. The Proseal LMA provides a good oropharyngeal seal with the provision of gastric drain.

SGAs can be used for neonates and premature infants for short cases, if the anaesthesiologist is well experienced with their use. However, SGA should be avoided in children undergoing surgery in head and neck area, suspected of having a full stomach, surgery in difficult position (e.g. prone) and when airway is either difficult and/or not freely accessible to the anaesthesiologist.

The method of insertion of different SGAs is more or less similar. A roll can be placed below the nape of the neck to provide stability to the head and open the short neck area with neck extension. The cuff of the SGA cuff can be either fully or partially deflated at the time of insertion. The tip and dorsal surface of the cuff of the selected SGA should be lubricated with water-soluble gel. After induction and attaining adequate depth of anaesthesia, the head is positioned in the 'sniffing' position; the left hand opens the mouth. The SGA is held in the right hand like a pen with the ventral side of the cuff facing downwards and tip of the index finger inserted into the 'pouch' at the junction of SGA cuff to the airway tube (Figs 8.7A to D). The SGA is inserted from the center of the mouth by pressing the tongue and then directed towards the hard palate in the oropharyngeal cavity till resistance is felt. The finger is then removed and the cuff inflated with air with minimal recommended volume to achieve optimal leak pressure. During insertion, if resistance is felt in between, then the SGA should be withdrawn slightly and direction of pressure should be changed for reinsertion. There are different techniques of SGA insertion, i.e. 180° rotation, partial inflation technique, thumb insertion technique, etc. Inflation of the SGA cuff leads to slight outward movement of SGA.

I-gel, SLIPA and air-Q SP do not need inflation due to inbuilt cuff design.

MAINTENANCE OF ANAESTHESIA

General anaesthesias for procedures projected to last more than an hour are usually managed with muscle relaxation to permit controlled ventilation. Procedures lasting less than an hour, especially peripheral orthopaedic procedures, herniotomies, urethral and ophthalmic procedures may be well managed with spontaneous ventilation through an appropriately placed supraglottic device, commonly a laryngeal mask airway, especially if an appropriate regional block is given. It must be remembered though, that minor movements, like uprolling of the eyeball, can be very irritating in small ophthalmic procedures and the child may be better off with relaxant

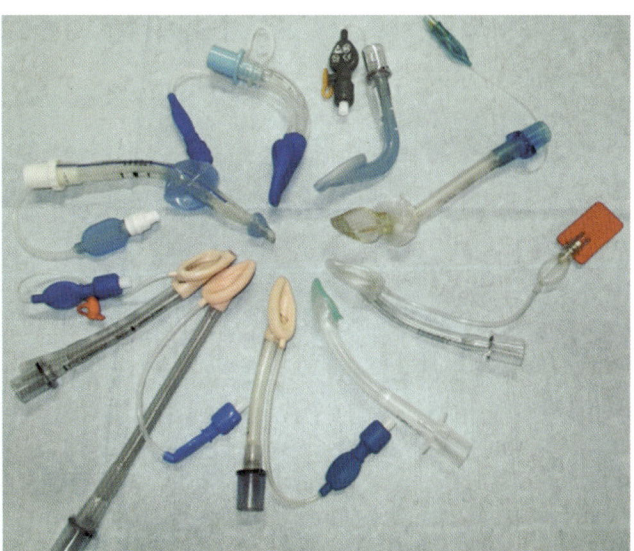

Fig. 8.6. Supraglottic airway devices

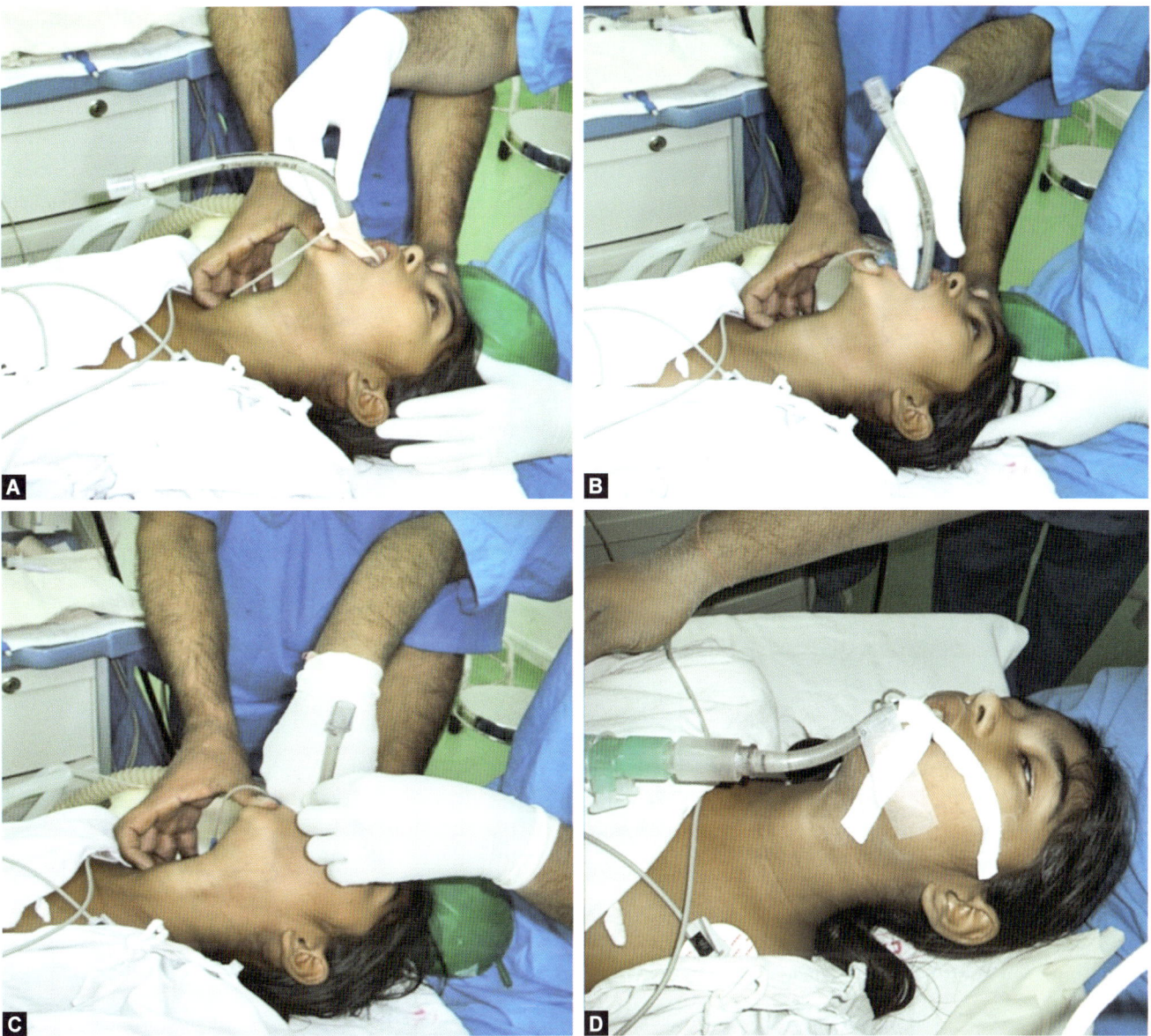

Figs 8.7A to D. Insertion of flexible LMA in a child

supplementation and controlled ventilation. Any of the commonly available inhalational agents is suitable for maintenance. Sevoflurane is preferable for children with cardiac disease on account of its cardio-stability.

The child's fluid requirements must be carefully met through the procedure. Blood transfusion is generally indicated for losses exceeding 10–15% of the estimated blood volume. This margin is reduced, if the child concomitantly has anaemia, cardiac and/or respiratory disease.

The body temperature needs careful monitoring and measures to warm the child should be readily available. It is good practice to keep the warming devices in position and use them, if needed.

Use of regional analgesia is increasing in children and confers analgesia of superior quality, as well as sparing intraoperative opioid and relaxant use. Children waking up without pain are easier to manage, reduce anxiety in parents and have a decreased incidence of adverse psychological conse-quences, like enuresis and behavioural problems. If a child is likely to present multiple times for surgery, e.g. staged urethroplasty, good analgesia in the first surgery results in atraumatic parental separation and reduces fear of the hospital and doctors in subsequent surgeries.

Intravenous analgesic supplementation should be provided judiciously throughout the procedure, especially if no neuraxial/regional block has been given. The incidence of postoperative delirium is

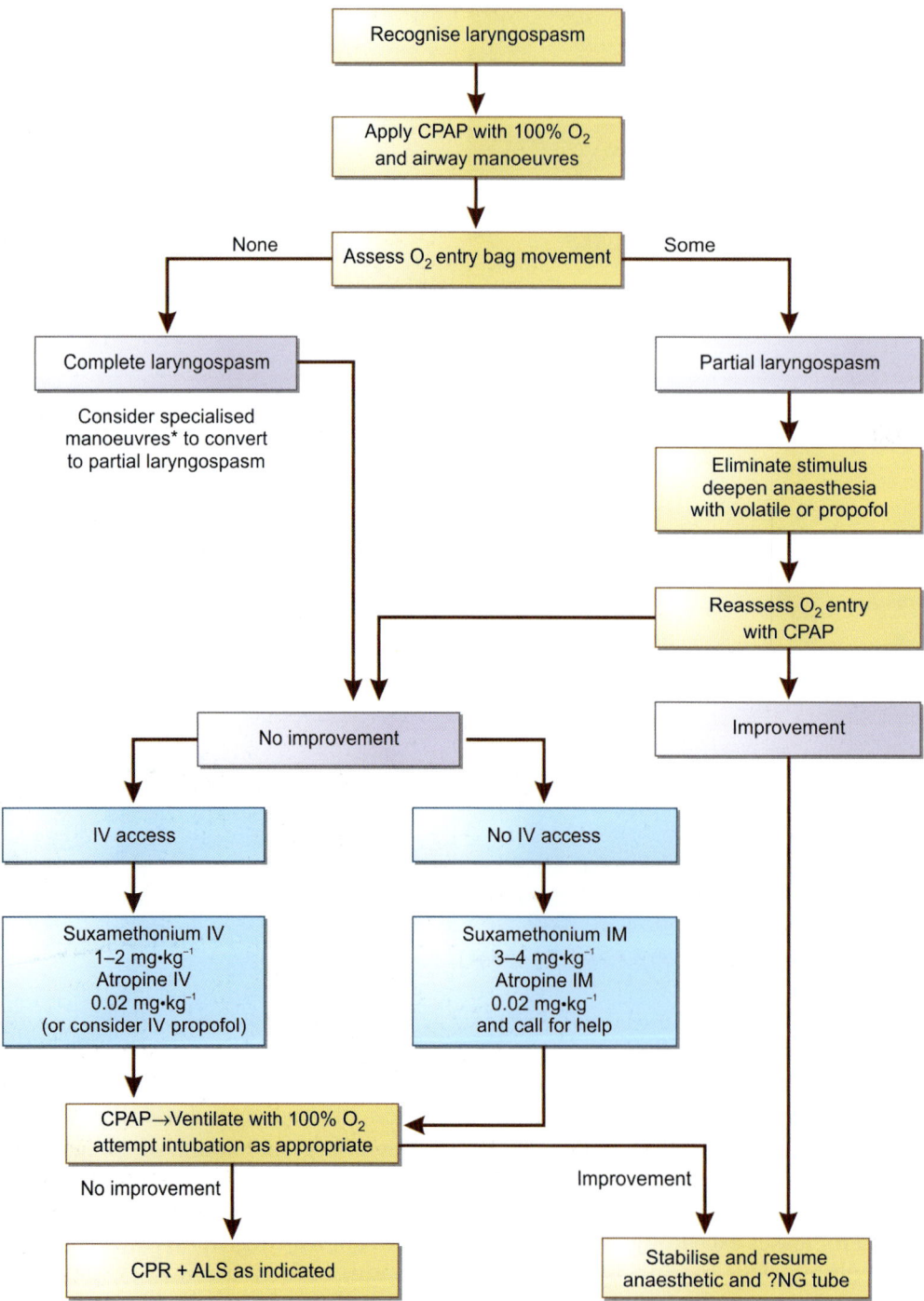

Fig. 8.8. Algorithm for treatment of laryngospasm[6]

high in children who are in pain at recovery from anaesthesia.

EXTUBATION AND POST-ANAESTHESIA CARE

Antiemetic prophylaxis should be routinely administered to all children at the end of the procedure. Intravenous ondansetron at 100 μg kg^{-1} is generally acceptable.

At the end of surgery, after dressings have been applied, inhalational agents are discontinued and the child ventilated with 100% oxygen. After airway reflexes have returned (child is swallowing, and coughing on the tube), residual neuromuscular blockade is reversed with neostigmine 60–70 μg kg^{-1} and atropine 20 μg kg^{-1}/glycopyrrolate 10 μg kg^{-1}. Supraglottic devices can be removed when the child is breathing regularly with a good tidal volume, and one should ideally not wait for the child to bite on the device. Removal of the endotracheal tube (ETT) requires more skill and accurate timing: extubating the trachea when the child is not fully awake may lead to breath-holding which can proceed to laryngospasm.

Laryngospasm at emergence is a medical emergency. It can range from mild to severe and is classified as partial or complete. Treatment options start from applying continuous positive airway pressure (CPAP) of 10–20 cm H$_2$O with 100% oxygen and airway repositioning, which terminates the condition in nearly 40% of cases. Painful stimuli, like forward mandibular pull or deep pressure on the 'laryngospasm notch' (immediately anterior to the mastoid process), may 'break' the laryngospasm if in early stages; however, nearly 40% proceed to require 10–15 mg suxamethonium or 20–30 mg propofol, and up to 25% may require re-intubation. A useful algorithmic approach has been proposed for managing laryngospasm (Fig. 8.8).

Children should preferably be nursed in the lateral position (Fig. 8.9A), receive oxygen by facemask or 'blow-by' and have their saturation monitored till they are awake, after which they can be returned to their beds. Very small babies can be nursed in their mother's lap with warming devices and monitoring on display (Fig. 8.9B).

It is a good practice to allow breastfed infants to feed as early as possible.

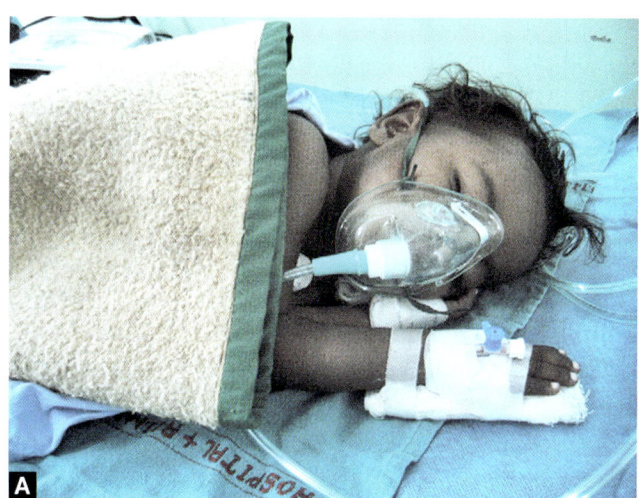

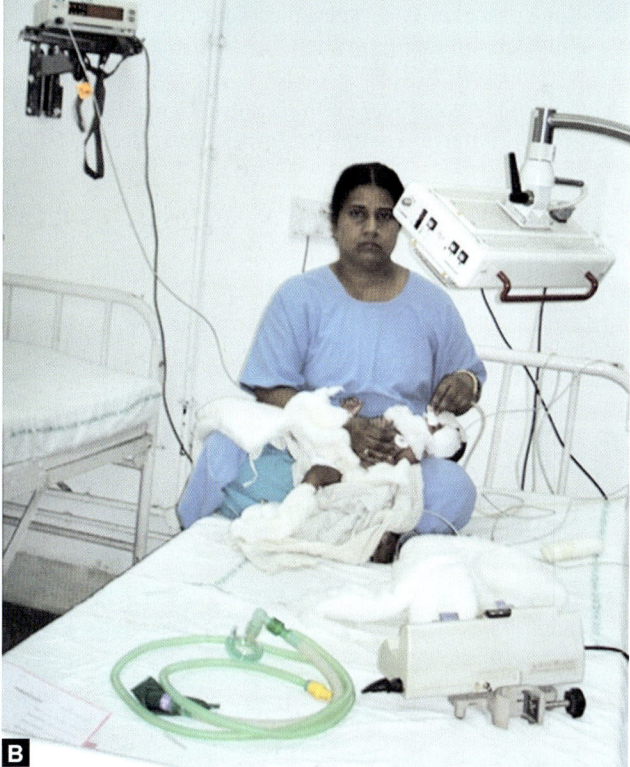

Fig. 8.9A and B. Idial positioning and monitoring for postoperative care

CONCLUSION

General anaesthesia in children is a gratifying exercise for the anaesthesiologist as well as the parent. Careful planning of induction technique keeping the age and mental conditioning of the child is paramount and sets the stage for the rest of the anaesthetics. Inserting IV cannulae in children, especially neonates, is an advanced skill mandatory for the paediatric anaesthesiologist. The airway needs careful assessment and good planning, specially in syndromic children with airway issues. It is important for the paediatric anaesthesiologist to familiarize oneself with as many supraglottic airway devices and video-laryngoscopes because possible as they can be very handy while managing a difficult airway. Extubation of the trachea and provision of good postoperative analgesia are both skills to be acquired by a paediatric anaesthesiologist. Postoperative care should be consummate with the severity of surgery.

REFERENCES

1. Tan L, Meakin GH. Anaesthesia for the uncooperative child. Continuing Education in Anesthesia, Critical Care & Pain J 2010;10(2):48–52.

2. Trapp LD. Techniques for Induction of General Anesthesia in the Pediatric Dental Patient. Anesth Prog 1992;39:138–141.

3. Shawky JEL. A New Friendly Approach to Pediatric Inhaled Induction. Anesth Analg 2005;100(3):901–902.

4. Scully SM. Parental presence during pediatric anesthesia induction. AORNJ 2012;96:26–33.

5. Cook-Sather SD, Schreiner MS. Pediatric anesthetia techniques. In: Katowitz JA (Ed). Pediatric Oculoplastic Surgery. Springer-Verlag: NY 2002;pp 64–69.

6. Hampson-Evans D, Morgan P, Farrar M. Pediatric laryngospasm. Pediatric Anesthesia 2008;18:303–307.

7. Gavel G, Walker RWM. Laryngospasm in anaesthesia. Continuing Education in Anaesthesia, Critical Care & Pain J 2013;7:1–5.

8. Chattopadhyay S, Rudra A, Sengupta S. Laryngospasm in Paediatric Anaesthesia: A Review. International Journal of Anesthesiology Research 2013;1:97–104.

9. Zeilinska M, Holtby H, Wolf A. Pro–con debate: intravenous vs inhalation induction of anesthesia in children. Pediatric Anesthesia 2011;21:159–168.

10. Hemmings JR HC. The pharmacology of intravenous anesthetic agents: a primer. Anesthesiology News 2010;10:9–16.

11. Nieminen K, WestereÁn-Punnonen S, Kokki H, et al. Sevoflurane anaesthesia in children after induction of anaesthesia with midazolam and thiopental does not cause epileptiform EEG. Br J Anaesth 2002;89(6):853–856.

12. Gecaj-Gashi A, Nikolova-Todorova Z, Ismaili-Jaha V, et al. Intravenous lidocaine suppresses fentanyl-induced cough in children. Cough 2013;9:20.

13. Gazal G, Fareed WM, Zafar MS. Effectiveness of gaseous and intravenous inductions on children's anxiety and distress during extraction of teeth under general anesthesia. Saudi J Anesth 2015;9(1):33–36.

14. Steur RJ, Perez RSJM, De Lange JJ. Dosage scheme for propofol in children under 3 years of age. Pediatric Anesthesia 2004;14:462–467.

15. Subhash A. Equipments For Paediatric Anaesthesia. Indian J Anaesth 2004;48(5):365–371.

16. Booker PD. Equipment and monitoring in paediatric anaesthesia. Br J Anaesth 1999;83:78–90.

17. Cote CJ. Pediatric anesthesia. In: Miller RD. Miller Textbook of Anesthesia, 8th edn. Elsevier Saunders: Philadelphia 2015;pp 2757–2598.

18. Holzman RS. Airway management. In: Davis PJ, Cladis FP, Motoyoma EK (Eds): Smith's Anesthesia for Infants and Children, 8th edn. Elsevier Mosby: Philadelphia, 2011; pp 344–364.

19. Polaner DM. Management of general anesthesia. In: Holzman RS, Mancuso TJ, Polaner DM (Eds): A Practical Approach to Pediatric Anesthesia, Lippincott-Williams Wilkins: Philadelphia 2008;pp 100–116.

20. Ferrari LR. General preoperative evaluation and consultative pediatric anesthesia. In: Holzman RS, Mancuso TJ, Polaner DM (Eds): A Practical Approach to Pediatric Anesthesia, Lippincott-Williams Wilkins: Philadelphia 2008;pp 100–116.

21. Ghazal EA, Mason LJ, Cote CJ. Preoperative evaluation, premedication and induction of anesthesia. In: Cote CJ, Lerman J, Anderson BJ(Eds): Cote and Lerman's A Practice of Anesthesia for Infants and Children, 5th edn 2013; pp 31–75.

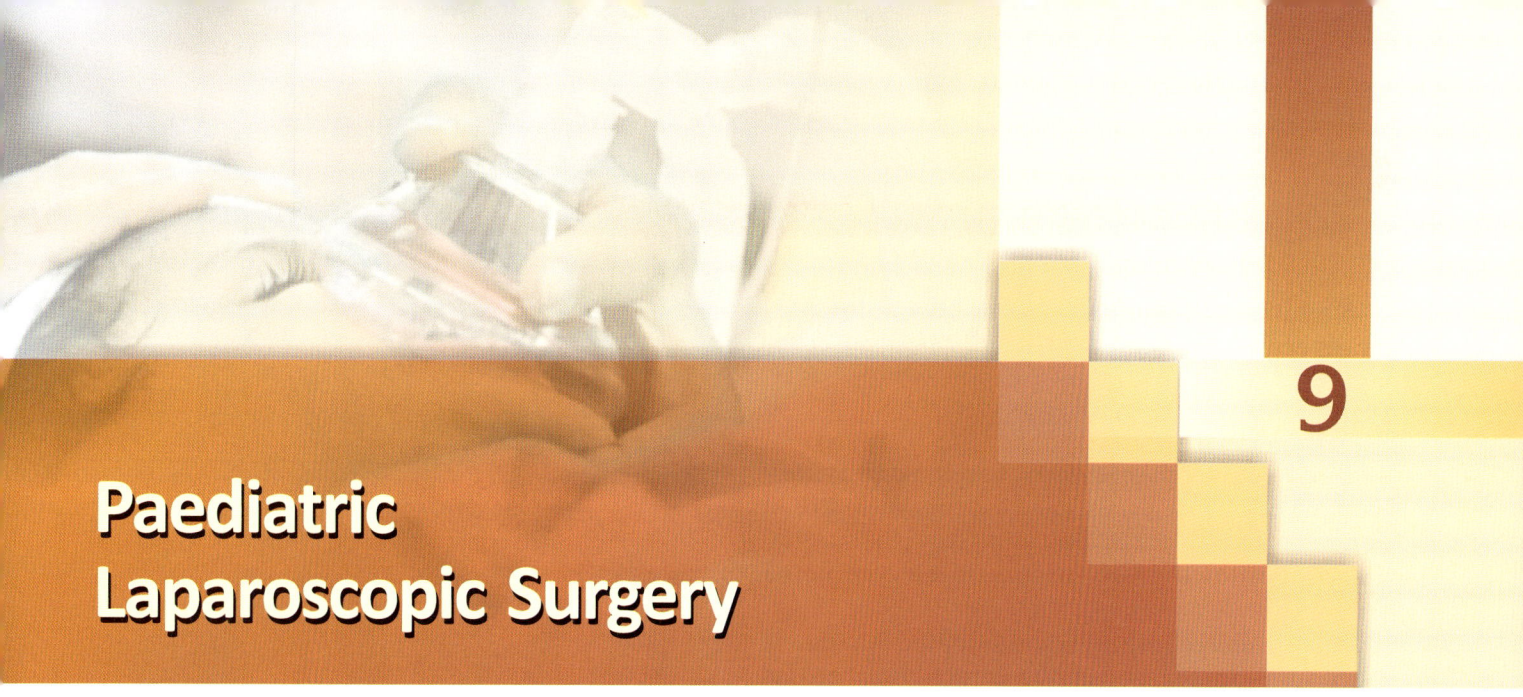

Paediatric Laparoscopic Surgery

Jayashree Sood

- **Patient position**
- **Insufflation of gas**
- **Anaesthetic management**

With the acceptance of minimal access surgery in adults, laparoscopy was initiated in the paediatric population as well. The first case of laparoscopy in paediatric surgery was reported by Stephen Gans in 1971, in his landmark publication "Advances in Endoscopy of Infants and Children,"[1] in which he endoscopically correctly verified a hernia on the contralateral side while the endoscope had been placed in the hernial sac being operated on the opposite side.[2] Simultaneously in 1971, Klimkovich et al. also reported several successful thoracoscopic procedures in children.[3]

There was a learning curve for both surgeons and anaesthesiologists in performing these procedures laparoscopically in the paediatric population. While the surgeon had to learn the laparoscopic skill, the anaesthesiologist had to understand the physiological changes of carboperitoneum and rise in intra-abdominal pressure. As the experience in paediatric laparoscopy increased and its advantages became well recognized, the laparoscopic approach in this patient population became popular and is well established now, so much so that contraindications to this approach are few.[4,5]

As in adults, paediatric laparoscopy was initially performed for simple surgical indications, e.g. diagnostic laparoscopy, appendicectomy and cholecystectomy; but now this approach is routinely used for advanced procedures, like Nissen's fundoplication, splenectomy and nephrectomy.[6]

The laparoscopic approach has become so popular that new techniques, like single incision laparoscopic surgery (SILS) are also now being used in the paediatric population.[7]

With the introduction of 'robot' in the surgical armamentarium, paediatric robot-assisted laparoscopic surgery is also gaining momentum.[8]

"Children are not small adults." This statement is true not only because of anatomical and physiological characteristics, but also because of psychological and emotional differences compared to the adult population.[9]

There are several perioperative concerns in this approach and awareness of complications likely to occur while performing paediatric laparoscopic surgery is mandatory.

Besides specific anatomic and structural changes, the pathophysiological changes associated with laparoscopy in infants and neonates are similar to those observed in the adults. These include:

- Patient position
- Insufflation of gas—CO_2 (carboperitoneum)
- ↑ intra-abdominal pressure (IAP)

In addition to insufflation, physiological disturbances can also be due to access or equipment.[10]

PATIENT POSITION

As in adults, paediatric laparoscopic surgery also necessitates positioning the child appropriately so that abdominal viscera are pushed away from the surgical site, thus allowing the surgery to be completed successfully.

The Trendelenburg position adopted for pelvic procedures increases venous return and cardiac output, while the reverse Trendelenburg position required during fundoplication and cholecystectomy reduces venous return and cardiac output.[11] These changes may be well tolerated in children with normal myocardial function, but can have serious consequences in children with compromised function.[12] This is of great significance in neonates and infants under 3 months of age, since they have a relatively fixed cardiac output due to immature myocardial fibers. They can increase cardiac output only by increasing the heart rate. These babies need extreme caution in positioning, insufflation of gas and resultant increase in intra-abdominal pressure.[11]

INSUFFLATION OF GAS

The ideal gas for insufflation should be non-combustible, inert and soluble. These properties minimize the adverse effects of systemic absorption and accidental entry into a blood vessel (Fig. 9.1).

Carbon dioxide is the insufflating gas of choice because it is inert, soluble and does not support combustion. After carboperitoneum, the systemic effects seen are due to the systemic absorption of CO_2 and the rise in intra-abdominal pressure.

According to Fick's law of diffusion, the diffusion of gas across a membrane is proportional to the area and thickness of the membrane and the difference in partial pressure across the membrane. Thus children absorb a larger volume of insufflating gas since their peritoneum is thinner and surface area larger as compared to body mass.[10]

Low quality of peritoneal fat and small distance between the vessels and the serous surface increases the permeability of the peritoneum to CO_2.[13]

The smaller and younger the baby, more significant are the physiological changes as in addition to

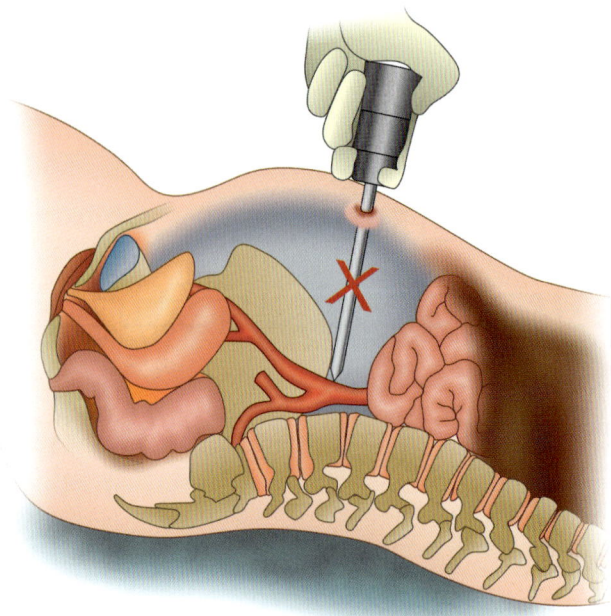

Fig. 9.1. Insertion of trochar

decreased peritoneal thickness there is lesser muscle mass, and reduced organ reserve.[10]

Carboperitoneum and ↑IAP produce several changes in the various systems of the body.

Cardiovascular System

Rise in intra-abdominal pressure compresses the inferior vena cava thus reducing preload. Increase in the systemic vascular resistance increases afterload and the mean arterial pressure, while the cardiac output falls.[14] There is a biphasic response to the rise in intra-abdominal pressure. An IAP <10 mm Hg squeezes blood from the splanchnic vasculature into the circulation thus increasing preload, while an IAP >15 mm Hg impedes venous return thus reducing preload.[6]

Respiratory System

The Trendelenburg position adversely affects the respiratory system, while the reverse Trendelenburg improves respiratory parameters.

Raised intra-abdominal pressure splints diaphragmatic movement and shifts it in a cephalad direction. This reduces lung compliance and functional residual capacity thus predisposing to atelectasis and enhanced ventilation perfusion mismatch.

Insufflation of CO_2 along with Trendelenburg position, reduces lung compliance and increases peak inspiratory pressure (PIP). Increased IAP further aggravates these parameters, however, they return to normal after exsufflation.[15]

Laparoscopy in infants less than 1 year reduces tidal volume, oxygen saturation and lung compliance; and increases the peak inspiratory pressure and $EtCO_2$. The ventilator settings have to be adjusted several times to restore tidal volume and achieve normocarbia.[16]

In neonates too, laparoscopy may reduce oxygen saturation and increase $EtCO_2$, but hyperventilation may not be able to correct the hypercarbia. It has been observed that cessation of insufflation quickly normalizes $EtCO_2$.[17] The $EtCO_2$ correlates with insufflation pressure (IAP) and the duration of insufflation.

Renal System

Pneumoperitoneum and increased IAP reduces renal blood flow and increases urinary excretion of N-acetyl-beta-glucosaminidase which indicates renal injury.[18]

Central Nervous System

Positioning (head low), carboperitoneum and raised IAP increase intracranial pressure and reduce cerebral perfusion pressure.[16]

A special subgroup of concern are the **neonates**. Some of the latest indications in neonates are laparoscopy and thoracoscopy.[13] Distinct physiological and anatomic characteristics in neonates makes them more susceptible to surgical complications.

Newborns have a higher peritoneal and pleural absorption surface per unit of weight.[19] They are very sensitive to insufflation and require meticulous monitoring. Neonates are more sensitive to thoracoscopy than laparoscopy.

Long duration insufflation and high insufflation pressure are risk factors for intraoperative acidosis.[20] Some of the risk factors identified for intraoperative acidosis requiring interruption of insufflation in neonates undergoing either laparoscopy or thoracoscopy are operative time more than 100 minutes, thoracic insufflation under pressure, high variation in $EtCO_2$, low preoperative temperature, high oxygen

requirement and high requirement of vascular expansion at the beginning of insufflation. More than 100 minutes of insufflation requires close follow up because of risk of hypothermia and delayed extubation.[17]

The respiratory consequences of thoracic insufflation in neonates are desaturation and an increase in the $EtCO_2$. These changes are more marked during thoracic insufflation rather than abdominal. All these changes revert to the normal range within 15 minutes of exsufflation. Hypothermia is a significant finding in all neonates undergoing these procedures. Occasionally bradycardia accompanies the hypothermia.

The incidence of surgical complications in paediatric laparoscopy is reported to be around 4–5%. In most cases, the complication can be managed laparoscopically. A conversion rate of 5–10% has been reported as acceptable.[21]

ANAESTHETIC MANAGEMENT

Preanaesthetic Assessment

A thorough preoperative history and examination is essential. Preoperative investigations are done according to the child's status and procedure going to be done.

Premedication may be given according to hospital protocol.

Induction of Anaesthesia

Induction may be done with either inhalational or intravenous route. Intubation with cuffed endotracheal tube and controlled ventilation is recommended. A nasogastric tube is inserted to decompress the stomach while urinary catheterization avoids bladder injury during trocar insertion.[22] Ventilation with ProSeal has also been found to be satisfactory in paediatric laparoscopy surgeries. It is effective in achieving an adequate oropharyngeal seal and pulmonary ventilation (Fig. 9.2).[23]

Atropine may be administered to prevent bradycardia, due to vagal stimulation on peritoneal stretching.[24] Neuromuscular block is achieved with short-acting neuromuscular blockers.

In neonates, an FiO_2 of 1 and lower body temperature at the start of insufflation predicts increased anaesthetic incidents.[25]

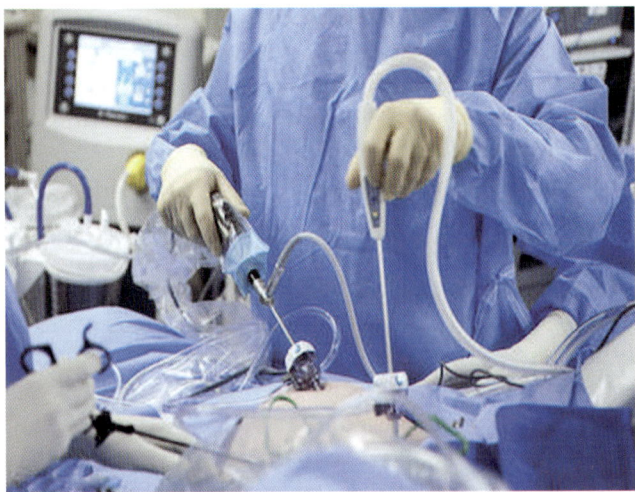

Fig. 9.2. Laparoscopic surgery in progress

Certain physiological changes affect the ventilatory parameters during laparoscopy. Newborns have a higher peritoneal and pleural absorption surface per unit of weight.[26] Small amount of peritoneal fat and small distance between vessels and the serous surface increase the diffusion of CO_2 into the peritoneum.[17]

Therefore, end tidal CO_2 has been found to be 33% higher in neonates and small children as compared to larger children and adults.[17]

Increased IAP along with increased duration of insufflation increases absorption of CO_2 and produces hypercarbia.[17]

To achieve normocarbia, an increase in minute ventilation by 25–30% may be required. PEEP may be required to counteract the effects of increased IAP on the lower lung zones.[11]

Nitrous oxide may be avoided as it has been implicated in postoperative nausea and vomiting, and bowel distension. Nitrous oxide even supports combustion in the presence of methane in the bowel. Complications pertaining to laparoscopy; pneumothorax, subcutaneous emphysema and gas embolism may be encountered in the children as well.

At the end of the procedure, the abdomen should be deflected and CO_2 expelled from the abdomen.

Pain in Paediatric Laparoscopy

Pain after laparoscopic procedures may be as severe as open ones. Meticulous attention should be given for perioperative pain management.

Local anaesthetic infiltration of port sites, regional blocks (caudal) and IV analgesics including paracetamol and NSAIDs are recommended.

CONCLUSION

There is a long learning curve for surgeons and anaesthesiologists dealing with laparoscopic surgery in children, particularly neonates.

Proper understanding of pathophysiology in the paediatric population is essential for successful laparoscopic surgery with minimal postoperative morbidity.

REFERENCES

1. Gans AL. Historical development of Paediatric endoscopic surgery. In: Holcomb, GW (Ed). Pediatric Endoscopic Surgery. East Norwalk, CO: Appleton and Lange 1994; pp. 1–7.
2. Gans SL, Berci G. Advances in endoscopy of infants and children. J Pediatr Surg 1971;6(2):199–233.
3. Klimkovich IG, Geldt VG, Okulov AD, et al. Thoracoscopy in Children. Khirurgiia (Mosk) 1971;47:19–24.
4. Lobe T. Laparoscopic surgery in children. Curr Probl Surg 1998;35:862–948.
5. Rothenberg SS, Chang JHT, Bealer JF. Experience with minimally invasive surgery in infants. Am J Surg 1998; 176:654–658.
6. Tobias JD. Anaesthesia for minimally invasive surgery in children. Best Pract Res Clin Anaesthesiol 2002;16(1):115–130.
7. Mahdi BD, Rahma C, Mohamed J, Riadh M. Single-port laparoscopic surgery in children: A new alternative in developing countries. Afr J Paediatr Surg 2015;12(2): 122–125.
8. Lee RS, Retik AB, Borer JG, Peters CA. Pediatric robot assisted laparoscopic dismembered pyeloplasty: comparison with a cohort of open surgery. J Urol 2006;175(2): 683–687.
9. Rodgers BM, Ryckman FC, Moazam F, Talbert JL. Thoracoscopy for intrathoracic tumors. Ann Thorac Surg 1981;31(5):414–420.
10. Esposito C, Montupet P. Complications of laparoscopic minimally invasive surgery. Pediatr Endosurg Innov Tech 2003;7:13–18.
11. Lasersohn L. Anaesthetic considerations for paediatric laparoscopy. S Afr J Surg 2011;49(1):22–26.
12. Tobias JD, Holcomb GW III. Anesthetic management for laparoscopic cholecystectomy in children with decreased myocardial function: Two case reports. J Pediatr Surg 1997;32:743–746.

13. McHoney M, Corizia L, Eaton S, Kiely EM, Drake DP, Tan HL, Spitz L, Pierro A. Carbon dioxide elimination during laparoscopy in children is age dependent. J Pediatr Surg 2003;38(1):105–110.

14. Kardos A, Vereczkey G, Pirot L, et al. Use of impedance cardiography to monitor haemodynamic changes during laparoscopy in children. Paediatr Anaesth 2001;11: 175–179.

15. Manner T, Aantaa R, Alanen M. Lung compliance during laparoscopic surgery in paediatric patients. Paediatr Anaesth 1998;8(1):25–29.

16. Bannister CF, Brosius KK, Wulkan M. The effect of insufflation pressure on pulmonary mechanics in infants during laparoscopic surgical procedures. Paediatr Anaesth 2003;13(9):785–789.

17. Kalfa N, Allal H, Raux O, et al. Tolerance of laparoscopy and thoracoscopy in neonates. Pediatrics 2005;116; e785–e791.

18. Koivusalo AM, Kellokumpu I, Ristkari S, Lindgren L. Splanchnic and renal deterioration during and after laparascopic cholecystectomy: a comparison of the carbon dioxide penumoperitoneum and the abdominal wall lift method. Anesth Analg 1997;85:886–891.

19. Hazebroek EJ, Haitsma JJ, Lachmann B, Steyerberg EW, de Bruin RW, Bouvy ND, Bonjer HJ. Impact of carbon dioxide and helium insufflation on cardiorespiratory function during prolonged pneumoperitoneum in an experimental rat model. Surg Endosc 2002;16:1073–1078.

20. Sefr R, Puszkailer K, Jagos F. Randomized trial of different intraabdominal pressures and acid-base balance alterations during laparoscopic cholecystectomy. Surg Endosc 2003;17:947–950.

21. Chen MK, Schropp KP, Lobe TE. Complications of minimal-access surgery in children. J Pediatr Surg 1996;31: 1161–1165.

22. Diemunsch PA, Torp KD, Dorsselaer TV, et al. Nitrous oxide fraction in the carbon dioxide pneumoperitoneum during laparoscopy under general inhaled anaesthesia in pigs. Anesth Analg 2000;90:951–953.

23. Sinha A, Sharma B, Sood J. ProSeal as an alternative to endotracheal intubation in pediatric laparoscopy. Paediatr Anaesth 2007;17(4):327–332.

24. Tobias JD. Anaesthesia for minimally invasive surgery in children. Best Pract Res Clin Anaesthesiol 2002;16(1): 115–130.

25. Kalfa N, Allal H, Raux O, Lopez M, Forgues D, Guibal MP, Picaud JC, Galifer RB. Tolerance of laparoscopy and thoracoscopy in neonates. Pediatrics 2005;116(6):e785–791.

26. McHoney M, Corizia L, Eaton S, et al. Carbon dioxide elimination during laparoscopy in children is age dependent. J Pediatr Surg 2003;38:105–110.

10

Regional Anaesthesia in Paediatrics

Mahesh Kumar Arora, Dalim Kumar Baidya

- **Pharmacokinetic and pharmacodynamics of local anaesthetics in children**
- **Central neuraxial blockade**
- **Peripheral nerve blocks**
- **Truncal blocks**
- **Upper extremity blocks**
- **Lower extremity blocks**

Inadequate perioperative pain relief in children may have adverse long-term physiological and psychological consequences, like altered sensory processing and abnormal response to future painful stimuli.[1,2] Moreover, adequate perioperative analgesia has been linked to improved metabolic and endocrine parameters and overall better postoperative outcomes after major surgery.[3] Intravenous opioid analgesia is effective, but there may be increased postoperative systemic complications. Therefore, regional anaesthesia may be used in routine paediatric anaesthesia practice whenever feasible.

The use of ultrasound guidance has facilitated the performance of several regional blocks and enhanced the inherent safety associated with these procedures. Recent evidences suggest that peripheral nerve blockade is assuming greater prominence in paediatric anaesthesia practice, and data from the Paediatric Regional Anaesthesia Network (PRAN) suggests that increased use of ultrasound guidance may be partly driving this trend.[4]

Safe and effective use of regional techniques in children requires thorough understanding of developmental anatomy of the neural structures, muscle and bone of the area to be blocked as well as pharmacology of local anaesthetics.

PHARMACOKINETICS AND PHARMACODYNAMICS OF LOCAL ANAESTHETIC IN CHILDREN

In neonates and small infants, enzymatic activity for metabolism and biotransformation of drugs is limited. Oxidation and reduction of drugs is immature. Conjugation reactions are limited at birth and do not reach adult rates until approximately 3 to 6 months of age.[5,6]

Clearance of drugs is also slower in neonates and small infants. Neonates do not metabolize mepivacaine, with most of it excreted unchanged in the urine.[7]

The nature of the epidural space in infants differs from that in the adult in various aspects. Epidural space in neonates has smaller absorptive surface for local anaesthetics. Therefore, absorption half-time of epidural LA is high in neonates and decreases steadily as the infant grows (for levobupivacaine, this is 0.36 hours at 1 month and 0.14 hours at 6 months of postnatal age). This, combined with reduced clearance, causes increased time to maximum plasma concentration (T_{max}) in neonates (2.2 hours at 1 month and 0.75 hours [80% of the adult value] by 6 months of postnatal age).[8] This implicates requirement of prolonged monitoring for LA systemic toxicity in small infants. Similarly, plasma concentrations at which lidocaine depresses cardiovascular and respiratory systems in neonates are about half of those for adults. Current pharmacokinetic and pharmacodynamic data suggest that increased caution should be exercised when local anaesthetic is used in infants. It is recommended that both the bolus and infusion doses of LA be reduced by approximately 30% for infants younger than 6 months of age (maximum infusion rate of bupivacaine 0.2 to 0.3 mg/kg/hr).[9]

CENTRAL NEURAXIAL BLOCKADE

Anatomic and Physiologic Considerations

Performance of regional anaesthetic techniques in children is affected by several differences in anatomy and physiology to those that exist in adults. The conus medullaris in neonates and infants is located more caudal at L3 vertebral level and reaches the adult level at L1 at approximately 1 year of age due to differential growth of spinal cord and vertebral column. Thus lumbar puncture in infants should be performed at the L4–5 or L5–S1 space to avoid direct needle injury to the spinal cord. Midline approach to subarachnoid blockade is preferable to a paramedian one. This is because: (a) needle is "walked off " the laminae in paramedian approach and vertebral laminae are poorly calcified at infancy, and (b) cephalad direction of needle required in paramedian approach is more likely to cause direct injury to intrathecal neural structures. Cerebrospinal fluid (CSF) volume as percentage of body weight is greater in infants and young children than in adults.[10] This accounts for the comparatively larger doses of spinal local anaesthetics required for surgical anaesthesia in infants and young children. Moreover, CSF turnover rate is also greater in infants and children, accounting for shorter duration of subarachnoid block than adults.

Sacrum is narrower and flatter than in adults. This coupled with low-lying dural sac make dural puncture more likely during an attempted caudal blockade in infants. Therefore, the needle must not be advanced deeply in neonates. Ligamentum flavum is thinner and less dense in infants and children than in adults. Therefore, engagement of the epidural needle is more difficult to detect and unintended dural puncture during epidural catheter placement is more likely in the hands of a novice.

Spinal and epidural blockade in infants and small children is not associated with haemodynamic instability as compared to older children and adults, even when the height of the block reaches upper thoracic dermatomes. Heart rate is preserved but heart rate variability, as determined by spectral analysis, is less as parasympathetic activity modulating heart rate appears to be attenuated in infants who receive spinal anaesthesia.[11] This attenuated vagal tone allows for heart rate compensation to preserve haemodynamic stability during spinal anaesthesia. This is important as other compensatory mechanisms are less developed: venous capacitance in the lower extremities in infants is relatively small and resting sympathetic peripheral vascular tone is relatively lacking.[12] However, very high levels of spinal blockade may cause significant bradycardia.

Epidural Anaesthesia

Epidural anaesthesia can be administered by the caudal, lumbar, or thoracic route used for various thoracic, abdominal or lower limb surgeries (Fig. 10.1A).

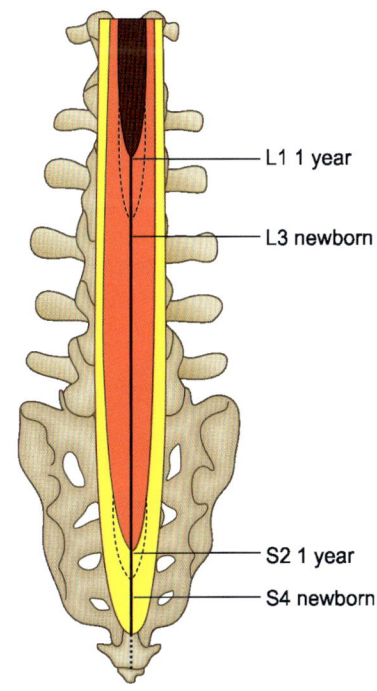

L1 1 year

L3 newborn

S2 1 year

S4 newborn

Fig. 10.1A. Termination of spinal cord at various ages

Caudal Epidural Anaesthesia

Caudal epidural anaesthesia is the most commonly used regional technique in children. First described in 1933,[13] it gained popularity since 1960s.[14] This is commonly used for lower abdominal and lower limb surgeries in children.

Technique: The child is placed in the lateral decubitus position. The cornua of the sacral hiatus are easily palpated as two bony ridges, about 0.5 to 1.0 cm apart. This may be located by first palpating the L4–5 intervertebral space in the midline, and then palpating in a caudal direction until the sacral hiatus is reached. Usually, the sacral hiatus forms an equilateral triangle with both the posterior superior iliac crests. Hiatus is often located just at the beginning of the crease of the buttocks. A 22-gauge short-bevel needle should be used because a long-bevel needle may increase the risk of intravascular injection.[15] A styletted needle may avoid introduction of a dermal plug into the caudal space. Alternately, an intravenous cannula may be used. The needle is initially directed cephalad at a 45° to 75° angle to the skin until the pop through the sacrococcygeal ligament is felt. Once the caudal-epidural space has been entered, the needle should be advanced only a few millimeters. Advancing the needle any further should not be attempted because the dural sac lies relatively caudad in infants (Figs 10.1B and C).[16] To rule out intravascular injection, the needle or the catheter should be simply observed for passive return of blood. Some clinicians aspirate the needle with a syringe; however, most veins collapse when negative pressure is applied, and bone marrow does not come out through such small diameter needles. An effective way to identify an intraosseous placement is that attempts to slide the catheter it

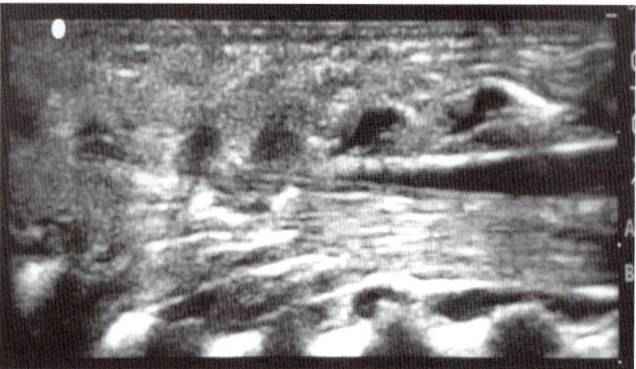

Fig. 10.1C. Caudal block—ultrasound-guided

buckles. On subarachnoid puncture, CSF will passively flow through the needle once the space has been breached. After the caudal epidural location has been confirmed, local anaesthetic should be slowly injected in an incremental fashion. Some clinicians recommend using a test dose of LA while others view the entire volume of LA as simply an aggregate of multiple small (1 to 2 ml) test doses and administer the entire volume in increments while observing the ECG for peaked T waves.

For continuous caudal catheter insertion, first the desired length of catheter to be advanced should be determined by measuring the distance from the sacral hiatus to the desired level. An 18-gauge Tuohy/Crawford needle or an 18 G IV catheter[17] is used to enter the epidural space. Epidural space is confirmed loss of resistance to a small volume of saline. After confirming the absence of blood or CSF, local anaesthetic is administered. Test dose containing 1:200,000 epinephrine may be administered before the entire LA volume is injected.

In infants and small children, the catheter can often be advanced successfully to the desired level. However, the catheter can exit through dural sleeve or get coiled or folded back in older children, particularly when advanced through lumbar route.[18] Epidurograms are performed by injecting 0.5–1 ml of iohexol and imaging by fluoroscopy. A characteristic "bubbly" pattern in the midline is observed. Other localization techniques include: (a) Tsui stimulating catheter, where stimulating electrode at the tip of advancing catheter produces motor twitches in the myotome at the catheter's tip, (b) Ultrasound hydro-dissection technique, where small amount of saline is injected and visualized by ultrasonography.[19] Catheter

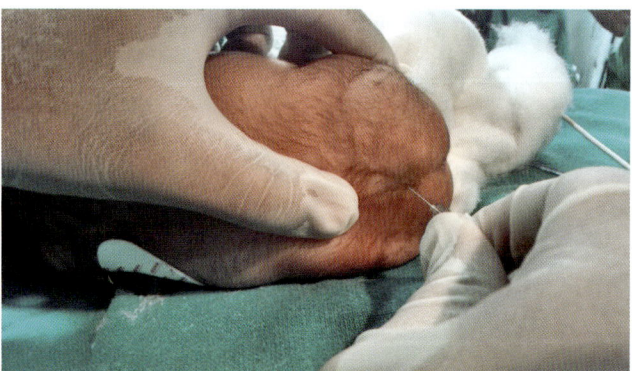

Fig. 10.1B. Caudal block

tip should be placed at a level near the midpoint of the dermatomes for vertical surgical incision and within two segment of a transverse incision. This allows better intraoperative anaesthesia and post-operative analgesia with less volume of LA. Although the routine use of an epidurogram is not standard practice, some method of localization technique should be used when a catheter is threaded cephalad for more than several centimetres. However, a catheter should never be forced or advanced against resistance. Since caudal catheters are at increased risk of faecal contamination, proper dressing should be done and adhesive clear dressing like Tegaderm (3M, St Paul, Minn.) will allow regular inspection as well.

Lumbar and Thoracic Epidural Anaesthesia

In thoracic or upper abdominal surgeries, it may be preferable to place epidural catheters at a lumbar or thoracic interspace (Fig. 10.2). Incision congruent placement allows enhanced analgesia using smaller volume of drug and avoids contamination by stool and urine. However, direct lumbar and thoracic epidural catheters should be placed in anaesthetized infants and children only by experienced anaesthesiologists.[20]

Technique: The technique for both lumbar and thoracic epidural catheters placement is similar to that in adults with few exceptions and the midline approach is preferred. The ligamenta flava are thinner and less dense in infants, thereby requiring extra care to avoid subarachnoid puncture. The LOR technique should be used with saline, as there are several reports of venous air embolism in infants and children when air was used to test for LOR.[21] A short length (5 cm) 18-gauge Tuohy needle and a 20- or 21-gauge catheter should be used. Thinner 23- and 24-gauge catheters

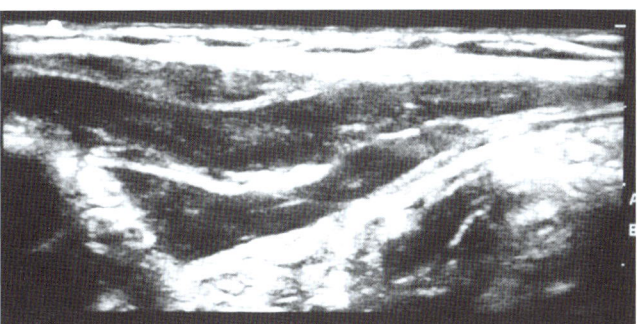

Fig. 10.2. Ultrasound image of epidural space

are more prone to kinking and offer higher resistance to flow giving rise to repeated occlusion alarms during continuous infusions.

Selection of drug: Bupivacaine, ropivacaine or levo-bupivacaine is usually used. For volume determination, simple method is to administer 1 ml/kg (up to 20 ml) of local anaesthetic (usually 0.125 to 0.2% bupivacaine with or without 1:200,000 epinephrine). This generally provides a sensory block with minimal motor block up to the T6 level. However, if repeated doses are anticipated, or in infants less than 6 months of age, concentration or volume should be reduced to avoid the risk of accumulation. Another simple regimen for a caudal block is Armitage Formula: 0.5 ml/kg for lumbosacral, 1 ml/kg thoracolumbar, and 1.25 ml/kg mid-thoracic.[22] If the total volume exceeds 20 ml, then reduce concentration of bupivacaine below 0.2%. Since the level of the block depends on the volume administered, the concentration of the LA should be changed depending on desired density of the block and on the risk of toxicity.

Continuous Epidural Infusions

Continuous epidural infusions of LA maintain a constant level of analgesia, leads to better pain score, overall less consumption of drugs and theoretically may reduce the risk of infection by fewer entries into the epidural catheter and risk of accidental administration of the wrong drug. However, strict adherence to dose is important to reduce toxicity. Maximum dose of bupivacaine is 0.4 mg/kg/hr, which should be reduced by approximately 30% for infants younger than 6 months of age.[9] Ropivacaine and levobupivacaine carry reduced risks of toxicity, thus may be preferred.

Adjunctive Drugs

Epidural opioids can be safely used to augment intraoperative anaesthesia or to provide postoperative analgesia. Intermittent epidural morphine 50 μg/kg Q8–12 hour with or without LA may be used. Otherwise, fentanyl at concentration of 1–3 μg/ml in epidural LA solution can be used as continuous infusion. However, the child should be observed for opioid-related side effects. Epidural administration of clonidine 2 μg/kg has found to cause significant prolongation of analgesia in several studies, including a meta-analysis. In neonates, however, neuraxial clonidine has been associated with apnoea. Sedation and bradycardia are other adverse effects reported with epidural clonidine.[23]

Complications

Several evidences have supported overall safety of epidural anaesthesia in children. The PRAN database reported from their first prospective cohort of 9087 epidural and caudal blocks (6210 single injection [mostly caudal] and 2946 continuous caudal or epidural anaesthesia) no complications of any kind lasting more than 3 months.[4] Commonest complication was catheter displacement or malfunction in the postoperative period in continuous blocks. The French-Language Society of Paediatric Anaesthesiologists (ADARPEF) published a prospective study on regional anaesthetics in children in which they reported on 10,098 epidural blocks.[24] There were no permanent sequelae seen in any child.

Intravascular or intraosseous injection into the marrow cavity may result in a rapid increase in the blood level of LA leading to cardiac toxicity and cardiac arrest. Epidural needle may pass through the sacrum and perforate bowel or the pelvic organs, particularly in infants in whom ossification of the sacrum is incomplete.

Infection (meningitis, epidural abscess) is an uncommon but grave complication. It rarely occurs, particularly in children with immunodeficiency syndromes and cancer who are receiving long-term infusions.[25] Epidural abscess, however, is a surgical emergency and failure to treat can lead to a permanent neurologic injury. *Staphylococcus aureus* is most common causative pathogen and mostly occurs when catheters are left in place more than 48 hours. If there is any question that the site is infected, the catheter should be removed. Although systemic infection is rare, catheter colonization is common (up to 35%) and rate of colonization is similar with both caudal and lumbar epidural approaches.[26] Fluid leak from the insertion site in caudal epidural catheters is common especially in the presence of presacral oedema. If a child develops fever of unknown origin with an indwelling caudal epidural catheter in place, then the catheter should be removed.

Epidural haematoma is also a rare complication. The presence of clinical coagulopathy or thrombocytopenia is an unacceptable risk and is a contraindication to central neuraxial blockade. One should follow ASRA guidelines for central neuraxial blockade in anticoagulated patients.[27] Optimal outcome depends on rapid diagnosis and prompt treatment and decompression.

Postoperative urinary retention may be associated with central neuraxial opioids in the blocks. Regional anaesthesia with LA does not cause urinary retention, and data shows the contrary.[28] Epidural morphine 50 µg/kg was associated with an 11% incidence of urinary retention with increased doses showing higher incidences.[29]

Long-term neurologic sequelae of central neuraxial blockade are rare in children. In a prospective study of more than 2,500 infants and children, no evidence of neurologic complications were found[30] although the first ADARPEF data revealed that 1 in 5000 infants younger than 3 months of age had MRI evidence of spinal cord ischaemia.[31]

Spinal Anaesthesia

Spinal anaesthesia has been successfully performed in children for more than one hundred years now.[32] Role of spinal anaesthesia in infants has been highlighted as an alternative to general anaesthesia to reduce the incidence of perioperative apnoea in preterm and ex-preterm neonates and infants (post-conceptional age less than 60 weeks). The finding has consistently been observed in both retrospective and prospective studies.[33,34] Concerns of adverse neurodevelopmental sequelae following general anaesthetics in infants have recently led to increased interest in spinal anaesthesia even in term infants.

Managing an awake infant under spinal anaesthesia may seem to be difficult (Fig. 10.3). However, when a successful block is achieved, majority of neonates fall asleep. This is due to diminished sensory input to the reticular activating system from the periphery leading to decreased consciousness (deafferentation). Significant decrease in sedation levels have been observed using bispectral index and spectral edge frequency analysis in infants undergoing spinal anaesthesia without the use of adjunctive agents.[35]

Technique

After routine monitors are attached, the child is placed in a sitting or lateral decubitus position. Excessive flexion of the neck should be avoided to prevent any

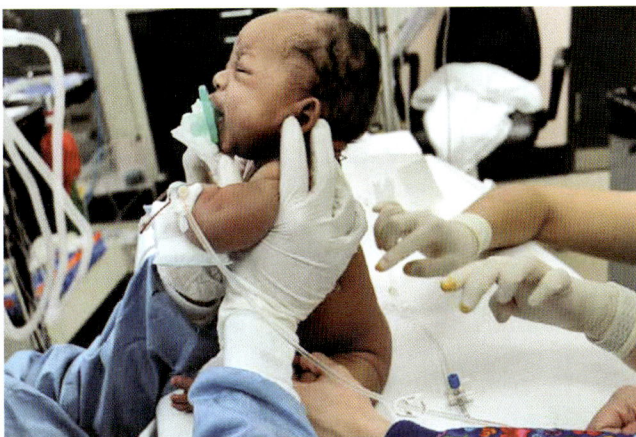

Fig. 10.3. Spinal anaesthesia in an infant

obstruction of the airway.[36] The sitting position may be beneficial as increased CSF hydrostatic pressure may lead to better flow of CSF through the spinal needle. The skin is infiltrated with a small amount of 1% lidocaine (with an insulin syringe), or EMLA cream applied to the infant's lumbar area at least 1 hour before spinal placement. The lumbar puncture is performed at the L4–5 or L5–S1 interspace using a midline approach with a 22-gauge or smaller, 1.5 inch styletted spinal needle. The depth of subarachnoid space in infants less than 60 weeks of post-conceptional age is approximately 1.5 cm from the skin.

Selection of Drug

Drug requirement per kilogram body weight is 5- to 10-fold greater in neonates as compared to adults, to reach a similar dermatomal distribution. However, the duration is only about one-third to one-half as long as in the adult. This appears to be due in part to the greater volume of CSF per kg and to more rapid turnover of CSF in this age group. Approximate dose requirement for 0.5% hyperbaric bupivacaine are:[37]

- Neonates and infants less than 5 kg: 0.5–1.0 mg/kg
- Infants and children 5–15 kg: 0.4 mg/kg
- Children more than 15 kg: 0.3 mg/kg

Complications

Complications after spinal anaesthesia include post-dural puncture headache, backache, neurologic sequelae, total spinal anaesthesia, and the risk of lumbar epidermoid tumours, if non-styletted needles are used for subarachnoid puncture.[38,39]

Total spinal anaesthesia has been reported in neonates. It is most commonly manifested by apnoea with no change in systemic blood pressure or heart rate. Post-dural puncture headache appears to be less frequent in infants and children, although the incidence in preverbal children is not known. Possible reasons may include increased rate of CSF production and reduced CSF pressure.[40]

PERIPHERAL NERVE BLOCKS

Peripheral nerve blocks (PNB) may be useful as adjuvants to general anaesthesia or as a sole anaesthestic for intraoperative and postoperative analgesia. In PNB, a target area is anaesthetized and therefore, side effects of central neuraxial blockade are avoided. Various PNBs, which are more frequently used in clinical practice of paediatric anaesthesia, are described here.

Selection of a Local Anaesthetic

Local anaesthetics commonly used are lidocaine, bupivacaine, levobupivacaine and ropivacaine. Longer-acting agents increase the duration of post-operative analgesia. Lidocaine can be combined with bupivacaine to have a rapid onset as well as long duration blockade. However, one must calculate the doses of the two drugs properly to avoid toxicity. Sodium bicarbonate (1 mEq of bicarbonate/10 ml of local anaesthetic) can be added to hasten the onset of action.[41] This alters the pKa of the solution and increases the active cationic form of the local anaesthetic in the solution.[42] The addition of epinephrine (1:200,000) may decrease vascular absorption and extend the duration of the block. Volume and concentration of local anaesthetic required for various blocks has not been adequately studied in children.

Infraorbital Nerve Block

Anatomy

The infraorbital nerve is the termination of the second division of the trigeminal nerve, the maxillary nerve. From pterygopalatine fossa, it enters the infraorbital groove and passes through the infraorbital canal and then emerges through the infraorbital foramen. The branches of the infraorbital nerve innervate the lower eyelid, the lateral inferior portion of the nose and its vestibule, the upper lip, the mucosa along the upper lip, and the vermilion. This block can be used for cleft lip repair,[43] reconstructive procedures on the nose (including septal reconstruction and rhinoplasty), and endoscopic sinus surgery.[44] There are two approaches to the infraorbital nerve block: intraoral and extraoral.

Technique

The infraorbital foramen is located by palpation of the infraorbital notch. After folding back the upper lip, a 27-gauge needle is inserted through the buccal mucosa parallel to the maxillary second molar and passed subcutaneously with the tip of the needle directed toward the infraorbital foramen. One finger is placed over the infraorbital foramen, which palpates the advancing needle beneath the skin and prevents passage of the needle into the orbit. When the needle tip reaches infraorbital foramen, 0.5 to 1.0 ml of local anaesthetic (bupivacaine 0.25%) is injected after careful aspiration.

In extraoral approach, the infraorbital ridge of the maxillary bone is palpated and the infraorbital foramen is identified. A 27-gauge needle is advanced toward the foramen at a 45-degree angle to the maxilla. After careful aspiration, 0.5 to 1.0 ml of bupivacaine 0.25% is injected.

Complications

Haematoma or ecchymosis can develop because of the loose adventitious tissue. Therefore, after injection, pressure should be applied to the infraorbital area to prevent spread of local anaesthetic into the periorbital area. Direct injection of LA into the orbit or eye and intravascular injection should be avoided. This block can be achieved with low volumes in infants and toddlers and hence only small volume of LA should be used.

TRUNCAL BLOCKS

Common truncal blocks include intercostal blocks, ilioinguinal block, penile block, rectus sheath block, and paravertebral block.

Intercostal Nerve Block

Although continuous epidural analgesia is considered gold standard for thoracotomy to reduce opioid requirements, optimize respiratory mechanics and encourage early ambulation, intercostal blocks may be useful as well.[45] The major disadvantage is the limited duration of analgesia. However, with the development of degradable bupivacaine microspheres and liposomal encapsulated bupivacaine, which significantly prolong analgesia, practice may change in the future.[46]

The uptake of LA after intercostal blocks is more rapid than following any other regional block. Moreover, plasma concentrations in children may increase more rapidly than in adults after identical blocks. Epinephrine (1:200,000) should, therefore, be added to 0.25% bupivacaine to reduce the absorption of local anaesthetic (total volume 1 to 5 ml for each nerve).

Anatomy

The intercostal nerves are derived from the ventral rami of the first through twelfth thoracic nerves. There are four branches—the first is the gray rami communicans to sympathetic ganglia; the second is the posterior cutaneous branch, which supplies the skin in the paravertebral area; the third, lateral cutaneous branch, arises anterior to the midaxillary line and sends subcutaneous branches both anteriorly and posteriorly; and the final branch provides cutaneous innervation to the midline of the chest and abdomen.

Technique

The site of injection may be either paravertebral or in the midaxillary line. The lower rib margin is located; the needle is inserted perpendicular to the skin over the rib and advanced until the rib is encountered. The needle is then walked off the lower edge of the rib for further 2–3 mm. A pop may be felt as the needle enters the neurovascular sheath. After negative aspiration for blood, LA is injected.

Complications

Pneumothorax has been reported after intercostal blockade, with an incidence of approximately 0.07% in adults.[47] Recently, with the use of ultrasound guidance, pleura can be visualized and puncturing the pleura can be avoided. Using smaller volumes of more dilute local anaesthetic may reduce the risk of systemic toxicity. The risk of intravascular injection may be reduced with incremental injection and frequent aspiration. High subarachnoid block may be another complication, usually associated with the posterior paravertebral approach.

Inguinal Block (Ilioinguinal and Iliohypogastric Nerves)

This block is used as an adjunct to general anaesthesia and for postoperative pain management for inguinal hernia repairs and is considered as effective as caudal anaesthesia[48] (Figs 10.4 and 10.5).

Anatomy

The inguinal area is innervated by the subcostal nerve (T12), iliohypogastric and ilioinguinal nerve (derived from L1). These nerves lie in close proximity to each

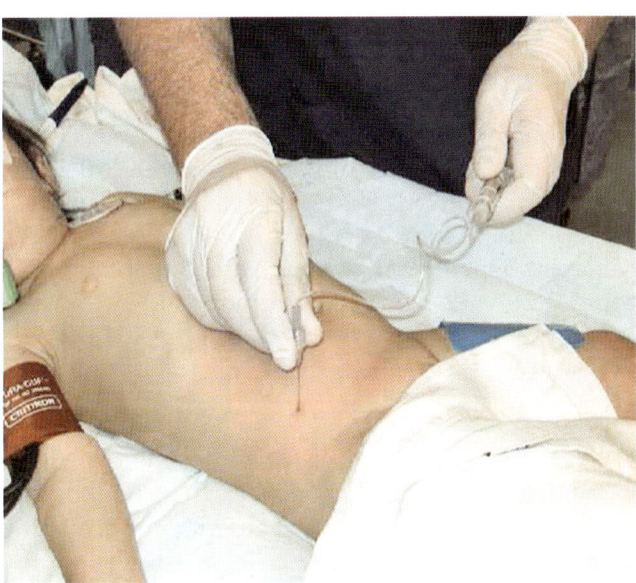

Fig. 10.4. Ilioinguinal nerve block

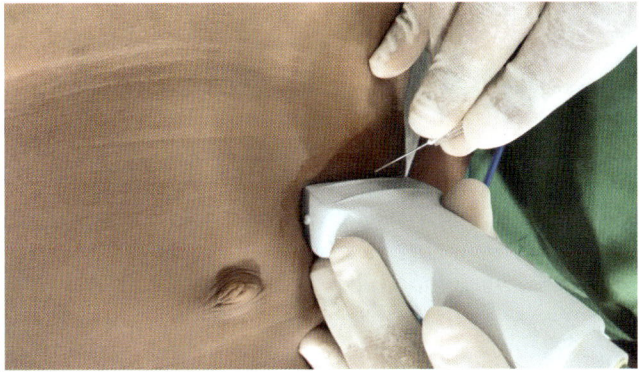

Fig. 10.5. Probe placement for ultrasound-guided ilioinguinal nerve block

other medial and superior to the anterior superior iliac spine. After piercing the internal oblique 2 to 3 cm medial to the anterior superior iliac spine, the nerve lies between the internal oblique and the external oblique aponeurosis.

Technique

A short-bevel 27-gauge needle is inserted at a 45° angle at a point one-fourth of the way toward the midline along a line drawn from the anterior superior iliac spine to the umbilicus. As the needle is advanced through the external and internal oblique muscles, two pops are elicited. After the second pop, a volume of 0.3 ml/kg of LA solution is injected in a fan-like fashion, cephalad toward the umbilicus, caudad toward the groin, and medially. While removing the needle, an additional 0.5 to 1.0 ml of local anaesthetic is injected to block the iliohypogastric nerve. Following orchidopexy or any other scrotal procedures, scrotal wound need to be separately infiltrated because this area is supplied by the genitofemoral nerve.

Complications

Complications are less common. Injection into the femoral vessels and potential femoral nerve block is a possibility. Care should be taken not to enter the peritoneal cavity. The use of ultrasound may also avoid the risk of bowel perforation.[49] Intravascular injection may be avoided by incremental injection with frequent aspiration.

Penile Block

A penile block (Fig. 10.6) is used for anaesthesia and postoperative analgesia for circumcision, urethral dilatation, and hypospadias repair. Caudal anaesthesia should be used for proximal shaft or penoscrotal hypospadias repair because penile block provides analgesia only for the distal two-thirds of the penis.[50] The block is easy to perform and has a high success rate. Epinephrine must never be used for this block because the dorsal artery of the penis is an end artery and vasospasm caused by epinephrine may cause necrosis.

Anatomy

The nerve supply of the penis is from the pudendal nerve and the pelvic plexus. Along the dorsal artery

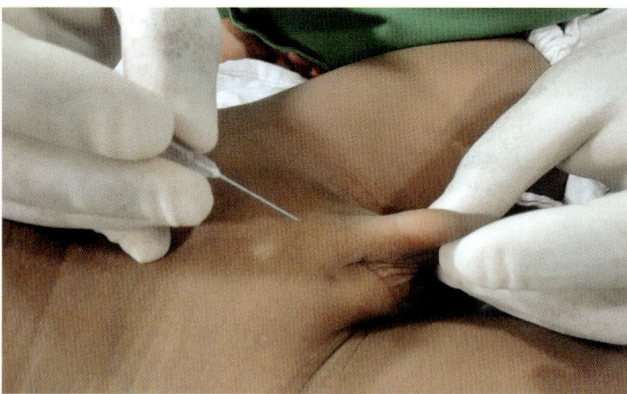

Fig. 10.6. Penile block

to the penis are two dorsal nerves of penis supplying the sensory innervation to the penis.

Technique

Penile block can be performed either as: (a) ring block or (b) blockade of the dorsal nerve. It has been found that the ring block provided analgesia of prolonged duration, although both techniques provided analgesia superior to EMLA cream.[51] The ring block is performed, by inserting a 27-gauge needle at the base of the penis, and injecting the local anaesthetic in a ring-shaped pattern around the base of the penile shaft. The needle may be inserted once in the midline and then redirected to each side. The alternate dorsal nerve block is performed, by inserting a 27-gauge needle 1 cm above the symphysis pubis in the midline, and directing it caudally at 30° angle. The needle is advanced 1 cm after it pierces the penile fascia and 1 to 4 ml of local anaesthetic is injected.

Complications

The major complication is compromise of organ blood flow and vasoconstrictors, such as epinephrine, must never be used for this block. There is a small risk of injury to the adjacent neurovascular structures. Applying pressure after the injection may minimize haematoma formation.

Rectus Sheath Block

This block has recently become popular for children undergoing umbilical hernia repair.[52] This provides excellent analgesia for most umbilical area surgery, including laparoscopic surgery.

Anatomy

The rectus sheath contains the thoracic intercostal nerves that can be blocked at the paraumbilical area (T10) using a small volume of local anaesthetic solution.

Technique

On either side of the umbilicus, about 1 cm from midline, a needle is inserted into the rectus sheath. A pop can be felt as the needle advances beyond the anterior rectus sheath, through the rectus abdominis muscle and then just anterior to the posterior rectus sheath. After negative aspiration, a volume of 0.1 ml/kg of local anaesthetic solution is injected. Use of ultrasound may facilitate performing this block.[53]

Paravertebral Block

Main advantage of paravertebral block is strict unilateral anaesthesia of one or more adjacent dermatomes. So, this is used for unilateral thoracic or abdominal surgical procedures. The level of the puncture depends on the surgical intervention; for a thoracotomy the block is performed at T5–6, for renal surgery at T9–10, for ureteric surgery at T11–12.

Anatomy

The paravertebral space is a triangular wedge-shaped area situated in the angle between the lateral border of the vertebral body and the anterior surface of the transverse process. The medial boundary of the paravertebral space is the lateral part of the vertebral body and disc, the dorsal limitation is the transverse process and costotransverse ligament, and the antero-lateral boundary is the parietal pleura. Structures that pass through the paravertebral space include the spinal nerve roots, intercostal nerve, the sympathetic chain, and the intercostal vessels. The paravertebral space should be considered as a "potential space" only because the pleura are very adhesive to the other structures. However, communication exists between different thoracic levels of the paravertebral space that allows spread of LA to multiple segments. In the lumbar region, each individual paravertebral space must be blocked separately because there are no communications between adjacent lumbar levels.[54]

Technique

Block can be performed either blindly by loss of resistance (LOR) technique or with the help of nerve stimulator or ultrasound guidance.

Loss-of-resistance technique: The skin is punctured lateral to the spinous process and the needle is advanced perpendicularly until transverse process is contacted. A Tuohy needle (19 to 20 gauge in infants and 18 gauge in older) is then "walked" below (underneath) the transverse process and with LOR technique the costotransverse ligament is pierced and the paravertebral space located.

Approximately, skin to paravertebral space distance[55] (mm)ranges from ??0.53 ??kg to ??21.2.

Once in the paravertebral space, the bolus dose of LA is injected after careful aspiration to exclude any blood or air. If a continuous technique is planned, a catheter can be introduced 1 to 2 cm into the paravertebral space through the Tuohy needle. The insertion of the catheter frequently needs manipulation of the Tuohy needle or injection of the bolus dose to "open up" the space. However, catheter should not be inserted more than 1 to 2 cm into the paravertebral space to avoid migration of catheter into the spinal canal through the intervertebral foramen (causing an epidural distribution of the block) or laterally, following the path of the intercostal nerve (giving a dense block of only one dermatome).

Nerve-stimulator-guided technique: A 21-gauge insulated needle of appropriate length, attached to a nerve stimulator (initial stimulating current: 2.5 to 5 mA, 1 Hz), is introduced perpendicular to the skin at 1–2 cm from the midline in the intervertebral space. Contractions of the paraspinal muscles are initially observed, and as the costotransverse ligament is reached, contraction of the paraspinal muscles disappear. After piercing the costotransverse ligament, muscle contractions of the corresponding level are sought and the needle tip is manipulated to achieve continued muscular contractions at 0.5 mA and LA is injected.[56]

Ultrasound-aided approach: With ultrasound guidance, the position of the transverse processes and the depth to the paravertebral space can be determined and pleural movement can be visualized in real time. With deposition of LA, downward (away) movement of pleura confirms proper placement of drug.

After a negative aspiration, 0.5 ml/kg of the local anaesthetic (levobupivacaine 0.25% or bupivacaine 0.25% or lidocaine 1%) with epinephrine 1:200,000 is injected in toddlers and older children. This dose usually covers five dermatomes. In neonates and infants, slightly modified dosage regimens are recommended.[57]

Complications

With LOR technique, overall failure rate is approximately 10% and the complications can be vascular puncture (4%), pleural puncture (1%), and pneumothorax (0.5%).[58] The risk for block failure is reduced to less than 5% and reduced risk for complications are observed when a nerve-stimulator–guided technique is used.[59] Use of ultrasound may further improve success while reducing complications.

UPPER EXTREMITY BLOCKS

Brachial Plexus Block

There can be four approaches to brachial plexus block (axillary, infraclavicular, supraclavicular, and interscalene). Among them, axillary approach is commonly used in children because it is easy to perform, has higher success rate and less chance of complications.[60] The infraclavicular block is preferred when a continuous catheter technique is planned for postoperative period.

Selection of drugs: Since larger volume of local anaesthetic is required, levobupivacaine or ropivacaine may be chosen to reduce the risk of toxicity. Longer-acting agents are usually preferred over lidocaine to prolong the duration of postoperative analgesia. Large volumes (up to 0.5 ml/kg) may be required particularly to ensure block of the musculocutaneous nerve, therefore, dose calculation must be done carefully not to exceed the maximal allowable doses. Adding epinephrine (1:200,000) may decrease vascular absorption and the potential for toxicity. Sodium bicarbonate (1 mEq/10 ml of local anaesthetic) added to the LA hastens the onset of blockade by increasing the pH of the solution; this is particularly the case with the premixed anaesthetic-epinephrine formulations that have a reduced pH.

Axillary Block (Fig. 10.7)

Anatomy: The brachial plexus arises in the neck from spinal nerves C5–C8, and T1, passes between the clavicle and first rib, and then goes into the axilla. The axillary artery is surrounded by a fascial sheath, containing median nerve anteriorly, ulnar nerve posteriorly, and the radial nerve on the posterolateral aspect.

Technique: Three different techniques are possible: paraesthesia technique, nerve stimulator guidance and ultrasound guidance. However, nerve stimulator and US guidance can be combined to increase precision. Eliciting sensory paraesthesia has little application in paediatric practice. With any of the techniques, a short of extension tubing attached between the needle and syringe facilitates precise handling of the equipment during procedure.

Arm should be abducted to 90 degrees. However, hyperabduction to be avoided as it may obscure the axillary pulse. The artery is palpated in the axilla, and a short-beveled needle is advanced. With a nerve stimulator, a distal motor response is elicited in each nerve distribution at 0.2–0.3 mA. Although divided doses of LA may be administered to each nerve locations by eliciting distinct motor response,

practically it is difficult to find subsequent response once some LA is injected for the first nerve. If nerve stimulator is not used, the needle is advanced until a distinct pop is felt as the needle pierces the axillary sheath and the drug is deposited. However, axillary sheath may be divided into separate fascial compartments for each nerve, and these may limit the spread of LA with single injection within the axillary sheath. Alternatively, the transarterial technique may be used. In this technique, the needle is aimed directly toward the axillary pulse. After blood is aspirated, the needle is advanced through the posterior wall of the artery. When blood can no longer be aspirated, half of the LA is deposited posterior to the artery. Then, the needle is withdrawn through the anterior wall of the artery, and the remainder of the dose is deposited anterior to the artery after reconfirming a negative aspiration for blood. Regardless of the technique, LA should always be administered in incremental quantities with repeated aspiration before each injection.

A tourniquet may be applied distally to promote proximal spread of LA and enhance the chances of a successful block of musculocutaneous nerve, which exits the brachial plexus proximal in the axillary fossa. Otherwise, musculocutaneous nerve may be blocked by infiltrating 1 to 3 ml of LA into coraco-brachialis muscle. An additional 1 to 3 ml of LA is injected subcutaneously in the medial aspect of upper arm to block the intercostobrachial nerve and its communications with the musculocutaneous nerve. These additional quantities of LA must be taken into account when calculating the total dose.

Complications: intravascular injection may occur. Intravascular injection may be avoided with incremental injection and frequent aspiration before each injection. A haematoma may form and compress the neurovascular bundle, causing limb ischaemia. Intraneural injection may be minimized by use of a nerve stimulator. When it is necessary to check the viability of the nerves at the end of surgery, block may be performed in the recovery room after surgery. All the three nerve functions can be checked by simple finger examination: the radial nerve (extension of the thumb), median nerve (flexion of the proximal interphalangeal joint of thumb), and ulnar nerve (scissoring of the fingers).[61]

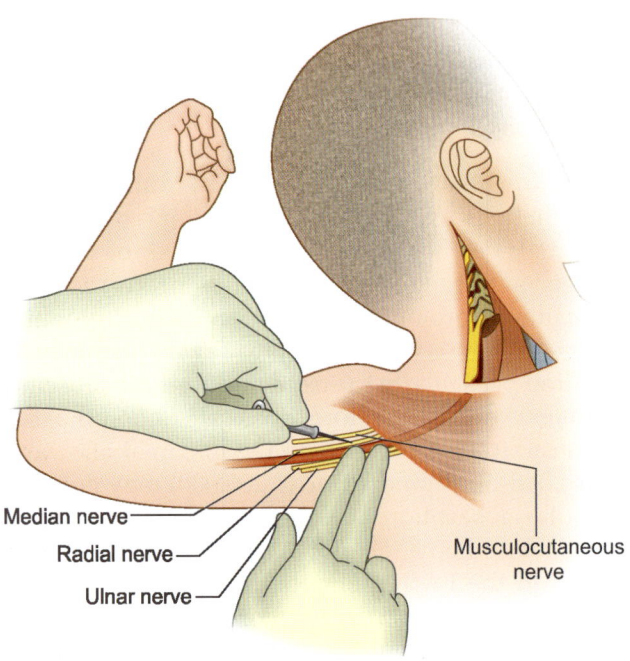

Median nerve

Radial nerve

Ulnar nerve

Musculocutaneous nerve

Fig. 10.7. Axillary approach to brachial plexus block

Infraclavicular Block

This approach is helpful when abduction of arm is painful or when continuous catheter technique is planned.[62]

Technique: With the arm in abduction or adduction, needle is introduced 2 cm below and medial to the coracoid process. Forearm flexion denotes stimulation of the musculocutaneous nerve and the needle is then re-directed to elicit stimulation of the brachial plexus. Any stimulation other than forearm flexion denotes brachial plexus response. An ultrasound-guided technique may also be used. Individual cords are usually visualized around the axillary artery.

Complications: There is the potential for intrapleural injection and pneumothorax, especially if the needle is directed medially. Because of the proximity of the plexus to the subclavian vessels, the procedure should not be attempted in children with coagulation abnormalities.

Supraclavicular Block (Fig. 10.8)

This block is performed for upper arm surgery as a single injection or catheter technique. This is an easy approach and can be readily performed. The entire brachial plexus, including the musculocutaneous and the axillary nerves, is located lateral to the artery.

Technique: A stimulating needle (1 mA) is passed above the clavicle lateral to the arterial pulsation and close to the inferior margin of the anterior scalene. The plexus is located superficially and if continued response to the stimulation is observed at 0.4 mA, 0.15 to 0.2 ml/kg of local anaesthetic solution is injected.

Ultrasound guidance is preferably used nowadays and needle introduced using the in-plane technique. US guidance has reduced the volume of LA required and can avoid accidental injection into vertebral artery.

Complications: Pleural puncture and intravascular injection can occur from misplacement of the needle. Cervical pleura is located close to the supraclavicular plexus; thus caution should be exercised while performing this block.

Interscalene Block

This technique is usually performed in older children undergoing shoulder surgery.

Anatomy: The interscalene groove is formed by the anterior and middle scalene muscles, lateral to the sternocleidomastoid muscle. In children, the lower nerve roots (C6 and C7) are close to the pleura, which may increase the potential for a pneumothorax. The vertebral artery is located in close proximity to the lower nerve roots (C7) and hence it is important to avoid intravascular injection. The phrenic nerve is also close to the nerve roots and may be unintentionally blocked.

Techniques: Dalens and associates reported parascalene technique of brachial plexus blockade for paediatric shoulder surgery. They used an extended head position and placed the puncture between the lower and middle thirds of a line, joining centre of the clavicle and the C6 transverse process.[63] This technique may avoid encountering the vertebral artery and pleura. With perpendicular needle direction, the lower roots (C8 and T1) are not blocked or require very large amounts of LA to be blocked. Ultrasound guidance helps in safe blockade of both these roots. With the use of a nerve stimulator, diaphragmatic stimulation may be observed when phrenic nerve is stimulated as a result of ventromedial needle position. In US-guided approach, the probe is initially placed

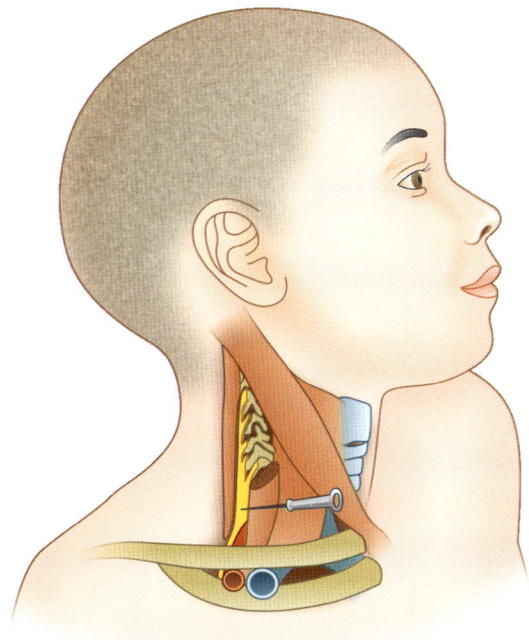

Fig. 10.8. Interscalene approach to brachial plexus block

medially to identify thyroid gland and the major vessels in the neck. Then the probe is moved along the lateral border of sternocleidomastoid muscle and moved in a caudal direction to visualize C5–C7 roots of the brachial plexus between the anterior and medial scalene muscles. In very small children, all C5–T1 roots can be simultaneously visualized. The needle is advanced in plane or tangentially. Total LA volume of 0.15 to 0.25 ml/kg is usually sufficient.

Complications: Unintentional blockade of the phrenic and recurrent laryngeal nerves can happen in young children as these nerves lie close to the site of injection. Some degree of phrenic nerve blockade is almost always present in children receiving interscalene blocks.[64,65] The risk of pneumothorax is also greater in children because the apex of the lung is situated more rostral in infants and small children. Total spinal anaesthesia is also more likely with the interscalene approach than axillary blockade.[66]

LOWER EXTREMITY BLOCKS

Lower extremity nerve blocks are mainly used in children for managing postoperative pain and as an adjunct to general anaesthesia in intraoperative period. Sciatic, femoral, and lateral femoral cutaneous blockade alone or in combinations can provide both excellent postoperative analgesia and surgical anaesthesia for selected operations. The fascia iliaca block produces anaesthesia of multiple nerves with a single injection.

Sciatic Nerve Block

Anatomy

The sciatic nerve arises from L4–S3 roots of the sacral plexus, passes through the pelvis, and becomes superficial at the lower margin of the gluteus maximus muscle. It then descends in the posterior aspect of the thigh and supplies sensory innervation to the posterior thigh and entire leg and foot below knee, except for the medial aspect, which is supplied by the femoral nerve. It can be combined with a femoral nerve block for most operations below the knee.

There are multiple approaches to the sciatic nerve.[67] All approaches should be performed with the nerve stimulator guidance to elicit motor response in the foot. Ultrasound guidance improves the performance.

A newer lateral approach to the sciatic nerve in the popliteal fossa has been described which offers the block to be performed in the supine position. An infragluteal approach is another easy method of providing a sciatic nerve block in children.[68]

Posterior Approach (Labat's Approach)

In this approach, the child is placed in the lateral position with site to be operated up. The upper leg is flexed and the lower leg is kept extended. A line is drawn from the posterior superior iliac spine to the greater trochanter of the femur. Another line is drawn from ischial tuberosity to the greater trochanter. The first line is bisected and a perpendicular line is drawn from that point to the second line. The point at which it intersects the second line is the site of needle insertion. A 22-gauge insulated needle attached to nerve stimulator is advanced in the perpendicular plane and motor response is elicited.

Anterior Approach

After emerging from the lower border of the gluteus maximus, sciatic nerve passes medial and deep to the lesser trochanter of the femur. With the child in the supine position, a line is drawn from the anterior superior iliac spine to the pubic tuberosity. A second line is drawn parallel to the first line from the greater trochanter. At the junction of medial one-third and lateral two-thirds of the first line, a perpendicular is drawn to the second line. The point of intersection of the perpendicular with the second line originating at the greater trochanter marks the point of needle entry. The needle is inserted in a perpendicular plane until bone is contacted. Then the needle is withdrawn a little and redirected medially and motor response is sought. This approach carries a greater risk of puncture of the femoral vessels.

For these two approaches, usually a dose of 0.2 ml/kg of bupivacaine (0.25% with epinephrine 1:200,000) is administered for children older than 6 months of age. When combined sciatic and femoral nerve block is used, consideration should be given to limiting the total dose.[69]

Lateral Popliteal Approach

This block is usually used for surgery to the foot and knee, such as clubfoot repair or triple arthrodesis, and in combination with a femoral nerve block for knee surgery.[70] The advantages are that it can be performed in the supine position,[71] and it preserves hamstring function to allow early ambulation with crutches.

Anatomy: The popliteal fossa is a diamond-shaped area located behind the knee. It is bordered by the biceps femoris laterally, medially by the tendons of the semitendinosus and semimembranosus muscles, and inferiorly by the heads of the gastrocnemius muscle. Here, the sciatic nerve divides into two branches, the larger tibial nerve medially and the common peroneal nerve laterally. However, at the apex of the popliteal fossa, they are in close proximity and enclosed in a common sheath.

Technique: After induction of general anaesthesia, the lower leg is kept elevated on a pillow. Biceps femoris tendon is palpated and the tendon is then traced upward for 3 to 5 cm. A 22-gauge needle is inserted anterior to the tendon in a horizontal plane and the foot is observed for plantar flexion or dorsiflexion while advancing the needle with cephalad angulation. On eliciting contraction, 5 to 8 ml of LA is injected. Continuous catheter techniques can also be used to provide effective analgesia in children in the postoperative period.[72] Ultrasound guidance may improve precision and safety with the technique.

Complications: Intraneural and intravascular injection should be avoided.

Infragluteal-parabiceps (Subgluteal) Approach

This is a simple approach and offers additional advantage of blocking the posterior cutaneous nerve supplying the posterior portion of the thigh.[68]

Technique: The child is placed in supine or a lateral position and the biceps femoris tendon is palpated and traced cephalad to the distal crease of the buttock. A stimulating needle is then inserted perpendicularly, beside the biceps femoris tendon until a twitch is obtained (either inversion or eversion of the foot). An ultrasound-guided approach may facilitate this block.[73] Usually 0.2 ml/kg of LA is injected.

Complications: Profound motor block can be seen in most children after a subgluteal block and caution should be exercised, if the child is discharged home.[74]

Femoral Nerve Block (Fig. 10.9)

This block may be used in trauma victims with fractured femoral shaft preoperatively for pain relief so that manipulations for transport or radiographic procedures are not painful.[75]

Anatomy: The femoral nerve is located lateral to the femoral artery and deep to both the fascia lata and fascia iliaca.

Technique: A 22-gauge blunt B-bevel needle is advanced perpendicularly lateral to the pulsation of the femoral artery below the inguinal crease. Two

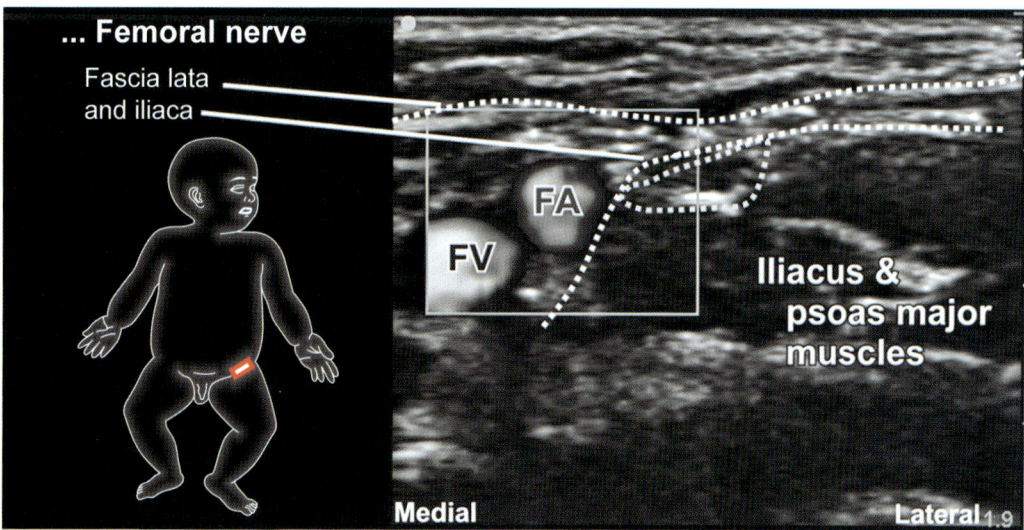

Fig. 10.9. Ultrasound image of femoral nerve

distinct pops can be felt as the needle traverses the fascial tissues. Approximately, 5 to 10 ml of LA is deposited lateral to the femoral pulse and deep to the fascia iliaca. Ultrasound guidance may be used to visualize femoral nerve[73] and catheter can be placed to provide continuous analgesia in the postoperative period.[75]

Complications: Haematoma may occur in children on anticoagulants or with blood dyscrasia, as the nerve lies in close proximity to the femoral artery. Intravascular injection may be avoided with frequent aspiration.

Fascia Iliaca Block

This block produces blockade of the femoral, lateral femoral cutaneous, and obturator nerves with a single injection of LA and is particularly useful in children to provide unilateral anaesthesia or analgesia of the lower extremity.[76]

Anatomy: This compartment is bounded superiorly by the iliac crest, superficially by fascia iliaca and iliacus muscle, and by the psoas muscle at deeper plane. There is no major nerve or blood vessels in close vicinity the needle. This block has been reported to be superior to the "3 in 1" block.[76]

Technique: The needle is inserted approximately 1 cm below the junction of the outer and middle thirds of the inguinal ligament and advanced at about 75 degrees angle to the skin. Two characteristic pops are felt as the needle pierces the fascia lata and then the fascia iliaca. Angulation of needle is subsequently decreased and the needle is directed cephalad as the local anaesthetic is incrementally injected. LA volume is massaged to promote proximal flow of the drug. Usually, a volume of 0.3 to 0.5 ml/kg is sufficient in most cases.

Complications: As volume required to achieve an adequate block is large, care has to be taken not to exceed the maximum dosage of the local anaesthetic.

CONCLUSION

To conclude, regional anaesthesia should be considered an integral part of routine paediatric anaesthesia practice today. Beneficial aspects of paediatric regional anaesthesia beyond pain relief in improving perioperative outcome need not be overemphasized.

Ultrasonography has improved safety and efficacy of the procedures and considerably enhanced the interest in paediatric regional blocks.

REFERENCES

1. Peters JW, Schouw R, Anand KJ, van Dijk M, Duivenvoorden HJ, Tibboel D. Does neonatal surgery lead to increased pain sensitivity in later childhood? Pain 2005;114:444–454.
2. Taddio A, Katz J. The effects of early pain experience in neonates on pain responses in infancy and childhood. Pediatr Drugs 2005;7:245–257.
3. Anand KJ, Sippell WG, Aynsley-Green A. Randomised trial of fentanyl anesthesia in preterm babies undergoing surgery: effects on the stress response. Lancet 1987;1: 62–66.
4. Polaner DM, Martin LD. Quality assurance and improvement: the Pediatric Regional Anesthesia Network. Paediatr Anaesth 2012;22:115–119.
5. Besunder JB, Reed MD, Blumer JL. Principles of drug biodisposition in the neonate. A critical evaluation of the pharmacokinetic- pharmacodynamic interface (Part I). Clin Pharmacokinet 1988;14:189-216.
6. Besunder JB, Reed MD, Blumer JL. Principles of drug biodisposition in the neonate. A critical evaluation of the pharmacokinetic-pharmacodynamic interface (Part II). Clin Pharmacokinet 1988;14:261–286.
7. Brown AK, Zuelzer WW, Burnett HH. Studies on the neonatal development of the glucuronide conjugating system. J Clin Invest 1958;37:332–340.
8. Chalkiadis GA, Anderson BJ. Age and size are the major covariates for prediction of levobupivacaine clearance in children. Paediatr Anaesth 2006;16:275–282.
9. Berde CB. Convulsions associated with pediatric regional anesthesia. Anesth Analg 1992;75:164–166.
10. Otila E. Studies on the cerebrospinal fluid of premature infants. Acta Paediatr Scand 1948;35:3–100.
11. Oberlander TF, Berde CB, Lam KH, Rappaport LA, Saul JP. Infants tolerate spinal anesthesia with minimal overall autonomic changes: analysis of heart rate variability in former premature infants undergoing hernia repair. Anesth Analg 1995;80:20–27.
12. Payen D, Ecoffey C, Carli P, Dubousset AM. Pulsed Doppler ascending aortic, carotid, brachial, and femoral artery blood flows during caudal anesthesia in infants. Anesthesiology 1987;67:681–685.
13. Campbell MF. Caudal anesthesia in children. J Urol 1933;30: 245–249.
14. Spiegel P. Caudal anesthesia in pediatric surgery: a preliminary report. Anesth Analg 1962;41:218–221.
15. Dalens B, Hasnaoui A. Caudal anesthesia in pediatric surgery: success rate and adverse effects in 750 consecutive patients. Anesth Analg 1989;68:83–89.

16. Desparmet JF. Total spinal anesthesia after caudal anesthesia in an infant. Anesth Analg 1990;70:665–667.

17. Owens WD, Slater EM, Battit GE. A new technique of caudal anesthesia. Anesthesiology 1973;39:451–453.

18. Baidya DK, Pawar DK, Dehran M, Gupta AK. Advancement of epidural catheter from lumbar to thoracic space in children: Comparison between 18G and 23G catheters. J Anesthesiol Clin Pharmacol 2012;28:21–27.

19. Chen CP, Tang SF, Hsu TC, et al. Ultrasound guidance in caudal epidural needle placement. Anesthesiology 2004;101:181–184.

20. Krane EJ, Dalens BJ, Murat I, Murrell D. The safety of epidurals placed during general anesthesia. Reg Anesth Pain Med 1998;23:433–438.

21. Saberski LR, Kondamuri S, Osinubi OY. Identification of the epidural space: is loss of resistance to air a safe technique? A review of the complications related to the use of air. Reg Anesth 1997;22:3–15.

22. Armitage EN. Caudal block in children. Anaesthesia 1979;34:396.

23. Ansermino M, Basu R, Vandebeek C, Montgomery C. Nonopioid additives to local anaesthetics for caudal blockade in children: a systematic review. Paediatr Anaesth 2003;13:561–573.

24. Ecoffey C, Lacroix F, Giaufre E, Orliaguet G, Courreges P. Epidemiology and morbidity of regional anesthesia in children: a follow-up one-year prospective survey of the French-Language Society of Paediatric Anaesthesiologists (ADARPEF). Paediatr Anaesth 2010;20:1061–1069.

25. Smitt PS, Tsafka A, Teng-van de Zande F, et al. Outcome and complications of epidural analgesia in patients with chronic cancer pain. Cancer 1998;83:2015–2022.

26. Kost-Byerly S, Tobin JR, Greenberg RS, et al. Bacterial colonization and infection rate of continuous epidural catheters in children. Anesth Analg 1998;86:712–716.

27. Horlocker TT, Wedel DJ, Benzon H, et al. Regional anesthesia in the anticoagulated patient: defining the risks (the second ASRA Consensus Conference on Neuraxial Anesthesia and Anticoagulation). Reg Anesth Pain Med 2003;28:172–197.

28. Fisher QA, McComiskey CM, Hill JL, et al. Postoperative voiding interval and duration of analgesia following peripheral or caudal nerve blocks in children. Anesth Analg 1993;76:173–177.

29. Krane EJ, Tyler DC, Jacobson LE. The dose response of caudal morphine in children. Anesthesiology 1989;71: 48–52.

30. Dalens BJ, Mazoit JX. Adverse effects of regional anaesthesia in children. Drug Saf 1998;19:251–268.

31. Flandin-Blety C, Barrier G. Accidents following extradural analgesia (in children. The results of a retrospective study. Paediatr Anaesth 1995;5:41–46.

32. Gray HT. A study of spinal anaesthesia in children and infants: from a series of 200 cases, part I. Lancet 1909;2: 913–937.

33. Sartorelli KH, Abajian JC, Kreutz JM, Vane DW. Improved outcome utilizing spinal anesthesia in high-risk infants. J Pediatr Surg 1992;27:1022–1025.

34. Welborn LG, Rice LJ, Hannallah RS, et al. Postoperative apnea in former preterm infants: prospective comparison of spinal and general anesthesia. Anesthesiology 1990;72: 838–842.

35. Hermanns H, Stevens MF, Werdehausen R, et al. Sedation during spinal anaesthesia in infants. Br J Anaesth 2006; 97:380–384.

36. Gleason CA, Martin RJ, Anderson JV, et al. Optimal position for a spinal tap in preterm infants. Pediatrics 1983;71: 31–35.

37. Dalens BJ. Regional Anesthesia in Children.In Miller's Anesthesia (7th edn) by Miller RD. Churchill Livingstone 2010.

38. Kokki H, Hendolin H, Turunen M. Postdural puncture headache and transient neurologic symptoms in children after spinal anaesthesia using cutting and pencil point paediatric spinal needles. Acta Anaesthesiol Scand 1998;42:1076–1082.

39. Bailey A, Valley R, Bigler R. High spinal anesthesia in an infant. Anesthesiology 1989;70:560.

40. Kachko L, Simhi E, Tzeitlin E, et al. Spinal anesthesia in neonates and infants—a single-center experience of 505 cases. Paediatr Anaesth 2007;17:647–653.

41. Curatolo M, Petersen-Felix S, Arendt-Nielsen L, et al. Adding sodium bicarbonate to lidocaine enhances the depth of epidural blockade. Anesth Analg 1998;86:341–347.

42. Wong K, Strichartz GR, Raymond SA. On the mechanisms of potentiation of local anesthetics by bicarbonate buffer: drug structure-activity studies on isolated peripheral nerve. Anesth Analg 1993;76:131–143.

43. Rajamani A, Kamat V, Rajavel VP, Murthy J, Hussain SA. A comparison of bilateral infraorbital nerve block with intravenous fentanyl for analgesia following cleft lip repair in children. Paediatr Anaesth 2007;17:133–139.

44. Higashizawa T, Koga Y. Effect of infraorbital nerve block under general anesthesia on consumption of isoflurane and postoperative pain in endoscopic endonasal maxillary sinus surgery. J Anesth 2001;15:136–138.

45. Kolvenbach H, Lauven PM, Schneider B, Kunath U. Repetitive intercostal nerve block via catheter for postoperative pain relief after thoracotomy. Thorac Cardiovasc Surg 1989;37:273–276.

46. Grant GJ, Barenholz Y, Bolotin EM, et al. A novel liposomal bupi- vacaine formulation to produce ultralong-acting analgesia. Anesthesiology 2004;101:133–137.

47. Moore DC. Intercostal nerve block for postoperative somatic pain following surgery of thorax and upper abdomen. Br J Anaesth 1975;47:284–286.

48. Casey WF, Rice LJ, Hannallah RS, et al. A comparison between bupivacaine instillation versus ilioinguinal/iliohypogastric nerve block for postoperative analgesia following inguinal herniorrhaphy in children. Anesthesiology 1990;72:637–639.

49. Amory C, Mariscal A, Guyot E, et al. Isilioinguinal/iliohypogastric nerve block always totally safe in children? Paediatr Anaesth 2003;13:164–166.

50. Chhibber AK, Perkins FM, Rabinowitz R, Vogt AW, Hulbert WC. Penile block timing for postoperative analgesia of hypospadias repair in children. J Urol 1997;158:1156–1159.

51. Choi WY, Irwin MG, Hui TW, Lim HH, Chan KL. EMLA cream versus dorsal penile nerve block for postcircumcision analgesia in children. Anesth Analg 2003;96:396–399.

52. Isaac LA, McEwen J, Hayes JA, Crawford MW. A pilot study of the rectus sheath block for pain control after umbilical hernia repair. Paediatr Anaesth 2006;16:406–409.

53. Willschke H, Bosenberg A, Marhofer P, et al. Ultrasonography- guided rectus sheath block in paediatrican aesthesia—a new approach to an old technique. Br J Anaesth 2006;97:244–249.

54. Lönnqvist PA, Hesser U. Location of the paravertebral space in children and adolescents in relation to surface anatomy assessed by computed tomography. Paediatr Anaesth 1992;2:285–289.

55. Lönnqvist PA, Hesser U. Depth from the skin to the thoracic paravertebral space in infants and children. Paediatr Anaesth 1994;4:99–100.

56. Naja ZM, Raf M, El Rajab M, et al. Nerve stimulator-guided paravertebral blockade combined with sevoflurane sedation versus general anesthesia with systemic analgesia for postherniorrhaphy pain relief in children: a prospective randomized trial. Anesthesiology 2005;103:600–605.

57. Cheung SL, Booker PD, Franks R, Pozzi M. Serum concentrations of bupivacaine during prolonged continuous paravertebral infusion in young infants. Br J Anaesth 1997;79:9–13.

58. Lonnqvist PA, MacKenzie J, Soni AK, Conacher ID. Paravertebral blockade. Failure rate and complications. Anaesthesia 1995;50:813–815

59. Naja ZM, Raf M, El-Rajab M, et al. A comparison of nerve stimula- tor guided paravertebral block and ilio-inguinal nerve block for analgesia after inguinal herniorrhaphy in children. Anaesthesia 2006;61:1064–1068.

60. Fisher WJ, Bingham RM, Hall R. Axillary brachial plexus block for perioperative analgesia in 250 children. Paediatr Anaesth 1999;9:435–438.

61. Suresh S, Sarwark JP, Bhalla T, Janicki J. Performing US-guided nerve blocks in the postanesthesia care unit (PACU) for upper extremity fractures: is this feasible in children? Paediatr Anaesth 2009;19:1238–1240.

62. Wilson JL, Brown DL, Wong GY, Ehman RL, Cahill DR. Infraclavicular brachial plexus block: parasagittal anatomy important to the coracoid technique. Anesth Analg 1998;87:870–873.

63. Dalens B, Vanneuville G, Tanguy A. A new parascalene approach to the brachial plexus in children: comparison with the supraclavicular approach. Anesth Analg 1987;66:1264–1271.

64. Ediale KR, Myung CR, Neuman GG. Prolonged hemidiaphragmatic paralysis following interscalene brachial plexus block. J Clin Anesth 2004;16:573–575.

65. Sala-Blanch X, Lazaro JR, Correa J, Gomez-Fernandez M. Phrenic nerve block caused by interscalene brachial plexus block: effects of digital pressure and a low volume of local anesthetic. Reg Anesth Pain Med 1999;24:231–235.

66. Tetzlaff JE, Yoon HJ, Dilger J, Brems J. Subdural anesthesia as a complication of an interscalene brachial plexus block. Case report. Reg Anesth 1994;19:357–359.

67. Dalens B, Tanguy A, Vanneuville G. Sciatic nerve blocks in children: comparison of the posterior, anterior, and lateral approaches in 180 pediatric patients. Anesth Analg 1990;70:131–137.

68. Sukhani R, Candido KD, Doty Jr R, Yaghmour E, McCarthy RJ. Infragluteal-parabiceps sciatic nerve block: an evaluation of a novel approach using a single-injection technique. Anesth Analg 2003;96:868–873.

69. McNicol LR. Sciatic nerve block for children. Sciatic nerve block by the anterior approach for postoperative pain relief. Anaesthesia 1985;40:410–414.

70. DeVera HV, Furukawa KT, Matson MD, Scavone JA, James MA. Regional techniques as an adjunct to general anesthesia for pediatric extremity and spine surgery. J Pediatr Orthop 2006;26:801–804.

71. McLeod DH, Wong DH, Claridge RJ, Merrick PM. Lateral popliteal sciatic nerve block compared with subcutaneous infiltration for analgesia following foot surgery. Can J Anaesth 1994;41:673–676.

72. Vas L. Continuous sciatic block for leg and foot surgery in 160 children. Paediatr Anaesth 2005;15:971–978.

73. Oberndorfer U, Marhofer P, Bosenberg A, et al. Ultrasonographic guidance for sciatic and femoral nerve blocks in children. Br J Anaesth 2007;98:797–801.

74. 396. van Geffen GJ, Scheuer M, Muller A, Garderniers J, Gielen M. Ultrasound-guided bilateral continuous sciatic nerve blocks with stimulating catheters for postoperative pain relief after bilateral lower limb amputations. Anaesthesia 2006;61:1204–1207.

75. Stewart B, Tudur SC, Teebay L, Cunliffe M, Low B. Emergency department use of a continuous femoral nerve block for pain relief for fractured femur in children. Emerg Med J 2007;24:113–114.

76. Dalens B, Vanneuville G, Tanguy A. Comparison of the fascia iliaca compartment block with the 3-in-1 block in children. Anesth Analg 1989;69:705–713.

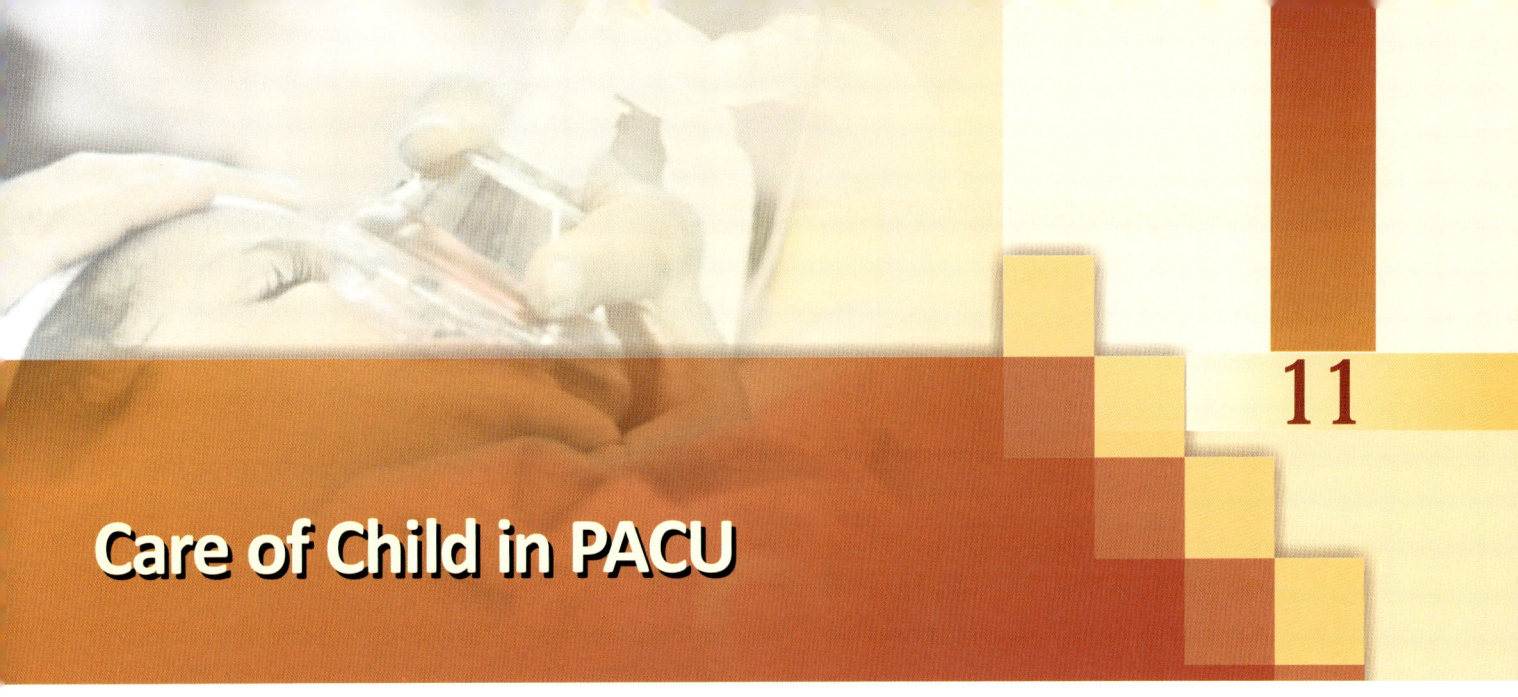

11

Care of Child in PACU

V Muralidhar

- ■ **Paediatric PACU**
- ■ **Alignment of pre-, intra- and postoperative strategies**
- ■ **Phases of recovery, support levels, and standards of clinical care**
- ■ **Management of common clinical problems and treatment**
- ■ **Flow of patients and criteria for discharge**

INTRODUCTION

The structure and function of a "Recovery Room" was a rudimentary concept in the 19th century. It made its debut as a bare room adjacent to the operating room, to allow patients to recover from the immediate effects of surgery and anaesthesia.[1–3] With the understanding on prevention of deaths in the immediate postoperative period, it has gradually evolved over time, to a modern post-anaesthesia care unit (PACU) with a controlled environment, design specifications and built-in processes for improved safety and outcomes (Tables 11.1 and 11.2).

PAEDIATRIC PACU

Intense focus on paediatric PACU has emerged only in the last few decades, with the realization that there are a number of problems unique to this group.[4,5] For example, paediatric patients, in comparison to adult patients, are shown to have a higher incidence of adverse events in the PACU, justifying a greater need for postoperative care. Gonzalez, et al. in a recent review, have re-emphasised the mandatory need for a well-organized PACU for paediatric patients.

Table 11.1	Structure of a modern paediatric PACU	
Modern PACU design	
Monitoring	ECG, SPO$_2$, NIBP, thermometer, invasive blood pressure equipment appropriate for paediatric patients.
Electrical	6–8 outlets, two connected to UPS for ventilator, infusion pumps as per standard guidelines
Medical gas	2–3 oxygen outlets, 3–5 suction outlets, compressed gas
Lighting	General, bed level, procedural, portable
Air-conditioning	Temperature 75°F with warming devices. Humidity 40–60%, air changes minimum 6 hour.
Communication	Code blue system, alarm system, broadcast system, paging, OT network, cordless telephone
Transport	Oxygen delivery, incubators, paediatric transport ventilators
Equipment	Paediatric resuscitation, difficult airway cart, warming devices, surgical thoracotomy, tracheostomy, etc.
Bed/building dimension	As per guidelines

Table 11.2	Building processes into paediatric PACU	
Schedule	**Processes**
▪ Staffing and education	▪ Performance based credentialling
▪ Quality assurance (clinical and other processes)	▪ Continuous quality improvement of structure, processes, outcomes
▪ Data management	▪ Integrated with hospital information system, computerized data management
▪ Resource allocation	▪ Paediatric surgical and anaesthetic needs

Further, even within the paediatric group, the pattern of problems need to be understood. For example, neonates and infants under one year of age have a greater mortality and morbidity as compared to older children. Only paediatric hospitals have dedicated paediatric PACUs. Most general hospitals have a combined PACU (adults and children), and in such cases, it is advisable to create some dedicated beds for paediatric patients. The specialized care in this area can help achieve the goals of paediatric PACU management which include: (a) Safe emergence, (b) Problem recognition and management, (c) Safe discharge, (d) Family orientation to allow acclimatization to the postoperative problems, (e) Appropriate resource utilization (time, beds, manpower, etc.).

ALIGNMENT OF PREOPERATIVE, INTRAOPERATIVE AND POSTOPERATIVE STRATEGIES

PACU management has to be seamless with preoperative assessment and intraoperative strategies. Recognition of potentially significant history, preoperative problems, intraoperative techniques, interventions and adverse events, help us anticipate PACU problems, plan postoperative strategies, special equipment and drugs needed, before the patient reaches the PACU.[6–13] Some of the common predictors of PACU problems in the paediatric age group are—congenital syndromes (Down's, Pierre Robin); comorbidities: Respiratory (OSA, asthma, chest infection); heart disease (CHD, failure, arrhythmias); bleeding diathesis (haemophilia); neuromuscular disorders (dystrophies); sepsis, electrolyte imbalance; bad anaesthetic history (difficult intubation, pain, vomiting); surgical risk factors (emergency surgery, long duration, blood loss, airway emergencies); intraoperative adverse events (pneumothorax); mediation risk factors (long-acting agents, overdose, narcotics).

PHASES OF RECOVERY, SUPPORT LEVELS AND STANDARDS OF CLINICAL CARE

Marshall and Chung identified 3 clear-cut phases of recovery (phases I, II and III) from the effects of surgery and anaesthesia. The patient, at the end of phase I recovers airway reflexes, can protect his/her airway and regains motor functions. At the end of phase II, patient has clinically recovered sufficiently to go home, and at the end of phase III, has returned to the preoperative physiological and psychological state. These levels of recovery are correlated with three levels of support which we need to provide: High support PACU-I, intermediate support (or step-down) PACU-II and low support (or ward/home) PACU-III, which require different levels of gradually decreasing infrastructure and manpower—monitoring, manpower and care designed for anticipated problems.[1–5,14]

Phase I postoperative care starts with the end of surgery, with the patient starting to emerge from the effects of anaesthesia and surgery. Phase I support is carried out in PACU-I, which is designed for high-level support for taking care during the period of highest risk. PACU-I standards include availability of beds in the ratio of 1:1 or 1:2 (OT:PACU bed), with the number of operating rooms, availability of trained nurse in the ratio of 1:1 or 1:2 in case of a sick patient (Patient : Nurse ratio). Supervision of coordination by a trained anaesthesiologist who is available near the patients, is recommended to be moved to PACU-II quickly to allow bed and manpower availability to sicker patients. PACU-II is the step-down and requires a lower support levels.[15–17]

The most commonly followed clinical processes of care, which must be adhered to, have been set and popularized by the American Society of Anesthesiologists (ASA). The ASA PACU standards of clinical care imply that these minimum standards of care (processes) are to be delivered in the PACU. It defines the way patients need to be transported from the OT to the PACU and by whom; the way handover is to be done and to whom, and further how they have to be sent out of the PACU:

▪ Standards I, II include mandatory levels of clinical care and must be delivered by a trained anaesthesiologist, during emergence and transportation to a dedicated area of care/PACU respectively.

Children are prone to airway obstruction during shifting and are generally transported in a lateral position.

- Standard III includes standards for detailed hand-over to the staff in the PACU in a predetermined manner.[18–22] A report by the anaesthesiologist to the PACU nurse including, but not necessarily limited to the following: Brief medical history, patient's name, age, sex, disability or barriers to communication (e.g. native language, deaf or blind, etc.), diagnosis, surgical procedure, surgeon's name, significant comorbidities, allergies and daily medications, anaesthetic course, complications, intraoperative fluid balance, pre-transfer laboratory data, time and dose of relevant medications administered intraoperatively that should be administered postoperatively (e.g. antibiotics and steroids), anticipated problems and postanaesthetic orders (e.g. oxygen administration, fluid administration, antiemetic and analgesic treatment).

- Standard IV includes standardized care (monitoring, documentation, treatment) in the PACU in a systematic manner. On accepting the patient, the PACU nurse evaluates and documents the patient's status at regular intervals. As noted above, several post-anaesthetic clinical evaluation scales are used for evaluating pain, respiration and ventilation, vomiting, haemodynamics, agitation, sedation, etc. to identify common and specific clinical problems mentioned below. Also, the patient is evaluated for the changing levels of recovery. Aldrete score is the most convenient and widely used PACU aid but has some limitations, because patients with cardiac dysrhythmias, oliguria, or severe nausea and vomiting can all score 10 but may not be suitably recovered. Appropriate monitoring equipment with paediatric accessories must be readily available. Normograms must be available for ready reference and diagnosis of respiratory and haemodynamic abnormalities. Continuous monitoring and documentation of SPO_2, ECG, intermittent non-invasive blood pressure, respiratory rate at the standard intervals recommended by the department is done in all patients. Timing of vital sign monitoring depends on the condition of the patient but is usually about once every 15 minutes for the first hour and half hourly thereafter. Temperature is measured and recorded on arrival and discharge. All patients require respiratory orders including delivery of oxygen by an appropriate device and rate of administration. Precautions must be taken in children who are at risk of oxygen toxicity. Other orders include appropriate equipment and drugs for paediatric usage, i.e. LMA or endotracheal tube, administration of bronchodilators, suctioning, positioning and administration of drugs, ventilation, NIV (Bi-PAP), etc. must be available at hand. Haemodynamic documentation also involves input and output (urine, drains). The volume, type of fluids, rate of administration and the delivery must be specified. Nausea and vomiting should be monitored and treated, as this can delay discharge. Investigations may be required, and paediatric patients often pose a challenge for blood sampling.[23]

MANAGEMENT OF COMMON CLINICAL PROBLEMS

Apnoeic Spells and Prematurity

Postoperative apnoea with cessation of breathing for more than 15 seconds can occur in the postoperative period and may be associated with cyanosis or pallor or desaturation and bradycardia up to 12 hours postoperatively. It is common in premature children with a postconceptual age of less than 44 weeks but may be seen in children with PCA up to 55 weeks. This is also associated with neurological abnormalities, necrotizing enterocolitis, etc. Apart from prematurity, other conditions which can lead to apnoeic spells include—anaemia, hypoglycaemia, infection and stress. Prevention is by avoiding surgery, which should be resorted to only if absolutely essential. All such babies must have a good intravenous access and general anaesthesia and sedatives must be avoided, if possible.[23] A subarachnoid block is preferred. Maintenance of temperature in the perioperative period is also important in these patients. Preoperative caffeine may be helpful 10 mg/kg.

Post-Intubation Croup (Post-Extubation Subglottic Oedema)

Contributing factors for this include using cuffed tubes, traumatic intubation, repeated intubations and trauma due to surgery, e.g. bronchoscopy, coughing on the tube, occult subglottic narrowing (e.g. Down syndrome, old tracheo-oesophageal fistula repair), non-implant tested tubes, lack of humidification, inappropriate size of ET, head and neck surgery and pre-existing tracheal irritation. Treatment depends on the severity and includes oxygenation, humidification, use of helium-oxygen mixtures, nebulised steroids or epinephrine (0.5 ml/kg of 1:1000 solution maximum 6 ml or diluted to 6 ml), and in severe cases, airway interventions, e.g. intubation.

Respiratory Obstruction

Respiratory obstruction may present as coughing, breath-holding or frank obstruction.[24–28] Minor obstruction may be corrected by re-positioning of the baby or placement of an oral or nasal airway. A major obstruction may require a chin-lift manoeuvre or placement of an LMA or an endotracheal tube. A laryngospasm may require clearance of the throat, CPAP or intervention with a relaxant. A difficult mask ventilation may require two practitioners to assess each other, or in some cases, there may be a complete inability to mask ventilate. A total obstruction needs immediate intervention. Airway problem occurs due to various reasons after airway surgery (e.g. cleft palate repair)—altered anatomy, numb palate, bleeding, obstruction, laryngospasm, packs placed by the surgeon, tongue sutures, other associated syndromes. A higher incidence of airway problems is seen in children with some of the syndromes.

Obstructive Sleep Apnoea

Seen commonly in obese children, and is diagnosed with more than ten episodes of obstructive apnoea or hyperpnoea per hour during sleep. This may be accompanied by PCO_2 50 mg Hg or higher, O_2 90% or less, episodes of desaturation of 80% or less. This may be treated with BiPAP, avoidance of sedation, then providing postoperative care in a high dependency area.

Hypothermia and Shivering

Children are prone to hypothermia and shivering as they are managed in adult PACUs where the temperature is low. Intraoperative and postoperative use of cold irrigating fluids, vasodilatory inhalational agents and improper warming techniques commonly lead to hypothermia. It can be prevented or treated by warming blankets, warmed IV fluids and use of certain drugs, such as intravenous pethidine 0.25–0.5 mg/kg and oxygenation.

Hypoxaemia and Hypercarbia

In addition to the airway problems mentioned earlier, hypoxaemia can occur due to—increased shunting (right to left), low FiO_2 (inadequate supply, diffusion hypoxia), hypoventilation due to drugs, upper abdominal surgery with raised abdominal pressure and pain. Children may need oxygenation or ventilation. But the FiO_2 has to be titrated so as not to cause oxygen toxicity in premature babies.

Negative Pressure Pulmonary Oedema (Type-I)

It is caused by a negative intrathoracic inspiration against a closed glottis leading to an increased venous return and increased hydrostatic pressure with fluid being drawn into the lung interstitium and/or alveoli. This is combined with a decreased return of fluid via lymphatics. Management is by removal of the cause of obstruction and by ventilatory support.

Postoperative Haemorrhage and Hypotension

This is a common cause of postoperative mortality and morbidity, although other causes of hypotension should be ruled out. This condition is difficult to diagnose in certain surgeries (e.g. tonsillectomy, palatal repair), when the child swallows the blood. Should be suspected when there is increased abdominal pain, pallor, restlessness, tachycardia or tachypnoea. Children are also prone to obstruction, vomiting, aspiration and layngospasm due to pressure of blood in the pharynx or regurgitated blood/clots. Requires a rapid control of the source of bleeding.

Hypertension

This uncommon problem in children is seen in those with pre-existing hypertension (renal disease, phaeo-chromocytomas), pain, hypoxaemia/hypercapnia, hypothermia. Treatment is with anti-hypertensives, pain, respiratory support, and temperature maintenance.

Arrhythmia

Arrhythmias are seen in children with electrolyte imbalances or hypoxaemic/hypercapnic and in acidotic patients. Treatment includes correction of electrolyte imbalance, respiratory support and treatment of the acidosis. In a study of perioperative cardiac arrests by Braz et al. (2006), over a 9-year period from a Brazilian Teaching Hospital, it was found that the major risk factors for cardiac arrests were neonates, children under one year and ASA grade III (poor physical status). All anaesthesia-related cardiac arrests were related to airway management and medication administration.[9,10,29]

Postoperative Nausea and Vomiting (PONV)

This is the most common complication seen in the PACU, leading to delayed discharge and unanticipated hospitalization after outpatient surgery.[30–33] It is commonly seen in the paediatric age group after strabismus surgery, middle ear surgery, orchidopexy and umbilical hernia repair. The causes are multifactorial, which include a predisposition, susceptibility to motion sickness, use of drugs, e.g. narcotics. The current practice is to stop oral fluids and maintain on intravenous fluids. Prophylaxis is very effective in decreasing its incidence. Treatment is usually multimodal and the commonly used drugs are—ondensetron 0.1–0.15 mg/kg, metoclopropamide 0.15 mg/kg, droperidol 0.02–0.5 mg/kg, decadron 0.2 mg/kg (tumour lysis syndrome in susceptible individuals). Occasionally, rectal promethazine 0.5 mg/kg (phenergan 12.5–25 mg) or prochlorperazine 0.1 mg/kg are administered.

Emergence Phenomenon (Agitation)

During emergence from anaesthesia, children are prone to disorientation, hallucinations, uncontrollable activity and this can be evaluated by various scales.[34,35] This hyperexcitable, hyperactive state is referred to as "Excitement delirium". It occurs most commonly, if a patient awakens in pain after receiving potent vapour anaesthetic, such as halothane, sevoflurane, isoflurane and desflurane. Other causes include sensory deprivation (eye bandage, eye lubricant), residual anaesthetic, awakening in a strange unfriendly environment (PACU) and perioperative use of ketamine. In most cases, it lasts only for a short while (few minutes to few hours), but occasionally, it may persist for 12–24 hours. It may be accompanied by transient neurological, symmetrical changes which include sustained and non-sustained ankle clonus, bilateral hyper-reflexia, Babinski's reflex and decerebrate posturing. Presence of focal neurological deficits goes against the diagnosis of excitement delirium. In any case of agitation, one should ascertain the adequacy of blood-gas exchange, evaluate pain/discomfort due to gastric or urinary distention. After ruling out these problems, a little sedation and parental pressure may quieten the child.

Management of Pain in PACU

Pain management in children is a challenge in terms of assessment and management, as it may occur along with sedation and delirium (paediatric anaesthesia delirium scale, Riker, Richmond, Michigan scale, etc.). There has been an improvement in pain scoring and evaluation by the introduction of a number of scoring systems.[36–41] Pain assessment scores which are most commonly used in newborns are the Premature Infant Pain Profile (PIPP), and the CRIES postoperative pain scales. In the two months to 7 years age group, the face, legs, activity, cry and consolability (FLACC) scale is a behavioural scale that has been designed for assessment by observing (1–5 minutes), reviewing the description of behaviour, and selecting the number that matches the observed behaviour. If the child can self report (describe, report, locate), it is the preferred strategy for pain assessment and this includes: The Poker Chip scale, Wong-Baker Faces scale, Faces Pain Scale Revised (FPS-R) and the Oucher scale can be used easily in children above six years of age (but may also be useful above 3–4 years). As the child learns the proportionality of numbers and colours (above 8 years), we can use the same scale as in adults (Visual Analogue Scale, Numeric Rating Scale).

A number of drugs, routes and delivery systems are available for management of paediatric patients. Some of the commonly used drugs in the paediatric age group are the following:

1. **Acetaminophen is one of the commonly used analgesics:** Oral dose—10–15 mg/kg at 6 hourly intervals; 20 mg/kg (single dose). Daily maximum oral dosing should not exceed 70 mg/kg for children, 60 mg/kg for term neonates, 45 mg/kg for premature infants >34 weeks gestational age. Rectal preparations of acetaminophen are as follows: First dose: 30–45 mg/kg; subsequent 20 mg/kg. With an interval of at least 6 hours after each dose. Intravenous—can be given in children not able to take oral preparations.

2. **The following non-steroidal analgesics (NSAIDs) are used:** Oral ibuprofen 10 mg/kg 6th hourly, parenteral ketorolac 0.25–0.5 mg/kg 6th hourly

with no loading dose, cox-2 inhibitor (celecoxib) 6 mg/kg twice daily, orally naproxen 7.5 mg/kg twice daily orally.

3. **Narcotics:** Drugs which have been used include—morphine, pethidine, fentanyl. These can be administered by different routes, although the most common route is intravenous. Intravenous delivery can be achieved by boluses, infusion or PCA.

4. **Regional blocks and continuous infusions:** Paediatric spinal, caudal, epidural and regional nerve blocks are commonly employed for anaesthesia and postoperative pain relief. This has greatly improved after the introduction of ultrasound and smaller probes.

FLOW OF PATIENTS AND CRITERIA FOR DISCHARGE (STANDARD V)

Four variations are seen in surgical patients in the PACU: In-patients; ambulatory; unanticipated admissions; and patients requiring intensive care. Neonates and some special groups of children are not advised to be operated on an OPD basis. Inpatients going to the ward are first taken to Phase I in the PACU where the patient emerges from anaesthesia. Then, in Phase II (step-down recovery area or pre-discharge area), the patient achieves the criteria for discharge to ward/home. Finally, in Phase III, the patient recovers completely from anaesthesia and the acute effects of surgery. Due to the increasing availability of very short-acting anaesthetic agents, some patients may be eligible to bypass phase I recovery in PACU, and be discharged directly from the operating room or procedure area to phase II recovery based on fast tracking criteria.[42]

Cost cutting and rapid turnover of patients in operating make it mandatory for PACU beds to be available quickly (flow) without diluting quality. A number of strategies, such as division of PACUs into 3 levels and use of objective criteria for moving patients from one area to another are used to improve efficiency, rapid flow and operational success. Standard V includes standards for discharge from the PACU using very objective criteria. Discharge criteria are followed to send patients out of the PACU, and the anaesthesiologist is generally responsible for the discharge. Further details on these standards may be found on the ASA website and the same standards are applicable to adult and paediatric patients.

Time Based Recovery

More recently, several studies have indicated that formal admission to the PACU for an hour or more may not be necessary, especially in view of the wide spread use of fast-acting agents. Patient is moved through the unit and discharged when he/she is haemodynamically stable, accepting oral intake, has voiding, is able to ambulate, has minimal pain, is able to maintain haemodynamics and saturation, has no vomiting.

Criteria/Score Based Recovery

A system that was based on the Apgar score was developed by Aldrete, and has been extensively used because it can be applied immediately and used again as a convenient means to evaluate safe discharge. A score of 9 achieved by the patient in the operating room or PACU enables a satisfactory move to phase II level of care. An Aldrete score 9/10 or 10/10 is required for patients to be moved from Phase I to Phase II. If they achieve this in OR, they can be moved directly to Phase II. The disadvantage is that it does not address pain, nausea and vomiting.

White and Song proposed fast tracking criteria that include pain, emetic scores, with a maximum score of 14. A score of 12, with no less than 1 in any category provides a criteria for bypassing PACU. This scoring system may offer advantages over the modified Aldrete system by effectively bypassing the PACU to phase II, but does not address the significant problems of postoperative nausea and vomiting that may occur hours after surgery and anaesthesia.[45–48] It also does not address postoperative pain that becomes problematic as the effects of intraoperative narcotics abate.

Post-Anaesthetic Discharge Scoring System (PADSS)

It is used to discharge patients home and see home readiness.[49,50] A score of 9/10 or 10/10 is required to be discharged home. This was later modified to include input and output criteria. In addition, other criteria were added and someone to escort and take care. The ASA also gives various age groups, surgeries, situations where children should not be discharged home and must be mandatorily admitted.

CONCLUSION

PACU for the paediatric age group has very unique problems. The infrastructure, processes and trained manpower have to be made specific to paediatric reuirements for maximum efficiency and clinical outcomes which are at par with International bench-marks.

The movement of patients into and out of a paediatric PACU is a dynamic process which forms a common pathway for inpatients, daycare patients and intensive care patients. Therefore, protocols determine the smoothness of flow of patients, as also the economy of manpower and resource utilization.

REFERENCES

1. Hannallah RS. Pediatric Issues for Ambulatory Surgery. Chap 6 in Day Surgery. Development and Practice. Lemos P, Jarrett P, Philip B, (Eds). International Association for Ambulatory Surgery (IAAS). Portugal 2006;139–156.
2. Douglas J. "The establishment and management of a recovery andresuscitation ward". BJA 1963;35:24–27.
3. Miller RD. "Millers Anaesthesia" 6th edn. SAJAA-SASA recovery room guidelines section V "Standards for Postanaesthesia Care" American Society of Anaesthesiologists 1996;395–396.
4. Murat I, Constant I, Maud'huy H. Perioerative Anaesthetic Morbidity in Children: A database of 24,165 anaesthetics over a 30 month period. Pediatr Anesth 2004;14:158–166.
5. Gonzalez LP, Pignaton W, Kusano PS, Modolo NSP, Braz JRC, Braz LG. Anesthesia-related mortality in pediatric patients: A systemic review. Clinics 2012; 67(4):381–387.
6. Marcus R. Human factors in pediatric anesthesia incidents. Pediatr Anesth 2006;16:242–250.
7. Tay CLM, Tan GM, Ng SBA. Critical incidents in paediatric anaesthesia: an audit of 10,000 anaesthetics in Singapore. Paediatr Anaesth 2001;11:711–718.
8. Practice guidelines for postanesthetic care. A report by the American Society of Anesthesiologists Task Force on Postanesthetic Care. Anesthesiology 2002;96:742–752.
9. White MC, Peyton JM. Anesthetic management of children wih congenital heart disease for non-cardiac surgery. Continuing Medical Education in Anaesthesia, Critical Care & Pain 2012;12(1):17–21.
10. Practice Guidelines for the Perioperative Management of Patients with Obstructive Sleep Apnea. A Report by the American Society of Anesthesiologists Task Force on Perioperative Management of Patients with Obstructive Sleep Apnea. Anesthesiology 2006;104:1081–1093.
11. Braz LG, Modolo NSP,do Nascimento Jr P, Bruschi BAM, Castiglia YMM, Garem EM, de Carvalho LR, Braz JRC. Perioperative cardiac arrest: A study of 53718 anaesthetics over 9 year from a Brazilian teaching hospital. BJA 2006;96(5):569–575.
12. Kain ZN, Mayes LC, Wang S-M, Hofstadter MB. Post-operative behavioural outcomes in children: effects of sedativepremedication. Anesthesiology 1999; 90:758-65.
13. Anand KJS, Soriano SG. Anesthetic agents and the immature brain: are these toxic or therapeutic? Anesthesiology 2004;101:527–530.
14. Dexter F. Analysis of strategies to decrease PACU costs Anaesthesiology 1995;82(1):94–101.
15. Merrill DG, Laur JL. Management by outcomes: efficiency and operational success in the ambulatory surgery center. Anesthesiol Clin 2010;28: 329–351.
16. American Society of Anesthesiologists. Standards for Postanesthesia Care. Available at: www.asahq.org/publicationsAndServices/standards/36.pdf (accessed September 25, 2007).
17. Association of Anaesthetists of Great Britain and Ireland. Immediate Postanaesthetic Recovery. London: AAGBI, 2002.
18. Anwari JS. Quality of handover to the postanaesthesia care unit nurse. Anaesthesia 2002;57: 488–493.
19. Smith AF, Pope C, Goodwin D, Mort M. Communication between anesthesiologists, patients and the anesthesia team: a descriptive study of induction and emergence. Can J Anaesth 2005;52:915–920.
20. Smith AF, Goodwin D, Mort M, Pope C. Adverse events in anaesthetic practice: qualitative study of definition, discussion and reporting. Br J Anaesth 2006;96:715–721.
21. Sexton JB, Thomas EJ, Helmreich RL. Error, stress and team work in medicine and aviation: cross-sectional surveys. Br Med J 2000;320:745–749.
22. Patterson ES, Roth EM, Woods DD, Chow R, Gomes JO. Handoff strategies in settings with high consequences for failure: lessons for health care operations. Int J Qual Health Care 2004;16:125–132.
23. Fullilove S, Fixsen J. Major limb deformities as compli-cations of vascular access in neonates. Paediatr Anaesth 1997;7:247–250.
24. Vlatten A, Soder C. Airtraq optical laryngoscope intuba-tion in a 5-month-old infant with a difficult airway because of Robin Sequence. Paediatr Anaesth 2009;19:699–700.
25. Dullenkopf A, Holzmann D, Feurer R, Gerber A, Weiss M. Tracheal intubation in children with Morquio syn-drome using the angulated video-intubation laryngo-scope. Can J Anaesth 2002;49:198–202.
26. Saxena S. The ASA difficult airway algorithm: Is it time to include video laryngoscopy and discourage blind and multiple intubation attempts in the nonemergency pathway? Anaesth Analg 2009;108:1052.
27. White C, Cook TM, Stoddart PA. A critique of elective paediatric supraglottic airway devices. Paediatr Aanaesth 2009;19(Suppl. 1):55–65.

28. Ramesh S, Jayanthi R. Supraglottic airway devices in children. Indian J Anaesth 2011;55:476–482.

29. Morray JP, Bhananker SM. Recent findings from the Pediatric Perioperative Cardiac Arrest (POCA) registry. ASA Newsletter June 2005;69(6).

30. Gan TJ, Meyer TA, Apfel CC, Chung F, Davis PJ, Habib AS, Hooper VD, Kovac AL, Kranke P, Myles P, Philip BK, Samsa G, Sessler DI, Temo J, Tramèr MR, Vander Kolk C, Watcha M; Society for Ambulatory Anesthesia. Society for Ambulatory Anesthesia guidelines for the management of postoperative nausea and vomiting. Anesth Analg 2007;105:1615–1628.

31. Apfel CC, Heidrich FM, Jukar-Rao S, Jalota L, Hornuss C, Whelan RP, Zhang K, Cakmakkaya OS. Evidence-based analysis of risk factors for postoperative nausea and vomiting. Br J Anaesth 2012; 109:742–753.

32. De Oliveira Jr GS, Castro-Alves LJ, Chang R, Yaghmour E, McCarthy RJ. Systemic metoclopramide to prevent postoperative nausea and vomiting: a meta-analysis without Fujii's studies. Br J Anaesth 2012;109:688–697.

33. Apfel CC, Philip BK, Cakmakkaya OS, Shilling A, Shi Y, Leslie JB, Allard M, Turan A, Windle P, Odom-Forren J, Hooper VD, Oliver C, Radke OC, Ruiz J, Kovac A. Who is at risk for postdischarge nausea and vomiting after ambulatory surgery? Anesthesiology 2012;117:475–486.

34. Sikich N, Lerman J. Development and Psychometric evaluation of the Paediatric Anesthesia Emergence Delirium Scale. Anesthesiology 2004;100:1138–1145.

35. Singh R, Kharbanda M, Sood N, Mahajan V, Chatterji C. Comparative evaluation of incidence of emergence agitation and postoperative recovery profile in paediatric patients after isoflurane, sevoflurane and desflurane. Anaesthesia 2012;56(2):156–161.

36. McNicol ED, Tzortzopoulou A, Cepeda MS, Francia MB, Farhat T, Schumann R. Single-dose intravenous paracetamol or propacetamol for prevention or treatment of postoperative pain: a systematic review and meta-analysis. Br J Anaesth 2011;106:764–775.

37. Ong CK, Seymour RA, Lirk P, Merry AF. Combining paracetamol (acetaminophen) with nonsteroidal anti-inflammatory drugs: a qualitative systematic review of analgesic efficacy for acute postoperative pain. Anesth Analg 2010;110:1170–1179.

38. Maund E, McDaid C, Rice S, Wright K, Jenkins B, Woolacott N. Paracetamol and selective and non-selective non-steroidal anti-inflammatory drugs for the reduction in morphine-related side-effects after major surgery: a systematic review. Br J Anaesth 2011;106:292–297.

39. Waldron NH, Jones CA, Gan TJ, Allen TK, Habib AS. Impact of perioperative dexamethasone on postoperative analgesia and side-effects: systematic review and meta-analysis. Br J Anaesth 2013;110:191–200.

40. Laskowski K, Stirling A, McKay WP, Lim HJ. A systematic review of intravenous ketamine for postoperative analgesia. Can J Anaesth 2011;58:911–923.

41. Giaufré E, Dalens B, Gombert A. Epidemiology and morbidity of regional anesthesia in children: a one-year prospective study of the French-language Society of pediatric anesthesiologists. Anesth Analg 1996;83:904–912.

42. Marshall S and Chung F. "Discharge Criteria After Ambulatory Surgery. Anaesth Analg 1999; 88:508–17.2.

43. Waddle JP, et al. "PACU length of stay: quantifying and assessing dependant factors". Anaesth Analg 1998; 87: 628–633.

44. Marshall S, Chung F. "Discharge criteria after ambulatory Surgery". Anaesth Analg 1999;88:508–517.

45. White PF, et al. "New criteria for fast tracking after out-patient anaesthesia: A comparison with the modified Aldrete's scoring system". Anaesth Analg 1999;88: 1069–1072.

46. Millar J. "Fast tracking in day surgery. Is your journey to the recoveryroom really necessary" Editorial II BJA 2004.

47. White PF, et al. "New criteria for fast tracking after out-patient anaesthesia: A comparison with the modified Aldrete's scoring system"Anaesth Analg 1999;88:1069–1072.

48. Heather EAD. "From Aldrete to PADSS: Reviewing Discharge criteriaafter Ambulatory Surgery" Journal of Perianaesthesia Nursing Aug 2006;21(4):259–267.

49. Chung F. "Recovery pattern and home readiness after ambulatory surgery" Anaesth Analg 1995; 80:896–902.

50. Jakobsson J. Assessing recovery after ambulatory anaesthesia, measures of resumption of activities of daily living. Curr Opin Anesthesiol 2011;24:601–604.

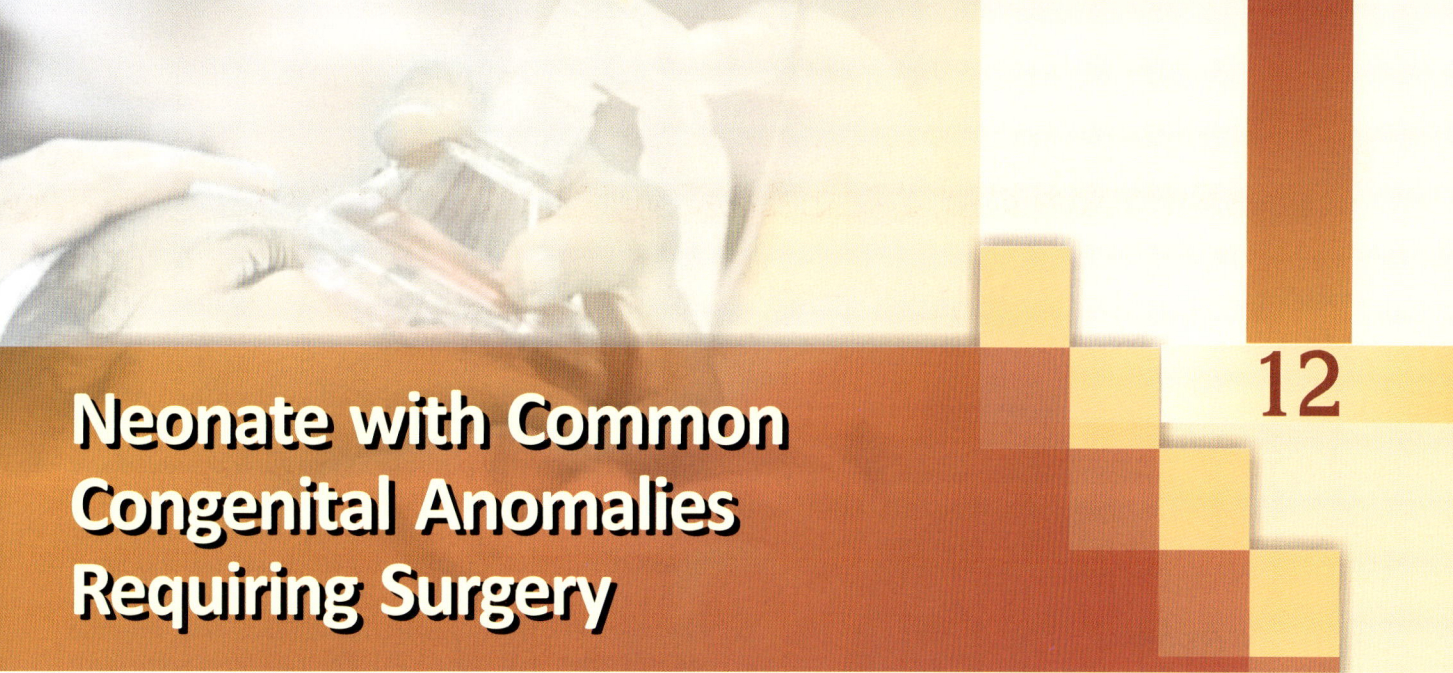

Neonate with Common Congenital Anomalies Requiring Surgery

12

Medha Mohta, Anup Mohta

- Oesophageal atresia with tracheo-oesophageal fistula
- Congenital diaphragmatic hernia
- Neural tube defects
- Hydrocephalus
- Idiopathic hypertrophic pyloric stenosis
- Abdominal wall defects: Omphalocele and gastroschisis

Neonates born with surgical anomalies present as a challenge to the anaesthesiologist. Surgical neonates differ from adults in their physiology, homeostasis, fluid and electrolyte requirements. Unstable physiology of the neonate leaves very little margin of error during anaesthetic management and the anaesthesiologist has to be very observant and careful.

Various surgical anomalies in a neonate include neural tube defects, hydrocephalus, oesophageal atresia with or without tracheo-oesophageal fistula, congenital diaphragmatic hernia, congenital lung malformations, idiopathic hypertrophic pyloric stenosis, intestinal atresia, abdominal wall defects, like gastroschisis or omphalocele, anorectal malformations, etc. Coexistence of many malformations as well as association with other defects, like cardiac anomalies, makes the task even more difficult. Each surgical anomaly has certain specific management requirements. An anaesthesiologist must know about the peculiarities of each anomaly and work as a team with the paediatric surgeon while the surgery is being performed.

Besides intraoperative concerns, pre- and post-operative management of the neonate undergoing surgery is very challenging. It is necessary to ensure preoperative stabilization of haemodynamic status; and correction of fluid and electrolyte imbalance, hypothermia, sepsis, and hypoglycaemia which may occur in a neonate in isolation or in varying combinations. The outcome of the neonate can be improved significantly by optimization of the preoperative condition. Similarly, postoperative management is very important and may require intensive care along with ventilation in many conditions. Thus, anaesthesiologist plays a very important role in improving the overall outcome of neonates undergoing surgery. This chapter aims to highlight surgical and anaesthetic considerations of some common congenital anomalies requiring surgical correction in neonates.

OESOPHAGEAL ATRESIA WITH TRACHEO-OESOPHAGEAL FISTULA

Oesophageal atresia encompasses a group of congenital anomalies characterized by an interruption of the continuity of the oesophagus combined with or without a persistent communication with the trachea. Oesophageal atresia (OA) and tracheo-oesophageal fistula (TOF) are relatively common birth defects with an incidence of approximately 1 in 2500 to 1 in 3000 live births,[1] and occur due to imperfect division of foregut during 4th–5th week of intrauterine life.[2]

Classification

The condition includes a spectrum of defects and includes, in the order of frequency, oesophageal atresia with distal tracheo-oesophageal fistula (86%), pure oesophageal atresia (7%), H-type tracheo-oesophageal fistula (4%), oesophageal atresia with proximal tracheo-oesophageal fistula (2%), and oesophageal atresia with both proximal and distal tracheo-oesophageal fistulae (<1%)[1] (Fig. 12.1).

Associated Anomalies

In about half the cases, there are congenital malformations in other organ systems, with cardiovascular system being the most commonly involved. Of several malformation associations involving OA/TOF, the best described is the VACTERL association which includes vertebral (17%), anorectal (12%), cardiac (20%), tracheo-esophageal, renal (16%), and limb malformations (10%).[3] It is, therefore, necessary to perform a thorough clinical examination and relevant radiological investigations to rule out these anomalies in any neonate suspected to have OA/TOF.

Diagnosis

The diagnosis of oesophageal atresia may be suspected prenatally by an ultrasound examination after 18th week of gestation which may show a small or absent fetal stomach bubble. Polyhydramnios also should arouse suspicion of obstruction of gastrointestinal tract.

Postnatally, OA/TOF should be suspected, if there is excessive salivation, repeated episodes of coughing, gagging, choking, regurgitation and cyanosis while feeding shortly after birth.[1] There may be sudden onset of respiratory distress following feeding attempts. Infants with oesophageal atresia are unable to swallow saliva and are noted to have excessive salivation requiring repeated suctioning. A stiff 10–12 French gauge catheter should be passed through the mouth into the oesophagus in such babies before the first feed. In oesophageal atresia, the catheter is seen to be arrested at about 9–10 cm from the lower alveolar ridge. A plain X-ray of chest and abdomen will show the tip of the catheter curled up in the upper chest or neck while gas in the stomach and intestine signifies the presence of a distal tracheo-oesophageal fistula. The absence of gastrointestinal gas is indicative of an isolated oesophageal atresia (Fig. 12.2).

Treatment

Surgical repair is the definitive treatment for OA and TOF. Surgery is generally performed within 24 to 72 hours in otherwise healthy neonates. Any delay in surgical repair predisposes the child to pneumonitis due to aspiration of saliva accumulated in upper pouch or reflux of gastric acid through the tracheo-oesophageal fistula.[4]

In the commonest variety, after stabilization, primary treatment includes right thoracotomy using extrapleural approach, division of tracheo-oesophageal fistula, and end-to-end anastomosis of two oesophageal ends. This procedure can also be done by thoracoscopic approach nowadays.[5] In pure atresia and wide gap oesophageal atresia, primary procedure includes cervical oesophagostomy with gastrostomy. Oesophageal continuity can be restored by different methods available when the child grows.[6]

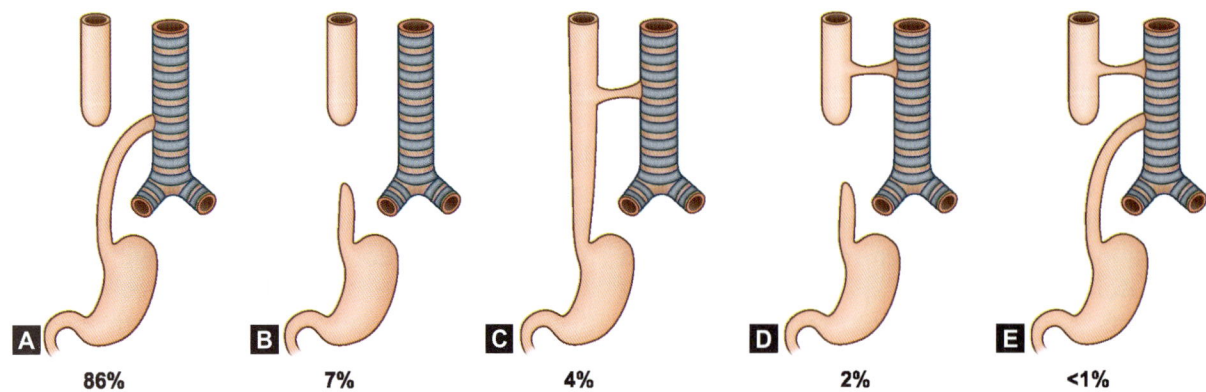

A 86%   **B** 7%   **C** 4%   **D** 2%   **E** <1%

Fig. 12.1. Types of oesophageal atresia with or without tracheo-oesophageal fistula

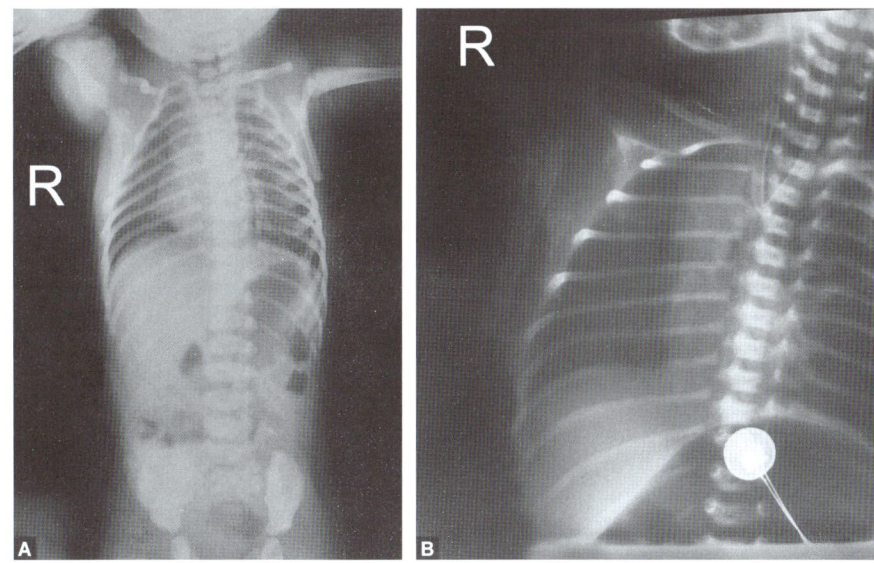

Fig. 12.2. Chest X-ray

Preoperative Preparation

The condition of the neonate should be stabilized before surgery. As oral feeding is not possible, intravenous fluids should be infused to prevent dehydration and hypoglycaemia. Prophylactic antibiotics reduce the risk of perioperative respiratory infection.[7] The neonate should be nursed in supine position with head raised. Continuous suction using Replogle tube or repeated suction of the upper oesophageal pouch and oropharynx is required to clear the secretions and thus reduce the risk of aspiration. Fluid-electrolyte and acid-base abnormalities should be corrected and chest condition should be optimized.

Echocardiography is important to diagnose any cardiac or vascular abnormality which could affect anaesthetic and surgical management and outcome. Haematological and biochemical profiles should be obtained and blood sample is sent for grouping and crossmatching.

Anaesthetic Management

The important concerns during anaesthetic management include ineffective ventilation due to inadvertent endotracheal tube placement in the fistula, massive gastric dilation, poor lung condition due to aspiration of gastric contents and/or respiratory distress syndrome of prematurity, and associated cardiac or other congenital anomalies.[4]

A major requirement is ability to ventilate lungs without ventilation of the fistula. To achieve this, either awake intubation or inhalation induction with spontaneous ventilation may be used to secure airway. To position the endotracheal tube properly, it is inserted as far as possible and then is slowly withdrawn until bilateral air entry is present on auscultation. If the fistula is large and just above the carina, various techniques can be used to prevent entry of the tip of the endotracheal tube into the fistula. A cuffed endotracheal tube may be used, the bevel may be directed anteriorly or a Fogarty catheter may be used to occlude the fistula until its ligation. Occasionally, the fistula may be at the carina or more distally. In these cases, bronchial intubation and one lung ventilation is required until ligation of the fistula. If facilities and expertise are available, a preoperative rigid bronchoscopy may be performed to define the position of the fistula and assess any other airway abnormality.[4]

Muscle relaxation with positive pressure ventilation can be started if, following endotracheal intubation, adequate ventilation can be achieved without gastric inflation.

The neonate is positioned in left lateral position with right arm raised across the head. This requires use of padding, tapes, and gel blocks. During the procedure, the surgeon usually compresses the lung to mobilize distal segment of oesophagus. This can result in desaturation which requires intermittent expansion of the lung. Other causes of intraoperative hypoxaemia include endobronchial intubation, endotracheal tube obstruction due to kinking, secretions or bleeding, kinking of bronchus or trachea, and atelectasis.[4]

The anaesthetist inserts a nasogastric tube which helps in identification of the upper oesophageal pouch. Later this tube is guided into the stomach by the surgeon before completing the oesophageal anastomosis. This is used to feed the baby in postoperative period.

Once the procedure is complete, the thoracic cavity is filled with saline. Absence of any bubbles on application of positive airway pressure confirms the integrity of the oesophageal repair.

Standard non-invasive monitors including pre-cordial stethoscope are used. Invasive arterial monitoring is indicated in patients with associated comorbid conditions, e.g. complex congenital heart disease or pulmonary disease, and during thoraco-scopic surgery.[8]

Postoperative Care

All these patients should be carefully monitored in neonatal intensive care unit. Neck of the neonate should never be extended while nursing or at the time of extubation otherwise the anastomosis can give way. Postoperative ventilation may be required in cases with poor preoperative lung condition or low birth weight. Analgesia is provided and intravenous fluids and antibiotics are continued. Feeding through nasogastric tube is usually started 48 hours after surgery.

Complications

Postoperative surgical complications include anastomotic leak, tracheomalacia, gastroesophageal reflux, recurrent TOF, dysmotility and stricture.[1]

CONGENITAL DIAPHRAGMATIC HERNIA

Congenital diaphragmatic hernia (CDH) is characterized by herniation of abdominal contents into thorax through a developmental defect in the diaphragm. It has an incidence of 1 in 2,000–4,000 live births and accounts for 8% of all major congenital anomalies.[9] Majority, approximately 90%, of diaphragmatic hernias are posterolateral with 80% left sided. Posterolateral diaphragmatic defects are known as Bochdalek hernia while the anterior defects are called Morgagni hernia.

Embryologically, the diaphragm develops during 8th to 12th weeks of gestation. Membranous septum transversum, pleuroperitoneal folds and muscle fibers from lateral thoracic wall join together to form diaphragm. Any failure of the process at any stage leads to a defect through which abdominal contents migrate into the thorax.[10]

Pathophysiology

Newborns with CDH have bilateral pulmonary hypoplasia, more severe on the affected side. Herniation of abdominal contents during gestation prevents growth of ipsilateral lung, whereas contra-lateral lung is affected due to mediastinal shift. The degree of pulmonary hypoplasia depends on the gestational age at which herniation occurs. Besides underdevelopment of airways, there is reduced arterial branching resulting in muscular hyperplasia of the pulmonary arterial tree. These changes result in increased pulmonary vascular resistance and pulmonary hypertension.[11] There is exaggerated response to hypoxia, hypercarbia and acidosis resulting in persistent pulmonary hypertension. This leads to persistent fetal circulation, right-to-left shunting (through the patent ductus arteriosus and foramen ovale) and intrapulmonary shunting, which exacerbates the hypoxia and hypercarbia.[12]

Associated Anomalies

CDH is associated with other congenital anomalies in about 40–50% cases.[13] These include cardiac defects mainly patent ductus arteriosus, septal defects, atrioventricular valve defects, and aortic arch hypoplasia; musculoskeletal; neural tube defects; duodenal atresia; renal anomalies; and chromosomal anomalies. Cardiac defects account for about half of all the defects.[14]

Diagnosis

Good quality ultrasound and fetal MRI can demonstrate congenital diaphragmatic hernia early in pregnancy.[10] Ultrasound at 20 weeks can show stomach or bowel loops in the chest with mediastinal shift, polyhydramnios and an absent intra-abdominal gastric bubble.[13] Fetal lung to head circumference ratio (LHR) less than 1.0 and herniation of left liver lobe in thorax indicate poor prognosis.[15]

The size of the diaphragmatic defect and the timing of migration of intra-abdominal structures into thorax is an important factor in early presentation with symptoms after birth. Clinically, the child presents with respiratory distress, cyanosis, reduced breath sounds and displaced apex beat to the contralateral side. Cyanosis, dyspnoea, and apparent dextrocardia constitute the classic triad of CDH.[16] Breath sounds are diminished or absent on the ipsilateral side, bowel sounds may be heard instead. The abdomen is scaphoid in shape.

A plain X-ray of chest confirms the diagnosis of CDH by demonstrating gas-filled bowel-loops in the thorax. A nasogastric tube shows mediastinal shift and defines the position of stomach. Compression of contralateral lung may be evident (Fig. 12.3).

Treatment

Fetal surgery has been described but is controversial. This involves *in utero* repair or plugging the trachea to encourage lung growth.[17]

After birth, the neonate requires surgical intervention. In contrast to previous practice of immediate

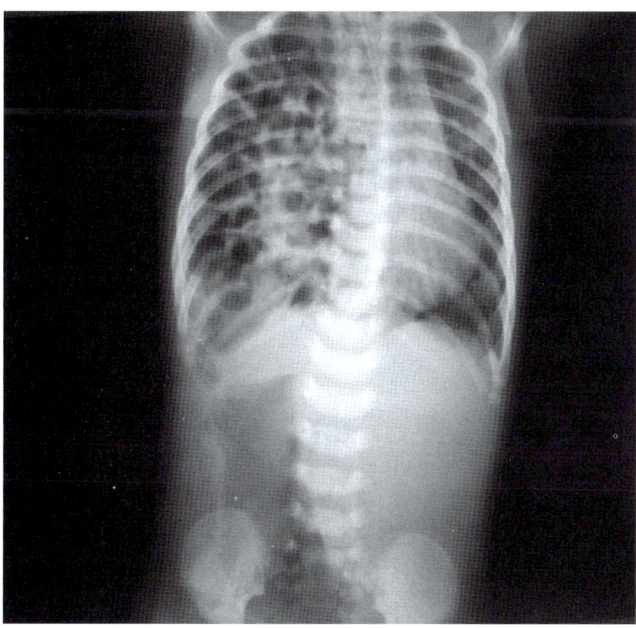

Fig. 12.3. CDH X-ray

surgery after birth, it is now recommended to delay the surgery until the neonate's condition has been stabilized. According to the CDH-EURO Consortium guidelines, surgery should be performed when the neonate has normal mean arterial blood pressure for the gestational age, pre-ductal saturation 85 to 95% at FiO_2 <0.5, lactate levels below 3 mmol/l and urine output more than 2 ml/kg/h.[18]

Surgical repair is typically carried out through the abdomen, with reduction of herniated contents and excision of sac before repair. The defect may be closed primarily by using locally available tissues or a muscle patch/inert graft may be needed. Right-sided CDH is preferably repaired through the thoracic approach. Nowadays, many surgeons repair the diaphragmatic defect by thoracoscopic approach with lesser morbidity and shorter hospital stay.[19]

Preoperative Care

The key to stabilization of neonates with congenital diaphragmatic hernia and severe respiratory distress is oxygenation with endotracheal intubation, paralysis and gentle ventilation. This can be done by conventional mechanical ventilation, high-frequency ventilation, inhaled nitric oxide or extracorporeal membrane oxygenation.[20]

Bag and mask ventilation should be avoided as distension of gut can further compress the intrathoracic contents and affect oxygenation. Therefore, early tracheal intubation and gastric decompression using a large bore nasogastric tube are recommended. Normovolaemia is aimed for and hypoxia, hypercarbia and acidosis are managed promptly.

Barotrauma must be avoided by limiting peak airway pressure to 25 cm H_2O and allowing permissive hypercapnia. The goals of oxygenation and mechanical ventilation are to achieve pre-ductal SaO_2 in the range of 85 to 95%, post-ductal SaO_2 above 70% and $PaCO_2$ 45–60 mm Hg.[18]

An echocardiography is needed to diagnose heart defects and to look for signs of pulmonary hypertension, shunting and left ventricular hypoplasia.[20] Inotropes may sometimes be necessary.

Anaesthetic Management

Intubation, if not already performed, should be done awake without bag and mask ventilation to prevent overdistension of stomach. If a child is vigorous, inhalational induction and intubation without muscle relaxant can be performed. Muscle relaxation and positive pressure ventilation is started after tracheal intubation. Nitrous oxide should not be used to avoid further bowel distension. Ventilation and oxygenation should be carefully controlled as hypoxaemia and hypercarbia can aggravate pulmonary artery hypertension. Therefore, PaO_2 should be maintained above 100 mm Hg and $PaCO_2$ below 40 mm Hg.[21] However, at the same time, care should be taken to avoid very high airway pressures during ventilation which can lead to barotrauma-induced pneumothorax. Haemodynamic stability should be maintained by adequate intravenous fluid management and avoiding anaesthetic agents with myocardial depressant action until herniated abdominal contents have been reduced and the chest has been decompressed. Analgesia is usually provided with high-dose fentanyl. Hypothermia increases oxygen consumption and should be avoided.

NEURAL TUBE DEFECTS

Neural tube defect (spinal dysraphism) is a common condition seen in neonates with a reported average incidence of 1 per 1000 live births.[22] This encompasses a spectrum of conditions which occur due to defective embryological development of neural arch during initial four weeks of gestation. There is protrusion of neural tissues and meninges on to the back. Neural tube defects can be classified into spina bifida occulta; and spina bifida aperta which includes meningocele, meningomyelocele, myelocele and rachischisis.

These conditions present with a lesion on the back, most commonly in the lumbosacral region. Meningomyelocele is the commonest presentation seen in clinical practice and is characterized by protrusion of meninges through a midline bony defect of the spine, forming a sac containing cerebrospinal fluid (CSF) with some components of neural tissues (Fig. 12.4). It is usually located in lumbosacral area. There is variable degree of neurological manifestations, like lower limb paresis, and bladder or bowel involvement. In meningocele, there is protrusion of meninges without any neural tissue in it. Damage to the covering meninges or skin could result in leakage of CSF and predisposition to meningitis.

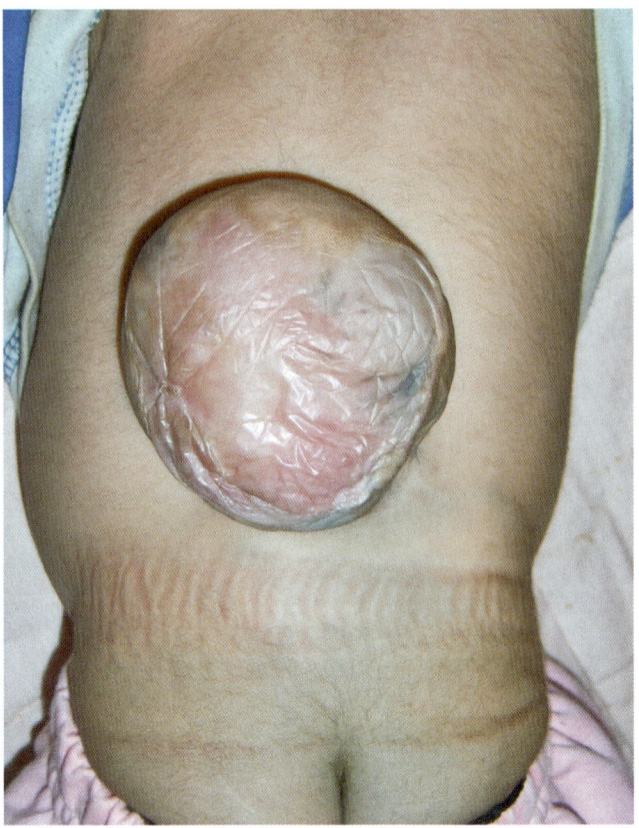

Fig. 12.4. Meningomyelocele

Associated Anomalies

Many cases with meningomyelocele have concomitant hydrocephalus. Arnold-Chiari malformation may be present which is characterized by downward displacement of cerebellar vermis into cervical spinal canal and elongation of brainstem and fourth ventricle. Other congenital malformations that may be associated with meningomyelocele include congenital heart disease, e.g. ASD or VSD, club feet, musculoskeletal defects, e.g. scoliosis or absent ribs, anorectal malformations, hip dislocation, facial clefts, umbilical hernia and VATER-L (vertebral, anal, tracheo-oesophageal fistula, renal and limb) anomalies.[23]

Diagnosis

The condition can be diagnosed by an antenatal ultrasound at about 18 weeks gestational age. Maternal serum or amniotic fluid alpha-fetoprotein levels are raised in open neural tube defects. Obstetrician should counsel the parents about the prognosis.

After birth, the anomaly is quite obvious; however, an ultrasound followed by magnetic resonance imaging (MRI) may be necessary to define the lesion.

Treatment

A multidisciplinary team is necessary for optimal management of such patients. Ruptured or leaking meningomyelocele needs emergent surgery within 24 hours. Otherwise also, this condition should be operated during initial 24 to 48 hours after birth as delayed surgery is associated with a higher rate of infection.[24] Aim of the surgery is to dissect and repose the neural tissue into the spinal canal and cover the defect with available tissue. If concomitant hydrocephalus is present, a shunt procedure is performed before or simultaneously with the repair of the lesion. Patients are followed up to assess the outcome, detect development of any neurological deficit and perform any corrective procedure as and when indicated. Mother is advised to take folic acid for few weeks before planning next pregnancy.

Preoperative Preparation

Good preoperative assessment is important to diagnose or rule out any associated congenital anomalies. For this, ultrasound, CT scan, MRI, echocardiography or urodynamic studies may be done as per the clinical indication. Besides haemoglobin, total leucocyte count in case of suspected infection and serum creatinine with urine examination in case of anomalies of urinary tract should be ordered. Blood grouping and crossmatching may be required in large defects.

Antisialogogue may be given as premedication.

Anaesthetic Management

Airway in these neonates may be particularly difficult as there may be associated hydrocephalus or facial clefts. Therefore, inhalational induction with sevoflurane is preferred. Special care should be taken in patients with Arnold-Chiari malformation as extension during intubation can lead to compression of cervical cord and brainstem.[25] These patients may have diminished response to hypoxia and may be more susceptible to postoperative apnoeic episodes.[26]

Position of the child during intubation is important. The swelling should be adequately padded and supported on a doughnut. The rest of the body should be placed on the pillows so as to avoid any pressure on the swelling. An alternative is to perform intubation in lateral position. Succinylcholine should be avoided in patients with neurological deficit. Nondepolarizing neuromuscular blocking agents, such as atracurium, can be used for muscle relaxation.

The surgical procedure is performed in prone position. Meticulous care is needed while positioning the child. Weight should be supported on bolsters kept under chest and pelvis with head well supported. Abdomen should be kept free. Eyes and all pressure points should be protected. Excessive flexion or extension of head should be avoided to prevent brainstem compression in patients with Arnold-Chiari malformation.

Blood loss assessment may be difficult due to simultaneous CSF loss. Sometimes there may be sudden blood loss from an abnormal vessel.[27] Unexplained hypotension could also occur due to sudden loss of CSF from sac leading to brainstem herniation.[28] All fluid deficits, including loss from the defect, should be replaced.

In many cases, spinal cord is tethered below the defect. These patients require intraoperative electromyography (EMG) monitoring to identify functional nerve roots. At the time of dural closure, the anaesthesiologist is asked to perform Valsalva manoeuvre to test the integrity of closure.[23]

Monitoring includes ECG, non-invasive blood pressure, pulse oximetry, capnography and temperature monitoring.

Although rare in India, patients having meningomyelocele may be allergic to latex, requiring precautions.[29]

HYDROCEPHALUS

Hydrocephalus can be defined broadly as a disturbance of cerebrospinal fluid (CSF) formation, flow, or absorption, leading to an increase in volume occupied by this fluid in the central nervous system (CNS).[30] This usually results in raised intracranial pressure (ICP). The normal ICP in neonates is 2–4 mm Hg. Presence of a large-sized head or a head that's growing very quickly in relation to the rest of the body is the main symptom of hydrocephalus. Other symptoms or signs could include vomiting, poor feeding, irritability, drowsiness, lethargy, bulging fontanelle, prominence of scalp veins and downward deviation of the eyes (setting sun sign).

The incidence of congenital hydrocephalus is 0.2–0.5 per 1000 live births.[31] An obstruction of the aqueduct of Sylvius is the most common cause of congenital hydrocephalus. This could occur due to blockage, infection, haemorrhage, tumour or arachnoid cyst. Other causes of congenital hydrocephalus include Arnold-Chiari malformations, neural tube defects or spina bifida, craniosynostosis, Dandy-Walker syndrome, etc.

Diagnosis

Antenatal diagnosis can be made in a fetus as early as the third or fourth month of pregnancy with the advancement in imaging techniques including ultrasound. Post-natal diagnostic modalities include ultrasound, computed tomography and magnetic resonance imaging (MRI) which can demonstrate the degree of ventricular enlargement and often the etiology of the hydrocephalus.[32]

Treatment

Medical treatment in hydrocephalus is used to delay surgical intervention. It may be tried in premature infants with post-hemorrhagic hydrocephalus. Normal CSF absorption may resume spontaneously during this interim period.

Acetazolamide, a carbonic anhydrase inhibitor, and osmotic diuretics decrease CSF secretion by the choroid plexus.[31] However, these drugs do not have sustained effects. These may induce metabolic consequences and thus should be used only as a temporizing measure.

Commonly available surgical options include shunt procedures and endoscopic third ventriculostomy (ETV). The principle of a shunt procedure is to establish a communication between the CSF—ventricular or lumbar; and a drainage cavity, i.e. peritoneum, right atrium or pleura. A ventriculo-peritoneal (VP) shunt is the most commonly performed procedure. Indian shunt systems in use include Upadhyaya shunt[33] or Chhabra shunt.[34]

Endoscopic fenestration of the floor of the third ventricle establishes an alternative route for CSF toward the subarachnoid space.

Anaesthetic Management

Care should be taken to maintain cerebral perfusion pressure (CPP) which is defined as the difference between mean arterial pressure (MAP) and sum of ICP and the central venous pressure (CVP). Therefore, measures should be taken to avoid fall in MAP and rise in ICP.

Anaesthesia can be induced by intravenous or inhalational route and airway is secured by tracheal intubation. Airway management may be difficult due to distorted anatomy of skull. As the head is large, a pillow kept under the body helps in proper alignment for laryngoscopy and intubation.

For VP shunt surgery, the patient is positioned supine with the head turned to the side opposite to the site of shunt placement. This allows good access to the surgeons. However, care should be taken to avoid endobronchial migration of tracheal tube and to maintain venous drainage by preventing obstruction of jugular vein.[35] Eyes should be carefully protected.

Hypotension should be avoided. Ketamine can increase ICP and thus should not be used. Non-depolarizing neuromuscular blocking agents are preferred for providing muscle relaxation. Succinyl-choline can be used, if risk of aspiration outweighs the risk of transient rise in ICP.[36] Normocarbia should be maintained as hypercarbia increases ICP by causing cerebral vasodilation and aggressive hypocarbia can cause brain ischaemia. A short-acting opioid, e.g. fentanyl is used, to provide analgesia.

As many neonates having hydrocephalus are premature with low birth weight, they may require ventilatory support in the postoperative period. Those who are extubated need intensive apnoea monitoring for 24 hours after surgery. Head up position should be avoided in postoperative period as it may result in subdural haemorrhage due to rapid collapse of ventricles.[36]

Postoperative analgesia can be provided by local infiltration with 0.25% bupivacaine and intravenous or rectal administration of paracetamol.

IDIOPATHIC HYPERTROPHIC PYLORIC STENOSIS

Idiopathic hypertrophic pyloric stenosis (HPS) is a condition characterized by thickening of pyloric portion of the stomach and manifests as obstruction to gastric emptying. Most infants present during initial month of life with forceful or projectile nonbilious vomiting after feeding. Occasionally, the vomitus may become blood-tinged because of gastritis. The condition is more common in males.

Associated Anomalies

Pyloric stenosis may be associated with cardiac anomalies, oesophageal atresia, Hirschprung's disease, intestinal malrotation, anorectal malformation, inguinal hernia and minor renal anomalies in 6–20% cases.[37]

Diagnosis

The diagnosis is initially suggested by the history. Palpation of a hypertrophied pyloric muscle, or "olive," is diagnostic in the majority of infants.[38] In doubtful cases, imaging can be used. Thickened prepyloric antrum can be demonstrated on ultrasound. The pyloric canal may range from 14 mm to more than 20 mm in length and the muscle thickness varies from 3 to 5 mm.[39] Contrast study can be performed in case of equivocal findings which demonstrates the "string" sign or "shoulder" sign.[40] The thickened muscle causes an external impression on the gastric antrum, termed the "shoulder sign".

Treatment

Vomiting of gastric contents leads to depletion of sodium, potassium, and hydrochloric acid, which results in severe dehydration and hypokalaemic, hypochloraemic metabolic alkalosis. Initially, urine is alkaline; however, in later stages, paradoxical aciduria can occur. The degree of dehydration can be estimated by clinical examination, urine output, and serum chloride and bicarbonate levels. Surgery should be deferred until the infant is appropriately resuscitated. Nasogastric tube helps to decompress and lavage the stomach. These infants require hospitalization and intravenous fluid replacement therapy which includes 0.9% saline in severely dehydrated and 5% dextrose in 0.45% saline in mild to moderate cases. When urine output has been demonstrated, 10 to 20 mEq/l of potassium chloride can be added to the fluids.[41] Serum electrolytes, skin turgor, moist mucous membranes, and urine output can be used as determinants of successful resuscitation and adequate hydration.

Surgery is performed once the child is stable and metabolic imbalance has been corrected. Classical surgical procedure of Ramstedt pyloromyotomy remains the gold standard. It can also be performed laparoscopically instead of open procedure. Recovery is generally uneventful.

Anaesthetic Management

These children are at a high risk for aspiration of gastric contents during induction of anaesthesia. Therefore, nasogastric suction using a wide-bore catheter should be performed with the infant in supine head down and both lateral positions immediately before induction.[37]

Either awake intubation or modified rapid sequence induction with cricoid pressure and gentle positive pressure ventilation can be used to secure the airway.[42] At the end of the surgery, trachea should be extubated in lateral position when neuromuscular recovery is complete and the infant is awake.

Good postoperative analgesia can be provided by infiltrating skin incision with 0.25% bupivacaine up to 1.0 ml/kg and paracetamol orally 10 to 15 mg/kg every 4 to 6 hours or rectally 40 mg/kg followed by 20 mg/kg every 6 hours.[21]

ABDOMINAL WALL DEFECTS: OMPHALOCELE AND GASTROSCHISIS (Figs 12.5 and 12.6)

Abdominal wall defects are congenital defects characterized by protrusion of intra-abdominal contents, like stomach, intestines, liver or other organs

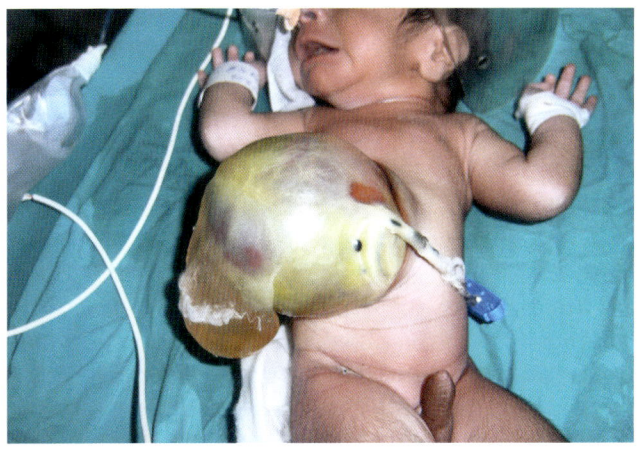

Fig. 12.5. Omphalocele

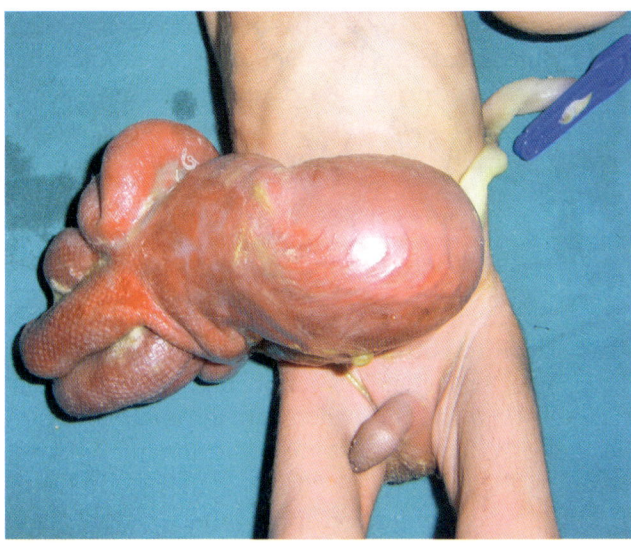

Fig. 12.6. *Gastroschisis*

out of the abdomen. These occur due to abnormal development of abdominal wall as a result of failure of various embryological components to fuse. The two main types of abdominal wall defects are gastroschisis and omphalocele (exomphalos). Gastroschisis develops when the abdominal wall does not completely close, and the abdominal organs are present outside the infant's body. Omphalocele occurs when some of the organs protrude through a para-umbilical defect in the abdominal wall. These organs are covered by a membrane consisting of Wharton's jelly, peritoneum, and amnion. Omphalocele can be classified as either minor or major on the bases of the size of defect and the sac.

The incidence of omphalocele is 1 in 13,000 live births; whereas the same for gastroschisis is 1 in 6,000 to 10,000 live births.[43]

Diagnosis

Gastroschisis and omphalocele can be differentiated on clinical examination. Gastroschisis occurs through a defect to the right of umbilicus, has no sac or covering and results in protrusion of stomach and intestines. It is usually not associated with other malformations or syndromes and has a good prognosis.[44] On the other hand, omphalocele occurs through an umbilical defect with a sac or membrane covering liver and intestines. It is associated with other malformations; can be part of syndromes and carries higher mortality.

Associated Anomalies

Cardiac anomalies, e.g. tetralogy of Fallot and atrial septal defect are the commonest (20%) malformations associated with omphalocele.[45] Some other associated anomalies include chromosomal trisomies, Beckwith–Wiedemann syndrome, pentalogy of Cantrell, extrophy of bladder or cloaca, imperforate anus, colonic atresia, vertebral anomalies and meningomyelocele.[43]

On the other hand, gastroschisis sometimes may be associated with other anomalies of gastrointestinal tract, e.g. intestinal atresia. Meckel's diverticulum and intestinal duplication.[45]

Management

While gastroschisis needs to be corrected immediately, surgical repair of omphalocele can be delayed till the patient is stabilized. In both the conditions, aim is to repose the protruded organs back into the abdominal cavity and close the abdominal wall with the locally available tissues with or without the help of prosthetic silos.

The newborns with either condition are kept nil orally, administered antibiotics and intravenous fluids. Loss of fluids and hypothermia is associated more with gastroschisis than omphalocele. The exposed bowel is covered with a moist dressing and the baby is nursed on side to prevent drag on the mesentery of the bowel. Nasogastric tube is inserted to decompress the bowel.

During surgery for gastroschisis, the protruded intestines are reposed back and the defect is closed. In omphalocele, the sac is excised and abdominal wall is closed after the protruded abdominal contents are reduced. In omphalocele major or some cases of gastroschisis, it may not be possible to attain primary closure of the abdominal wall. In such situations, a silo is created with prosthetic material. This is reduced gradually till abdomen can be closed.[46]

In some cases where the omphalocele is very large or is associated with other congenital malformations precluding primary repair, the sac is left intact. It gradually epithelializes leading to formation of ventral hernia that can be repaired at a later date.[47]

Preoperative Preparation

Considering the high incidence of associated congenital cardiac defects, patients with omphalocele should have an echocardiogram before receiving anaesthesia. In infants with gastroschisis and omphalocele, fluid and electrolyte imbalance must be corrected in the preoperative period.

Anaesthetic Management

Inherent tendency of neonates to be susceptible to hypothermia is exaggerated in these children due to exposure of bowel to environment. Therefore, it is necessary to take precautions to prevent heat loss. Nasogastric tube should be placed to decompress bowel before induction of anaesthesia. Besides preventing aspiration, it also facilitates subsequent abdominal closure. Nitrous oxide should not be used to avoid further distention of bowel. Intraoperative analgesia can be provided by fentanyl or morphine, if postoperative elective ventilation is planned. Single shot caudal block; or epidural or caudal catheter can be very useful to provide intraoperative and postoperative analgesia.[43] Third space fluid loss may be significant and should be adequately replaced using crystalloids or colloids. Any significant blood loss needs to be replaced by blood components.

After the protruded organs have been reduced, abdominal closure can proceed. The communication between the surgeon and the anaesthesiologist is of paramount importance at this stage as increased intraabdominal pressure due to forced closure can result in respiratory, haemodynamic and renal compromise. Respiratory compromise is indicated by significant rise in peak airway pressure and decrease in tidal volume or oxygen saturation. It is better to create a silo or ventral hernia rather than forced primary abdominal closure in such circumstances. Re-opening of abdomen and silastic pouch formation may be required in postoperative period, if the patient develops signs of compartment syndrome after primary closure. Therefore, close monitoring of the neonate after surgery is mandatory. A nasogastric tube with a saline column may be used to measure intra-gastric pressure. This pressure should be below 20 mm Hg for the primary closure to be successful.[48]

Postoperative ventilation may be indicated in some cases. Delayed motility of bowels is common with gastroschisis and the baby may need to be kept on intravenous fluids and parenteral nutrition for few days after surgery.

SUMMARY

Anaesthetic management of neonates undergoing surgery for congenital anomalies is a challenging task. The management of patients with one anomaly is made more complex due to coexisting anomalies in other organ systems which may have an impact on anaesthetic management. Anaesthesiologists need to be extra-vigilant due to labile physiology of the neonate which can change rapidly at any stage of management. Neonates require stabilization of haemodynamics and correction of fluid-electrolyte imbalance, hypothermia, hypoglycaemia, and sepsis, etc. They also need vigilant postoperative monitoring and care including good postoperative pain relief. Some of the neonate may require postoperative ventilation and intensive care management. There are certain specific perioperative management requirements for each surgical condition. It is imperative for the anaesthesiologist to be well aware of them so as to be able to efficiently manage this special patient group. Working in tandem with the surgeon is essential to improve the overall outcome.

The common congenital anomalies requiring surgery in neonates are oesophageal atresia with or without tracheo-oesophageal fistula, congenital diaphragmatic hernia, neural tube defects, hydrocephalus, idiopathic hypertrophic pyloric stenosis, abdominal wall defects, like gastroschisis or omphalocele, etc.

Oesophageal atresia encompasses a group of congenital anomalies characterized by an interruption of the continuity of the oesophagus combined with or without a persistent communication with the trachea. Oesophageal atresia with distal tracheo-oesophageal fistula (TOF) is the commonest defect. TOF may be associated with other congenital malformations. The best described is the VACTERL association which includes vertebral, anorectal, cardiac, tracheo-esophageal, renal, and limb malformations. The primary treatment includes right thoracotomy using extrapleural approach, division of tracheo-oesophageal fistula, and end-to-end anastomosis of two oesophageal ends. Preoperative preparation in a case of TOF includes correction of fluid-electrolyte and acid-base abnormalities and optimization of chest condition by intravenous fluids, antibiotics and regular suction of upper oesophageal pouch and oropharynx. Important concerns during anaesthetic management include ineffective ventilation due to inadvertent endotracheal tube placement in the fistula, massive gastric dilation, poor lung condition due to aspiration of gastric contents and/or respiratory distress syndrome of prematurity, and associated cardiac or other congenital anomalies. Either awake intubation or inhalation induction with spontaneous ventilation may be used and the tip of the tracheal tube should be positioned beyond the fistula. In postoperative period, neck of the neonate should never be extended while nursing or at the time of extubation. Postoperative ventilation may be required in cases with poor preoperative lung condition or low birth weight.

Congenital diaphragmatic hernia (CDH) is characterized by herniation of abdominal contents into thorax through a developmental defect in the diaphragm. These newborns have bilateral pulmonary hypoplasia, more severe on the affected side. There may be increased pulmonary vascular resistance and pulmonary hypertension. The exaggerated response to hypoxia, hypercarbia and acidosis results in persistent pulmonary hypertension. This can lead to persistent fetal circulation, right-to-left shunting and intrapulmonary shunting, which exacerbates hypoxia and hypercarbia. Surgery for CDH should be delayed until the neonate's condition has been stabilized with normal mean arterial blood pressure for gestational age, pre-ductal saturation 85 to 95% at FiO_2 <0.5, lactate levels below 3 mmol/l and urine output more than 2 ml/kg/h. Bag and mask ventilation should be avoided. Early tracheal intubation and gastric decompression using a large bore nasogastric tube are recommended. For ventilation, conventional mechanical ventilation, high-frequency ventilation, inhaled nitric oxide and extracorporeal membrane oxygenation have been used. Normovolaemia is aimed for and hypoxia, hypercarbia and acidosis are managed promptly. Intraoperatively, nitrous oxide should not be used. PaO_2 should be maintained above 100 mm Hg and $PaCO_2$ below 40 mm Hg. Very high airway pressures during ventilation can lead to barotrauma-induced pneumothorax and, therefore, should be avoided. Haemodynamic stability should be maintained by adequate intravenous fluid management and avoiding anaesthetic agents with myocardial depressant action.

Meningomyelocele is the commonest type of neural tube defect and is characterized by protrusion of meninges through a midline bony defect of the spine, forming a sac containing cerebrospinal fluid (CSF) with some components of neural tissues. It is usually located in lumbosacral area. Many cases with meningomyelocele have concomitant hydrocephalus or Arnold-Chiari malformation. Many other congenital anomalies may be present. Meningo-myelocele should be operated within initial 24 to 48 hours after birth. Position of the child during intubation is important. Special care should be taken in patients with Arnold-Chiari malformation as extension during intubation can lead to compression of cervical cord and brainstem. Also, these patients may have diminished response to hypoxia and may be more susceptible to postoperative apnoeic episodes.

Patients with hydrocephalus require shunt procedures or endoscopic third ventriculostomy (ETV). A ventriculoperitoneal (VP) shunt is the most commonly performed procedure. Cerebral perfusion pressure (CPP) should be maintained by avoiding fall in mean arterial pressure and rise in intracranial pressure (ICP).

Idiopathic hypertrophic pyloric stenosis (HPS) is a condition characterized by thickening of pyloric portion of the stomach and manifests as obstruction to gastric emptying. These infants may have severe dehydration and hypokalaemic, hypochloraemic metabolic alkalosis. Surgery should be deferred until the infant is appropriately resuscitated. Classical surgical procedure of Ramstedt pyloromyotomy remains the gold standard. Patients with HPS are at a high risk for aspiration of gastric contents during induction of anaesthesia. Therefore, nasogastric suction using a wide-bore catheter should be performed with the infant in supine head down and both lateral positions immediately before induction. Either awake intubation or modified rapid sequence induction with cricoid pressure and gentle positive pressure ventilation can be used to secure the airway.

The two main types of abdominal wall defects are gastroschisis and omphalocele. In gastroschisis, the abdominal wall does not completely close and the abdominal organs are present outside the neonate's body. Omphalocele occurs when some of the organs protrude through a paraumbilical defect in the abdominal wall. These organs are covered by a membrane consisting of Wharton's jelly, peritoneum, and amnion. Gastroschisis needs to be corrected immediately, whereas, surgical repair of omphalocele can be delayed till the patient is stabilized. These newborns are kept nil orally, administered antibiotics and intravenous fluids to correct fluid and electrolyte imbalance. The exposed bowel is covered with a moist dressing and the baby is nursed on side to prevent drag on the mesentery of the bowel. Nasogastric tube is inserted to decompress the bowel. Precautions should be taken to prevent heat loss. Bowel should be decompressed before induction of anaesthesia by nasogastric suction. Nitrous oxide should not be used to avoid further distention of bowel. Third space fluid loss may be significant and should be adequately replaced. In some cases, it may not be possible to attain primary closure of the abdominal wall. In such situations, a silo is created with prosthetic material. Some cases may require postoperative ventilation.

REFERENCES

1. Spitz L. Oesophageal atresia. Orphanet J Rare Dis May, 2007;11(2):24.

2. Gupta A. Tracheo-oesophageal fistula, oesophageal atresia & anaesthetic management. Indian J Anaesth 2002;46(5): 353–355.

3. Brown AK, Roddam AW, Spitz L, Ward SJ. Oesphageal atresia, related malformations and medical problems: a family study. Am J Med Genet 1999;85(1): 31–37.

4. Gayle JA, Gómez SL, Baluch A, Fox C, Lock S, Kaye A. Anesthetic considerations for the neonate with tracheo-oesophageal fistula. MEJ Anesth 2008;19(6):1241–1254.

5. Rothenberg SS. Management of associated anomalies of oesophageal atresia and tracheo-oesophageal fistula. J Laparoendosc Adv Surg Tech A 2012;22:195–199.

6. Ron O, De Coppi P, Pierro A. The surgical approach to esophageal atresia repair and the management of long-gap atresia: results of a survey. Semin Pediatr Surg 2009; 18:44–49.

7. Al-Rawi O, Booker PD. Oesophageal Atresia and Tracheoesophageal Fistula. Continuing Education in Anaesthesia, Critical Care & Pain 2007;7(1):15–19.

8. Broemling N, Campbell F. Anesthetic management of congenital tracheoesophageal fistula. Pediatr Anesth 2011; 21(11):1092–1099.

9. King H, Booker PD. Congenital diaphragmatic hernia in the neonate. Continuing Education in Anaesthesia, Critical Care & Pain 2005;5(5):171–174.

10. Waag KL, Loff S, Zahn K, Ali M, Hien S, Kratz M, Neff W, Schaffelder R, Schaible T. Congenital diaphragmatic hernia: a modern day approach. Semin Pediatr Surg 2008;17:244–254.

11. Bloss RS, Aranda JV, Beardmore HE. Congenital diaphragmatic hernia: pathophysiology and pharmacologic support. Surgery 1981;89(4):518–524.

12. Graves ED, Redmond CR, Arensman RM. Persistent pulmonary hypertension in the neonate. Chest 1988;93(3): 638–641.

13. Doherty C, MacKinnon RJ. Congenital diaphragmatic hernia—an update. Infant 2006;2(6):244–248.

14. Mielniczuk M, Kusza1 K, Brzeziński P, Jakubczyk M, Mielniczuk K, Czerwionka-Szaflarska M. Current guidelines on management of congenital diaphragmatic hernia. Anaesthesiology Intensive Therapy 2012;44(4):232–237.

15. Brown RA, Bosenberg AT. Evolving management of congenital diaphragmatic hernia. Paediatr Anaesth 2007; 17:713–719.

16. Brett CM, Davis PJ, Bikhazi G. Anesthesia for neonates and premature infants. In: Motoyama EK, Davis P (Eds.) Smiths Anesthesia for infants and children. 7th edn. Philadelphia, Mosby 2005;pp.5456.

17. Bosenberga AT, Brown RA. Management of congenital diaphragmatic hernia. Curr Opin Anaesthesiol 2008;21: 323–331.

18. Reiss I, Schaible T, van den Hout L, Capolupo I, Allegaert K, van Heijst A, et al. Standardized postnatal management of infants with congenital diaphragmatic hernia in Europe: The CDH EURO Consortium consensus. Neonatology 2010;98(4):354–364.

19. Gourlay DM, Cassidy LD, Sato TT, Lal DR, Arca MJ. Beyond feasibility: a comparison of newborns undergoing thoracoscopic and open repair of congenital diaphragmatic hernias. J Pediatr Surg 2009;44(9):1702–1707.

20. Tonks A, Wyldes M, Abhyankar A, Bagchi I, Dent K, Kilby M, et al. West Midlands. Congenital Anomaly Register. Congenital Diaphragmatic Hernia. 1995-2000. Available at www.perinatal.nhs.uk/car/reports/CDH%20report. pdf. Accessed on 15th May 2015.

21. Cote CJ. Pediatric anesthesia. In: Miller RD (Ed). Miller's Anesthesia, 7th edn. Philadelphia, Churchill Livingstone, 2010;2559–2596.

22. Salih MA, Murshid WR, Seidahmed MZ. Epidemiology, prenatal management, and prevention of neural tube defects. Saudi Med J 2014;35(Suppl 1):S15–28.

23. Bakshi S, Myatra S. Meningomyelocele. In: Kulkarni AP, Divatia JV, Patil VP, Gehdoo RP (Eds). Objective Anaesthesia Review: A Comprehensive Textbook for the Examinees 3rd edn. New Delhi. Jaypee 2013;141–145.

24. Herman JM, McLone DG, Storrs BB, Dauser RC. Analysis of 153 patients with myelomeningocele or spinal lipoma operated upon for a tethered cord: Presentation, management and outcome. Paediatric Neurosurgery 1993;19: 243–249.

25. Chand MB, Agrawal J, Bista P. Anaesthetic challenges and management of myelomeningocele repair. Postgraduate Medical Journal of NAMS 2011;11(1):41–46.

26. Bell WO, Charney EB, Bruce DA, Sutton LN, Schut L. Symptomatic Arnold-Chiari malformation: review of experience with 22 cases. J Neurosurg 1987;66:812–816.

27. Rath GP, Dash HH. Anaesthesia for neurosurgical procedures in paediatric patients. Indian J Anaesth 2012; 56(5):502–510.

28. Afroza S, Ali Z, Prabhakar H. Severe systemic hypotension during repair of leaking large meningomyelocele. J Anesth 2008;22:59–60.

29. Yassin MS, Sanyurah S, Lierl MB, Fischer TJ, Oppenheimer S, Cross J, et al. Evaluation of latex allergy in patients with meningomyelocele. Ann Allergy 1992;69(3):207–211.

30. Rekate HL. A contemporary definition and classification of hydrocephalus. Semin Pediatr Neurol 2009;16:9–15.

31. Venkataramana NK. Hydrocephalus Indian scenario—A review. J Pediatr Neurosci 2011;6(Suppl 1):S11–22.

32. Dinçer A, Özek MM. Radiologic evaluation of pediatric hydrocephalus. Childs Nerv Syst 2011;27:1543–1562.

33. Upadhyaya P, Bhargava S, Dube S, Sundaram KR, Ochaney M. Results of ventriculoatrial shunt surgery for hydrocephalus using Indian shunt valve: evaluation of intellectual performance with particular reference to computerized axial tomography. Prog Pediatr Surg 1982; 15:209–222.

34. Chhabra DK, Agrawal GD, Mittal P. "Z" flow hydrocephalus shunt, a new approach to the problem of hydrocephalus, the rationale behind its design and the initial results of pressure monitoring after "Z" flow shunt implantation. Acta Neurochir (Wien) 1993;121(1–2):43–47.

35. Nienaber J. Anaesthesia for ventriculoperitoneal shunts. South Afr J Anaesth Analg 2011;17(1):73–75.

36. Myatra S, Bakshi S, Bhosale S. Hydrocephalus. In: Kulkarni AP, Divatia JV, Patil VP, Gehdoo RP (Eds). Objective Anaesthesia Review: A Comprehensive Textbook for the Examinees, 3rd edn. Jaypee, New Delhi 2013;132–140.

37. Fell D, Chelliah S. Infantile pyloric stenosis. BJA CEPD Reviews 2001;1(3):85–88.

38. Irish MS, Pearl RH, Caty MG, Glick PL. The approach to common abdominal diagnosis in infants and children. Pediatr Clin North Am 1998;45:729–772.

39. Cohen HL, Zinn HL, Haller JO, Homel PJ, Stoane JM. Ultrasonography of pylorospasm: findings may simulate hypertrophic pyloric stenosis. J Ultrasound Med 1998; 17(11):705–711.

40. Hernanz-Schulman M. Infantile hypertrophic pyloric stenosis. Radiology 2003;227(2):319–331.

41. Aspelund G, Langer JC. Current management of hypertrophic pyloric stenosis. Semin Pediatr Surg 2007;16(1): 27–33.

42. Roberts JD, Romanelli TM, Todres ID. Neonatal emergencies. In: Coté CJ, Lerman J, Todres ID (Eds): A Practice of Anesthesia for Infants and Children, 4th edn, Elsevier Health Science, Philadelphia 2008;pp.747–766.

43. Poddar R, Hartley L. Exomphalos and gastroschisis. Continuing Education in Anaesthesia, Critical Care & Pain 2009;9(2):48–51.

44. Holland AJ, Walker K, Badawi N. Gastroschisis: an update. Pediatr Surg Int 2010;26(9):871–878.

45. Bruch SW, Langer JC. Omphalocele and gastroschisis. In: Prem P, (Ed). Newborn Surgery, 2nd edn. London: Arnold 2003;605–613.

46. Marven S, Owen A. Contemporary postnatal surgical management strategies for congenital abdominal wall defects. Semin Pediatr Surg 2008;17:222–235.

47. van Eijck FC, Aronson DA, Hoogeveen YL, Wijnen RM. Past and current surgical treatment of giant omphalocele: outcome of a questionnaire sent to authors. J Pediatr Surg 2011;46(3):482–488.

48. Yaster M, Buck JR, Dudgeon DL, et al. Hemodynamic effects of primary closure of omphalocele/gastroschisis in human newborns. Anesthesiology 1988;69:84–88.

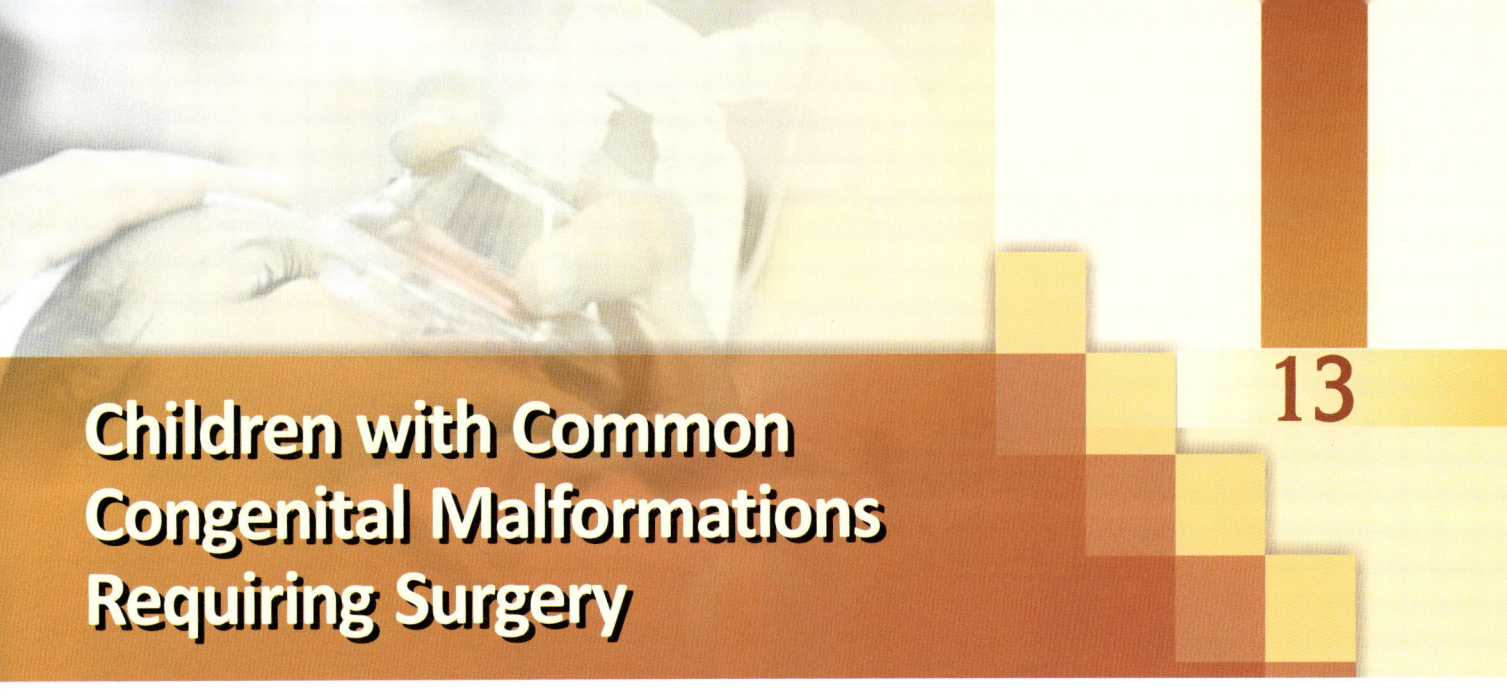

Children with Common Congenital Malformations Requiring Surgery

13

Medha Mohta, Priyanka Khurana

- ■ **Cleft lip and cleft palate**
  - ● Classification
  - ● Embryology
  - ● Associated congenital anomalies
  - ● Problems associated with cleft lip/palate
  - ● Anaesthetic management
- ■ **Congenital inguinal hernia**
  - ● Anaesthetic considerations
  - ● Regional anaesthesia techniques for Inguinal hernia
- ■ **Congenital Talipes Equinovarus**
  - ● Perioperative considerations
  - ● Tourniquet application
  - ● Caudal block
  - ● Postoperative management

A large number of children are born with congenital anomalies which require correction during early childhood. Some common anomalies include cleft lip, cleft palate, inguinal hernia and congenital talipes equinovarus. The anaesthesiologists in most of the centres encounter these patients quite often and, therefore, should be familiar with the anaesthetic management of all these conditions. The general principles of the management remain same as that for any other paediatric patient. However, each of these anomalies has certain specific considerations. This chapter discusses in brief the anaesthetic concerns with their management in these common congenital anomalies.

CLEFT LIP AND PALATE

Cleft lip and palate is one of the most common congenital anomalies seen in children. The overall incidence of cleft lip/palate is 1 in 800 live births, with cleft palate alone occurring in 1 in 2000 live births.[1] Cleft lip alone or in association with cleft palate is more common in males; however, isolated cleft palate is more common in females.[2] Both genetic and environmental factors may contribute to the aetiology of this congenital anomaly.

Cleft lip and palate may present as a sole anomaly or may be a part of various syndromes. If left uncorrected, children develop feeding, speech, hearing, dentition development and psychological problems. Surgical correction aims to restore both function and cosmesis.

Classification (Figs 13.1to 13.3)

1. **Isolated cleft lip:** Cleft lip can be unilateral or bilateral, complete or incomplete. Unilateral cleft lip is more common on left side. Complete cleft lip extends from the lip to the base of the nostril.
2. **Isolated cleft palate:** Cleft palate can also be unilateral or bilateral; complete or incomplete. Incomplete cleft palate has defect in the secondary palate which is posterior to the incisive foramen whereas complete cleft palate has defect in both primary and secondary palate.
3. **Cleft lip with cleft palate:** Cleft lip can present in combination with cleft palate.

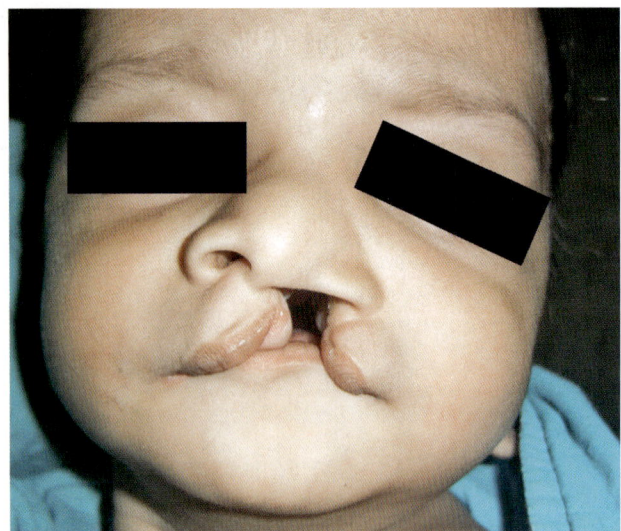

Fig. 13.1. Unilateral complete cleft lip

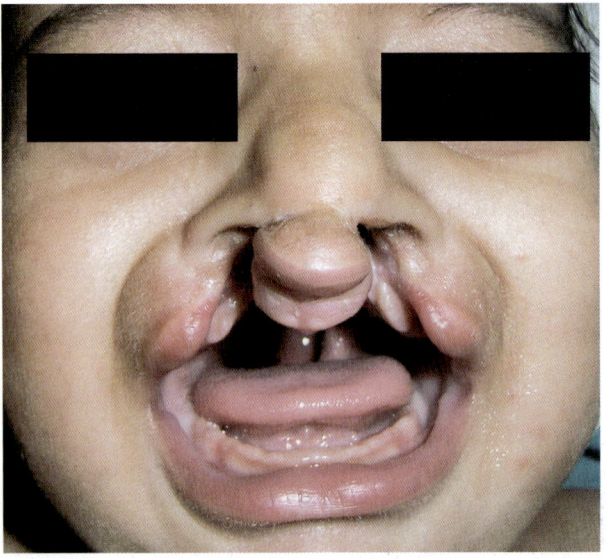

Fig. 13.2. Bilateral complete cleft lip

4. Submucosal cleft: Submucosal cleft has defect in the bone without any defect in the mucosa.

Embryology/Aetiology

Lip and primary palate develop from fusion of bilateral maxillary processes with the midline frontonasal process at around 6 weeks. Few weeks later, secondary palatal shelves fuse in the midline to separate the oral cavity from the nasal cavity. Any defect in the fusion of these processes leads to cleft lip and palate.

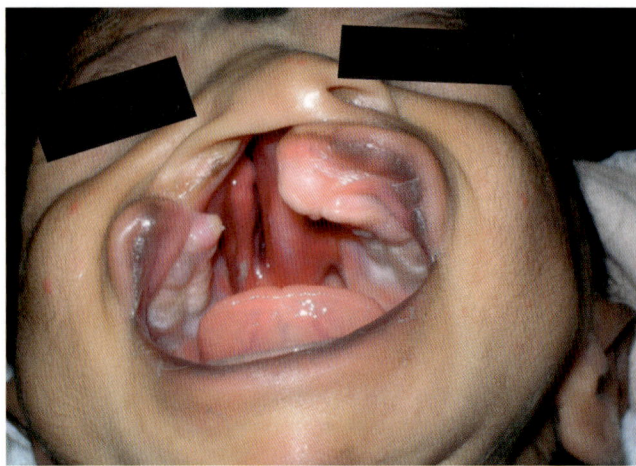

Fig. 13.3. Cleft palate (From Difficult Airway chapter)

Cleft may develop due to chromosomal aberrations or maternal factors, like high maternal age or intake of alcohol, benzodiazepines, anticonvulsants, salicylates or cortisone. The role of folic acid in prevention of cleft lip and palate is controversial.[3]

Associated Congenital Anomalies

Cleft lip and palate is commonly associated with various syndromes. This condition may be associated with other anomalies without any recognized syndrome. Craniofacial anomalies, congenital heart diseases, skeletal and renal anomalies are most frequently associated.

Following are the common syndromes associated with cleft lip and palate:

a. *Velocardiofacial syndrome (22q11 deletion)*
   - Most common associated syndrome
   - Velopharyngeal incompetence
   - Congenital cardiac disease
   - Immune deficiency

b. *Pierre Robin syndrome*
   - Cleft palate in 80% of cases
   - Micrognathia
   - Glossoptosis
   - Deafness
   - Hypermobility of joints

c. *Treacher Collins syndrome*
   - Cleft palate in ~30% of cases
   - Hypoplasia of zygomatic bones and mandible
   - Eye and ear abnormalities

- Deafness
- Choanal stenosis or atresia
- Significant risk of airway obstruction in neonatal period

d. *Down's syndrome*
- Macroglossia
- Microstomia
- Atlantoaxial subluxation and instability
- Small stature
- Mental retardation
- Congenital cardiac disease

e. *Goldenhar syndrome (hemifacial microsomia)*
- Incomplete development of palate, lip, nose, ear and mandible on one side of the face
- Scoliosis
- Renal and lung abnormalities

f. *Foetal alcohol syndrome*
- Small palpebral fissures
- Smooth philtrum
- Thin upper lip
- Growth deficiency
- CNS abnormalities, microcephaly.

In Pierre Robin syndrome, intubation becomes easier with age due to mandibular growth; whereas in Treacher Collins and Goldenhar syndromes, intubation may become more difficult with increasing age.

Problems Associated with Cleft Lip/palate

Upper Respiratory Tract Infection

These children have regurgitation of milk into nasal cavity leading to recurrent rhinorrhoea. Associated velopharyngeal incompetence may cause difficulty in swallowing, leading to regurgitation and aspiration. Eustachian tube dysfunction is present in all children with cleft palate causing chronic serous otitis media.[4] The incidence of infection increases with the severity of defect.[5]

Feeding Difficulty

Infants have difficulty in sucking due to inability to make an effective seal and create negative pressure. Feeding should be done in upright position so that gravity helps in swallowing. A long-handled spoon or a bottle with specially designed Haberman nipple is helpful. This nipple has a one-way valve which does not allow the milk to flow back and a slit valve near the tip which prevents baby from being overwhelmed with milk. It minimizes baby's efforts for sucking and also decreases chances of regurgitation and aspiration.[6]

Nutrition

Because of feeding problems, these children are usually malnourished and dehydrated. Increased effort for feeding leads to fatigue and impaired weight gain. Nutritional deficiencies, like anaemia, are common.

Dentition (Fig. 13.4)

These children have abnormal dentition, like missing, rotated or supernumerary teeth. Abnormality of dentition may also contribute to speech difficulty.

Speech Problems

Children with cleft palate have hypernasal speech as they are unable to build up air pressure in the mouth due to escape of air out of nose. They have difficulty in making plosive sounds, like p/k/t/d and s/sh.

Chronic Airway Obstruction

Upper airway obstruction is common in patients with cleft palate. These children are usually snorers and may develop apnoea during feeds, have prolonged feeding time and failure to thrive because of inability to coordinate feeding and breathing. Recurrent airway

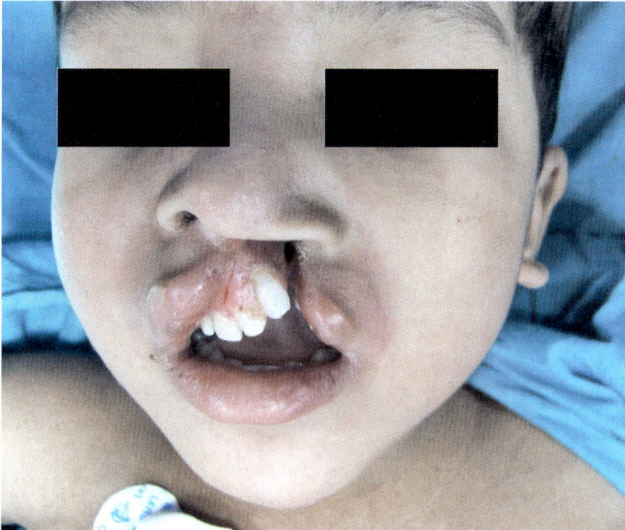

Fig. 13.4. Unilateral cleft lip with abnormal dentition

obstruction may cause chronic hypoxia, right ventricular hypertrophy and cor pulmonale.[7]

Treatment

Treatment is by surgical correction, but a team approach with involvement of surgeons, anaesthesiologist, speech therapist, orthodontist and lactation consultant is required for the overall development of the child.

Surgical repair of cleft lip is done between 6 and 12 weeks but at various centres, early repair during neonatal period is done to facilitate bonding and feeding.[8] Cleft lip repair has also been performed *in utero* and has been shown to minimize scarring.[9] Cleft palate repair is most commonly performed as a single stage procedure at 6 to 12 months. However, if it is associated with cleft lip, primary palate may be repaired along with cleft lip followed by repair of secondary palate at a later age.

In case of syndromic patients, multiple surgeries may be required for correction of associated craniofacial anomalies. Pharyngoplasty is needed in patients with cleft palate for co-existent velopharyngeal insufficiency. Velopharyngeal insufficiency leads to feeding and breathing problems and development of hypernasal speech due to inability of soft palate to approximate with posterior pharynx and close nasopharynx.

Anaesthetic Management

Preoperative Assessment and Preparation

Detailed history and physical examination should be done in all patients. In patients with other congenital conditions, respective systemic evaluation should also be performed. Availability of bank blood should be ensured in cases of large cleft palates. Complete haemogram is routinely done in all cases. Chest X-ray and ECG are required only in cases with cardiac and pulmonary involvement. Echocardiography may be done in patients with congenital heart anomalies.

Patient should be in good general condition and nutrition and hydration status should be taken care of in preoperative period. These patients usually have chronic rhinorrhoea; however, any evidence of acute infection should be treated as it reduces the incidence of postoperative respiratory complications. Surgical repair itself reduces the incidence of infections and thus risk and benefits of postponing surgery should be weighed individually.

These children frequently have difficult airway and thorough airway assessment should be performed preoperatively. Syndromic patients have associated airway problems due to other craniofacial anomalies. In non-syndromic patients, laryngoscopy and intubation may be difficult due to retrognathia and presence of maxillary protrusion in cases of bilateral cleft lip.

In very young patients (less than 6 months), there is no requirement of sedation. In older children, sedation should be advised, if there is no risk of airway obstruction. Oral midazolam in the dose of 0.25 to 0.5 mg/kg is most commonly prescribed.

Atropine or glycopyrrolate have an important role, if there is anticipated difficult airway. These should not be used routinely as tachycardia may obscure intraoperative hypovolaemia and inadequate depth of anaesthesia.

All anaesthetic equipment including suction and equipment for difficult airway should be checked and kept ready before induction. Pulse oximetry, non-invasive blood pressure, capnography, ECG, temperature and, wherever available, end tidal gases should be monitored.

Intraoperative Management

All these cases are conducted under general anaesthesia with endotracheal intubation and controlled ventilation. Inhalational induction with sevoflurane or halothane is routinely performed. In cases where preoperative intravenous access is available, intravenous induction with propofol or thiopentone is a safe alternative. Neuromuscular blocking agents are not administered until adequate ventilation with mask is ensured.

With increase in the severity of cleft palate, chances of airway obstruction decrease. However, in children with very wide cleft and hypoplastic mandible, tongue can prolapse into nasopharynx causing obstructed airway.[2] In such cases, the patient can be turned in lateral or semiprone position and nasopharyngeal and oropharyngeal airways or laryngeal mask airway (LMA) can be used to maintain a patent airway. Laryngoscopy may be difficult due to tendency of the laryngoscope blade to fall into the cleft. A piece of gauze can be placed within the gap to avoid this problem or a straight laryngoscope blade may be used.[10]

Intubation is performed with RAE (Ring, Adair, Elwin) south polar or reinforced tube. Endotracheal tube is always fixed in the midline on the lower lip. This fixation maintains facial symmetry in case of cleft lip and allows placement of mouth gag in case of cleft palate. Special care should be taken in tube fixation as due to sharing of airway with the surgeons, accidental dislodgment of endotracheal tube can occur during the procedure.

In patients with difficult airway, other adjuncts, like gum elastic bougie, LMA or fibreoptic bronchoscope, can be used to secure the airway. Pharyngeal pack is inserted by the anaesthesiologist or the surgeon to absorb blood and secretions intraoperatively. Head is placed on a ring and neck extension is achieved by placing a roll under the shoulders. Eyes should be adequately protected. During palate surgery, the surgeon applies Dingman mouth gag which has a slot for the tracheal tube in the midline. Final position of the tube should be confirmed after positioning and application of mouth gag. Any displacement or compression of the tube by mouth gag can be observed by leak or increase in airway pressure. Surgeons usually inject local anaesthetic with adrenaline to reduce surgical bleeding and improve surgical plane. Careful monitoring is required at this time as volatile anaesthetic agents sensitize the myocardium to the arrhythmogenic effects of adrenaline.

Opioids are most commonly used to attain intraoperative analgesia. Supplemental analgesia can be provided with intravenous or rectal paracetamol. Bilateral infraorbital nerve block is an effective means of providing analgesia in children undergoing cleft lip repair.[11] Infraorbital nerve can be blocked at its point of emergence from the infraorbital foramen which lies in line with the supraorbital notch and mental foramen. The needle is inserted perpendicular to the skin until bony resistance is felt and 1 to 2 ml of 0.5% bupivacaine with 1:200000 adrenaline is injected.

Greater palatine nerve provides the sensory supply to the mucous membrane of hard palate and gums. Bilateral greater palatine nerve block can provide analgesia in cleft palate repair. One to 1.5 ml of local anaesthetic is administered at point of emergence of the nerve from its foramen which lies medial and anterior to 2nd and 3rd molars.[12]

Before reversal throat pack is removed and oropharynx suctioned to remove pooled blood and secretions. Suctioning should be gentle to avoid trauma to surgical repair.

The tracheal extubation should be performed in awake state because partial or complete airway obstruction is common after cleft palate repair. After extubation, child is placed in lateral position to minimize risk of aspiration. In patients with preoperative airway obstruction, a tongue stitch is often placed by the surgeons at the end of the procedure which pulls the tongue forward away from the posterior pharyngeal wall.

Transfusion is rarely required in cases of cleft lip but blood loss may be significant in large palates requiring transfusion.

Postoperative Management

Postoperative airway obstruction is common after palatal surgery. It can occur due to reduction in size of airway after surgery and oedema of tongue due to application of mouth gag. Residual effect of anaesthesia and laryngeal oedema due to endotracheal intubation are other factors which can contribute to airway obstruction. The child should also be observed for postoperative bleeding and aspiration.

The analgesic effect of intraoperative nerve blocks may be supplemented with oral or rectal paracetamol and non-steroidal anti-inflammatory drugs.

CONGENITAL INGUINAL HERNIA

Inguinal hernia repair is a very common surgical procedure performed in children. The incidence of congenital inguinal hernia is 3–5% with greater preponderance in males.[13] In majority of children, it is indirect and arises from patent processus vaginalis. Inguinal hernia should be repaired shortly after diagnosis otherwise it can lead to entrapment of viscera resulting in obstruction or even strangulation. Congenital hernia repair is usually done as a day care procedure. The open procedure still remains the common approach but these days laparoscopic technique has also become popular (Figs 13.5 and 13.6).

Anaesthetic Considerations

Balanced general anaesthesia using LMA or endotracheal intubation is the most frequently used

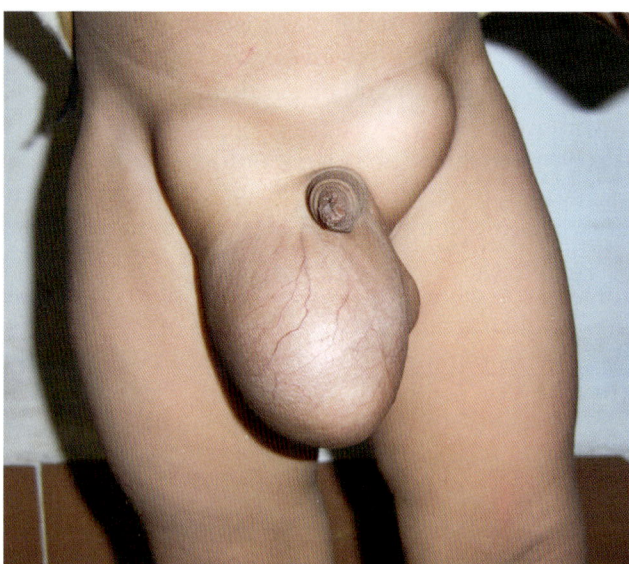

Fig. 13.5. Bilateral inguinal hernia

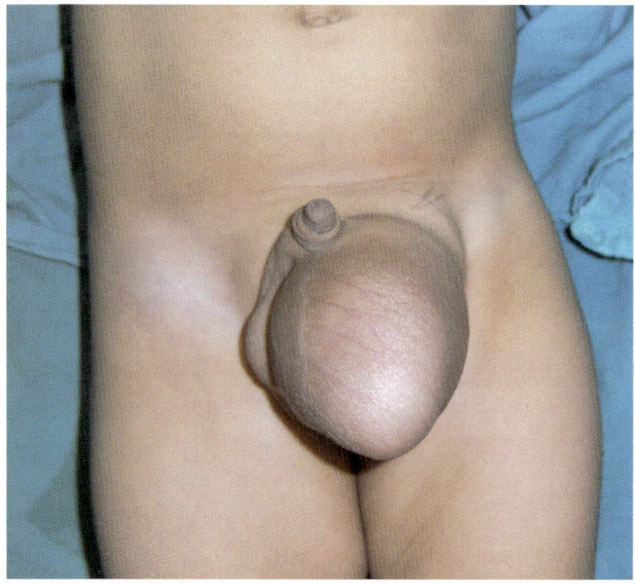

Fig. 13.6. Inguinal hernia with hydrocele

technique. Intravenous induction is preferred but in cases where intravenous access is not available, inhalational induction is equally acceptable. Spontaneous ventilation with intermittent support may be used for maintenance. Apart from systemic agents, perioperative analgesia can be supplemented with various regional anaesthetic techniques, like ilioinguinal iliohypogastric nerve block, caudal block or transversus abdominis plane (TAP) block.

The incidence of inguinal hernia escalates with increasing prematurity.[13] The preterm neonates undergoing general anaesthesia are very prone to cardiac and respiratory complications, particularly apnoea. Although former preterm infants up to 60 weeks postconceptual age can develop post-anaesthetic apnoea, those younger than 46 weeks are at the greatest risk.[14] Postanaesthesia apnoea in preterm infants can be due to multiple reasons which include immature respiratory drive, diaphragmatic fatigue, anaemia, obstructed airway, hypothermia and residual effect of anaesthetic drugs.[13]

In this group of high-risk patients, regional anaesthesia, especially central neuraxial blockade, is advocated. However, the risk of apnoea cannot be completely eliminated by regional anaesthesia. General anaesthesia can be administered in such infants but use of opioids and muscle relaxants should be avoided.[15] In infants with postconceptual age less than 46 weeks, continuous postoperative respiratory monitoring for 12 hours is recommended. In those between 46 and 60 weeks, respiratory monitoring for 12 hours should be done if history of apnoeic episodes, anaemia or neurological disease is present.[15]

Regional Anaesthesia Techniques for Inguinal Hernia

Caudal Block

Caudal block is the commonest regional technique used to provide perioperative analgesia in children undergoing hernia repair. Bupivacaine or ropivacaine in a volume of 1 ml/kg provides adequate analgesia. Various adjuvants, e.g. magnesium, ketamine and tramadol, etc. have been recently studied to improve the quality and duration of caudal analgesia in children undergoing inguinal hernia repair and have shown good results.[16,17]

Ilioinguinal and Iliohypogastric Nerve Block

These nerves provide sensation to the skin above the inguinal ligament and scrotum and can be blocked using anatomical landmarks or ultrasonography. The landmark for this block is a point 1 cm medial and caudal to the anterior superior iliac spine. Bupivacaine 0.25% in the dose of 1 mg/kg up to a maximum of 10 ml provides good analgesia.

Transversus Abdominis Plane Block

Transversus abdominis plane (TAP) block can be performed either by blind technique or under ultrasound guidance. Local anaesthetic is injected in the plane between internal oblique and transversus abdominis muscles. In blind technique, the entry point for the needle is lumbar triangle of Petit which is formed by latissimus dorsi posteriorly, external oblique muscle anteriorly and iliac crest inferiorly with the apex of the triangle at lower costal margin. After needle insertion, two pops are felt as the needle pierces through the external and internal oblique muscles. Local anaesthetic is injected after the second pop. Ultrasound guidance improves the efficacy of the block. In this the probe is kept in transverse plane to lateral abdominal wall in midaxillary line.[18] Bupivacaine 0.25% 0.5 ml/kg has been used with good results.[19]

CONGENITAL TALIPES EQUINOVARUS

The congenital talipes equinovarus (CTEV), also known as clubfoot, is a common developmental disorder of lower limb. It occurs in 1 in 1,000[20] to 1 in 400[21] live births and is more common in boys. The deformity has four components: ankle equinus, i.e. the foot points downward, hindfoot varus, i.e. inward turning of foot, forefoot adductus, i.e. the forefoot curls toward the heel, and midfoot cavus, i.e. increase in height of midfoot. It can be unilateral or bilateral. The condition is easily diagnosed at birth but can also be detected during prenatal ultrasound. Approximately one fourth of these patients have a family history of idiopathic CTEV (Fig. 13.7).[22]

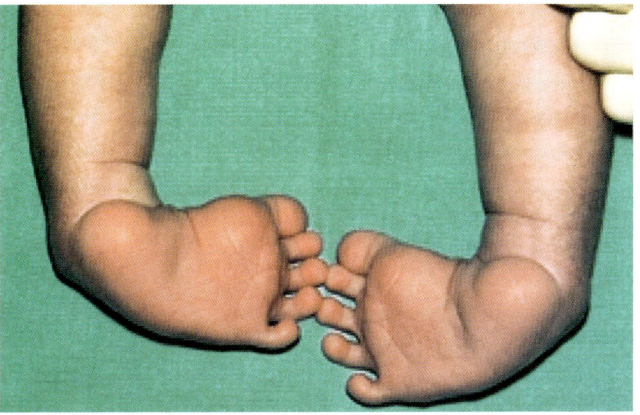

Fig. 13.7. Congenital talipes equinovarus

Most of the affected children have no associated anomalies. However, in some cases, CTEV may occur in association with neuromuscular disorders, such as arthrogryposis, spina bifida, myelodysplasia, cerebral palsy and muscular dystrophy, etc.[23]

Initial treatment is non-operative with serial careful manipulations and immobilization with strapping or casts. The most commonly used technique is Ponseti method.[20] Surgical treatment is required, if disability persists despite non-operative management.

The surgical procedures performed to correct CTEV include posteromedial release (PMR) of the soft tissue and percutaneous Achilles tenotomy. In refractory cases, triple arthrodesis or talectomy may be required.

Perioperative Considerations

The surgery is performed in either supine or prone position, with a tourniquet applied on the thigh. After the surgery, a cast is applied from foot to mid-thigh. Good postoperative analgesia is required.

Balanced general anaesthesia with controlled ventilation is used. Inhalational or intravenous induction is done depending on the age of the child and presence of IV cannula. Endotracheal tube is mandatory in procedures performed in prone position, whereas, LMA may be used if the patient is to be operated in supine position. Minor procedures, like tenotomy or change of cast, can be performed with mask and spontaneous ventilation.

If a surgery is to be performed in prone position, all precautions should be taken to avoid complications and injuries associated with this position.

In patients with associated neuromuscular disorders, concerns specific to the particular disorder must be addressed. These patients may also be at a risk of aspiration, prolonged muscular weakness and delayed recovery from anaesthesia.[24]

Tourniquet Application

Widest suitable cuff should be used and good working condition of all the components of the equipment must be ensured.[25] Before tourniquet application, the limb is exsanguinated by elevation and application of Esmarch's bandage. The tourniquet is applied over a smooth padding and then inflated. Limb occlusion pressure (LOP) is the pressure in the tourniquet at which the distal arterial blood flow is occluded. It can be measured by Doppler probe or pulse oximeter. A safety margin is added to cover intraoperative fluctuations in arterial pressure. This margin is usually 50 mm Hg for a normotensive paediatric patient. Therefore, the tourniquet should be inflated to a pressure 50 mm Hg higher than the LOP.[26] If arterial flow is present at this pressure, the tourniquet pressure should be increased in increments of 25 mm Hg until the flow stops. The tourniquet time should be minimized.[26,27] These precautions reduce the chances of damage to the underlying tissues.

Great care is needed at the time of deflation of tourniquet. Occlusion of blood supply to the limb results in progressive cellular hypoxia, acidosis, and cooling. At the time of deflation, the arterial pressure may fall due to decrease in peripheral vascular resistance and release of metabolites from the ischaemic limb into the circulation. There may be a transient increase in end tidal carbon dioxide with fall in temperature and central venous oxygen tension.[28] Therefore, end tidal carbon dioxide should be closely monitored and minute ventilation should be increased before and after deflation. Although the changes at the time of tourniquet deflation are usually well tolerated; these can result in development of reperfusion injury in severe cases.

Caudal Block

Caudal epidural block is a simple and very useful block for children undergoing CTEV surgery. When given immediately after induction of anaesthesia, it decreases intraoperative analgesic requirement and also provides postoperative pain relief. The most commonly used local anaesthetic is bupivacaine 0.25% in a volume of 0.5–0.75 ml/kg.

Postoperative Management

In postoperative period, the vital functions of the child should be carefully monitored and oxygen should be administered. The pain should be assessed and analgesia supplemented, if required. Options to provide postoperative pain relief include intravenous opioids, e.g. fentanyl or tramadol; diclofenac; or IV, rectal or oral paracetamol.

SUMMARY

Cleft lip and palate, congenital inguinal hernia and congenital talipes equinovarus (CTEV) constitute a substantial portion of paediatric anaesthesia practice. The major concerns during cleft lip and palate surgery include difficult laryngoscopy and intubation; problems due to shared airway; positioning; risk of postoperative airway obstruction; and issues related to co-existing anomalies. In patients undergoing inguinal hernia repair, regional anaesthesia techniques have an important role in providing perioperative analgesia. The risk of postanaesthesia apnoea in former preterm infants can be reduced by use of central neuraxial blocks. The issues which need to be addressed during CTEV surgery are implications of prone position, tourniquet application and postoperative pain relief.

REFERENCES

1. Kulkarni KR, Patil MR, Shirke AM, Jadhav SB. Perioperative respiratory complications in cleft lip and palate repairs: An audit of 1000 cases under 'Smile Train Project'. Indian J Anaesth 2013;57:562–568.

2. Deshpande JK, Kelly K, Baker MB. Anesthesia for pediatric plastic surgery. In: Motoyama EK, Davis PJ (Eds). Smith's Anesthesia for Infants and Children, 7th edn. Philadelphia, Mosby Elsevier 2006;723–736.

3. Johnson CY, Little J. Folate intake, markers of folate status and oral clefts: is the evidence converging? Int J Epidemiol 2008;37:1041–1058.

4. Schindler E, Martini M, Messing-Jünger M. Anesthesia for plastic and craniofacial surgery. In: Gregory GA, Andropoulos DB (Eds). Gregory's Pediatric Anesthesia, 5th edn. Oxford, Wiley-Blackwell, 2012.

5. Sharma A. Cleft palate. In: Yao FF, Fontes ML, Malhotra V (Eds). Yao and Artusio's Anesthesiology: Problem-Oriented Patient Management, 7th edn. London, Lippincott Williams & Wilkins, 2012.

6. Campbell AN, Tremouth MJ. A significant advance in the feeding of infants with cleft palates. Archives of Disease in Childhood 1987;62:1292–1293.

7. Law RC, de Klerk C. Anesthesia for cleft lip and palate surgery. Updat Anesth 2002;14:27–30.

8. Sandberg DJ, Magee WP, Denk MJ. Neonatal cleft lip and cleft palate repair. AORN J 2002;75:490–498.

9. Lorenz HP, Longaker MT. In utero surgery for cleft lip/palate: minimizing the "Ripple Effect" of scarring. J Craniofac Surg 2003;14:504–511.

10. Somerville N, Fenlon S. Anaesthesia for cleft lip and palate. Contin Educ Anaesth Crit Care Pain 2005;5:76–79.

11. Ahuja S, Datta A, Krishna A, Bhattacharya A. Infraorbital nerve block for relief of postoperative pain following cleft lip surgery in infants. Anaesthesia 1994;49:441–444.

12. Kamath MR, Mehandale SG. Comparative study of greater palatine nerve block and intravenous pethidine for postoperative analgesia in children undergoing palatoplasty. Indian J Anaesth 2009;53:654–661.

13. Zavras N, Christou A, Misiakos E, Salakos C, Charalampopoulos A, Schizas D, Machairas A. Current trends in the management of inguinal hernia in children. Int J Clin Med 2014; 5:770–777.

14. Cote CJ. Pediatric anesthesia. In: Miller RD (Ed). Miller's Anesthesia, 8th edn. Philadelphia, Elsevier Saunders 2015, 2757–2798.

15. Walther-Larsen S, Rasmussen LS. The former preterm infant and risk of post-operative apnoea: recommendations for management. Acta Anaesthesiol Scand 2006;50:888–893.

16. Kim EM, Kim MS, Han SJ, Moon BK, Choi EM, Kim EH, Lee JR. Magnesium as an adjuvant for caudal analgesia in children. Paediatr Anaesth 2014;24:1231–1238.

17. Choudhuri AH, Dharmani P, Kumarl N, Prakash A. Comparison of caudal epidural bupivacaine with bupivacaine plus tramadol and bupivacaine plus ketamine for postoperative analgesia in children. Anaesth Intensive Care 2008;36:174–179.

18. Mukhtar K. Transversus abdominis plane (TAP) block. J NYSORA 2009;12:28–33.

19. Alsadek WM, Al-Gohari MM, Elsonbaty MI, Nassar HM, Alkonaiesy RM. Ultrasound guided TAP block versus ultrasound guided caudal block for pain relief in children undergoing lower abdominal surgeries. Egyptian J Anaesth 2015;31:155–160.

20. Dobbs MB, Gurnett CA. Update on clubfoot: etiology and treatment. Clin Orthop Relat Res 2009;467:1146–1153.

21. Kyzer SP, Stark SL. Congenital idiopathic clubfoot deformities. AORN J 1995;61:492–506.

22. Lochmiller C, Johnston D, Scott A, Risman M, Hecht JT. Genetic epidemiology study of idiopathic talipes equinovarus. Am J Med Genet 1998;79:90–96.

23. Cummings RJ, Davidson RS, Armstrong PF, Lehman WB. Congenital clubfoot. J Bone Joint Surg Am 2002;84-A: 290–308.

24. Diu MW, Mancuso TJ. Pediatric diseases. In: Hines RL, Marschall KE (Eds). Stoelting's Anesthesia and Co-existing Disease, 6th edn. Philadelphia, Elsevier Saunders 2012; 583–640.

25. Reilly CW, McEwen JA, Leveille L, Perdios A, Mulpuri K. Minimizing tourniquet pressure in pediatric anterior cruciate ligament reconstructive surgery: a blinded, prospective randomized controlled trial. J Pediatr Orthop 2009;29:275–280.

26. Tredwell SJ, Wilmink M, Inkpen K, McEwen JA. Pediatric tourniquets: analysis of cuff and limb interface, current practice, and guidelines for use. J Pediatr Orthop 2001; 21:671–676.

27. Association of Perioperative Registered Nurses (AORN). Recommended practices for use of the pneumatic tourniquet in the perioperative practice setting. 2007 Standards, Recommended Practices and Guidelines, AORN. 2007.

28. Sharma JP, Salhotra R. Tourniquets in orthopedic surgery. Indian J Orthop 2012;46:377–383.

14

Anaesthesia in Special Situations

Anaesthesia for Radiological Procedures

Poonam Motiani

- Definition of sedation
- Five safety goals for sedation
- Risks of sedation and anaesthesia
- Guidelines for patient selection
- Guidelines for monitoring and personnel
- Concerns in specific locations
  - MRI
  - Computed tomography suite
- Common medications used in paediatric sedation

INTRODUCTION

The provision of anaesthesia outside the operating room provides a unique set of challenges. The standards and principles that underlie the care of the patient should not be abandoned in satellite locations. However, patients who are referred for procedures in satellite locations may present with minimal preoperative information, possess challenging physical and anaesthetic histories, and be scheduled in such a manner as to limit preparation time. The layout and special requirements of the satellite location can create unexpected barriers and may limit access to the patient and the availability of the anaesthesia equipment.

The challenges for the anaesthesiologists include an unfamiliar environment, inadequate anaesthesia support and insufficient number of trained personnel, and cramped, dark quarters and variability of monitoring modalities. In radiation oncology, MRI and occasionally the GI suite problems with noise and suboptimal positioning of the patient may be an issue. Sedation is the most common technique of ensuring immobility in infants, children, and the developmentally compromised who are unable to remain motionless on their own.

DEFINITION OF SEDATION

The Joint Commission, American Academy of Paediatrics (AAP)[1] and American Society of Anaesthesiologists (ASA)[2] define sedation as a sedation continuum that one can pass through escalating depths, described as minimal, moderate, and deep[3,4] [cote: Kaplan]. The term "Conscious Sedation" is no longer acknowledged as appropriate terminology nor is it recognized as an indicator of depth of sedation (Fig. 14.1). These depths of sedation rely on a subjective assessment of the patient's response to verbal, tactile, and painful stimuli to predict the patient's risk of respiratory and cardiovascular compromise.

The associated risks with each level of the sedation continuum are assumed but have never been validated.

The word "sedation" carries a deceptive meaning because it conveys the perception of a safe and pleasant state, even though sedation, particularly deep sedation (monitored anaesthesia care), can have potentially disastrous outcomes for patients as well for practitioners. Therefore, deep sedation requires the

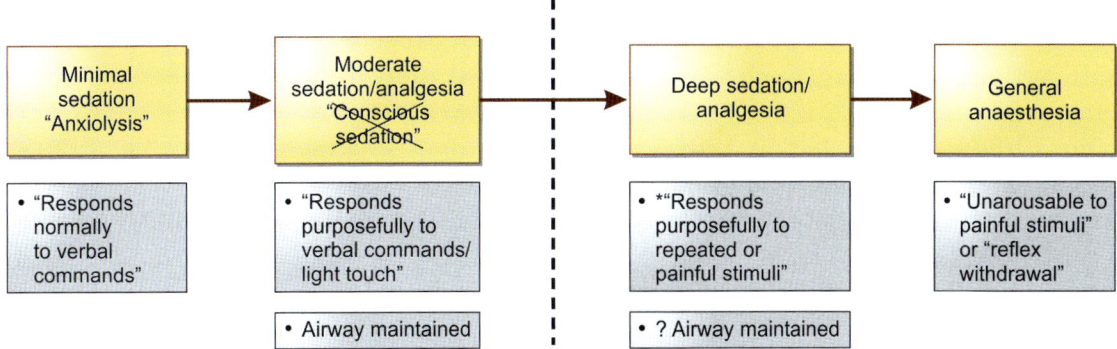

Fig. 14.1. ASA and JCAHO definition of sedation (from Kaplan et al.[4] with permission).
*Reflex withdrawal from a painful stimuluis is NOT considered a purposeful response

same level of competency and care as general anaesthesia.

The Joint Commission[5] in 2007, established recommendations:

- Minimal training and qualifications expected of sedation providers: "Individuals administering moderate or deep sedation and anaesthesia must be qualified and have the appropriate credentials to manage patients at whatever level of sedation or anaesthesia is achieved, either intentionally or unintentionally" (Fig. 14.1).[5]

- With respect to deep sedation, the Joint Commission specified that: "Individuals must be qualified to rescue patients from general anaesthesia and are competent to manage an unstable cardiovascular system as well as a compromised airway and inadequate oxygenation and ventilation".[5] The Joint Commission does not specify the methods required to validate a provider's rescue skills but instead states that "each organization is free to…determine that the individuals are able to perform the required types of rescue".[5]

FIVE SAFETY GOALS FOR SEDATION

The American Academy of Pediatrics[1] advocates five safety goals for sedation:

1. Guard the patient's safety and welfare
2. Minimize physical discomfort and pain
3. Control anxiety, minimize psychological trauma, and maximize the potential for amnesia
4. Control behaviour and/or movement to allow the safe completion of the procedure

5. Return the patient to a state in which safe discharge is possible.[3]

In general, the relative contraindications to sedation include an allergy to the sedatives utilized, a prior adverse reaction to sedation, history of a difficult endotracheal intubation or difficulty providing positive pressure ventilation via mask, uncontrolled gastroesophageal reflux, and a patient who has significant cardiac or respiratory compromise.[6]

RISKS OF SEDATION AND ANAESTHESIA

The risks of sedation and anaesthesia include hypoventilation, apnoea, airway obstruction, cardiopulmonary arrest, and the morbidity and mortality associated with these events.[7,8] These adverse responses during and after sedation for a diagnostic or therapeutic procedure may be minimized, but not completely eliminated, by: (1) a careful pre-procedure review of the patient's underlying medical conditions and consideration of how the sedation process might affect or be affected by these conditions, (2) presence of an individual with the skills needed to rescue a patient from an adverse response, (3) appropriate physiologic monitoring and continuous observation to accurately and rapidly diagnose complications and initiate of appropriate rescue interventions, and (4) appropriate drug selection for the intended procedure.[3]

GUIDELINES FOR PATIENT SELECTION

A focused patient history and sound clinical examination are essential in the stratification of patients and in safe planning of sedation/GA.

The main points which need to be addressed in history taking:

- Allergies and previous allergic or adverse drug reactions
- Medication/drug history, including dosage, time, route and site of administration for prescription, over-the-counter, herbal, or illicit drugs
- Relevant diseases, physical abnormalities and neurological impairments that might increase the potential for airway obstruction, such as a history of snoring or obstructive sleep apnoea
- A summary of previous relevant hospitalisations
- History of previous sedation or general anaesthesia and any complications or unexpected responses
- Relevant family history, particularly that related to anaesthesia

Children in ASA classes III and IV, those with special needs, anatomic airway abnormalities, or extreme tonsillar hypertrophy, often require general anaesthesia (as opposed to sedation). These and other patients with complicated medical histories may also warrant prior consultation with other specialties' such as cardiology, otolaryngology, pulmonary, or neurology.

GUIDELINES FOR MONITORING AND PERSONNEL

A. Monitoring Equipment

Part of the safety net of sedation is to use a systematic approach so as not to overlook having an important drug or a piece of equipment immediately available at the time of a developing emergency.

For both moderate and deep sedation, patients' level of consciousness, ventilatory and oxygenation status, and hemodynamic variables should be assessed and recorded at appropriate intervals. If recording is performed automatically, device alarms should be set to alert the care team to critical changes in patient status.

Monitoring should include (data to be recorded at appropriate intervals before, during, and after procedure):

For minimal and moderate sedation:

- Pulse oximetry
- Response to verbal commands when practical
- Pulmonary ventilation (observation, auscultation)

- Exhaled carbon dioxide monitoring considered when patients separated from caregiver
- Blood pressure and heart rate at 5-min intervals unless contraindicated
- Electrocardiograph for patients with significant cardiovascular disease.

For deep sedation:

- Response to verbal commands or more profound stimuli unless contraindicated
- Exhaled CO_2 monitoring considered for all patients
- Electrocardiograph for all patients

A commonly used acronym that is useful in planning and preparation for a procedure is SOAPME:[1]

- S (suction)—size-appropriate suction catheters and a functioning suction apparatus (e.g. Yankauer-type suction).
- O (oxygen)—adequate oxygen supply and functioning flow meters/other devices to allow its delivery.
- A (airway)—size-appropriate airway equipment [nasopharyngeal and oropharyngeal airways, laryngoscope blades (checked and functioning), endotracheal tubes, stylets, face mask, bag–valve–mask or equivalent device (functioning)]
- P (pharmacy)—all the basic drugs needed to support life during an emergency, including antagonists as indicated.
- M (monitors)—functioning pulse oximeter with size appropriate oximeter probes and other monitors as appropriate for the procedure [e.g. non-invasive blood pressure and end-tidal carbon dioxide monitors, electrocardiography (ECG) machines, stethoscopes].
- E (equipment)—special equipment or drugs for a particular case (e.g. defibrillators-with size-appropriate defibrillator paddles).

In those cases where remote observation of patients is needed, telemetry, clear observation windows, or a remote camera system may be used. The facilities required for the safe administration of anaesthesia and sedation are identical. A full range of paediatric equipment is necessary.[9]

B. Personnel

As would be expected, complications are more common in inexperienced hands and where there is a lack of attention to detail. There is a growing breed of paediatric anaesthesiologists to provide this specialist service. However, sedation/GA for radiological investigations worldwide is delivered by different specialists. For example, in the United Kingdom (UK), oral sedation requires the presence of two trained healthcare professionals and is usually carried out by sedation nurses who are skilled and competent in administrating sedation, and have knowledge of the pharmacology of the medications, airway management and advanced life support.

Nevertheless, nurse-led sedation is not without limitations and is not provided to certain groups of patients, namely neonates, infants and children with anticipated sedation or airway difficulties, in which cases an anaesthetic team is contacted. Deep sedation or anaesthesia with the help of propofol, ketamine, thiopental or sevoflurane is provided only by an anaesthetic team.[9,10]

During moderate sedation:[2]

- A designated individual, other than the practitioner performing the procedure, should be present to monitor the patient throughout procedures performed with sedation/analgesia.
- This individual may assist with minor, interruptible tasks once the patient is stable.

During deep sedation:[2] The monitoring individual may not assist with other tasks.

C. Training of Personnel

Individuals responsible for patients receiving sedation–analgesia should understand the pharmacology of the sedative and analgesic agents, as well as the pharmacology of antagonists. At least one individual capable of establishing a patent airway and positive pressure ventilation, as well as a means for summoning additional assistance, should be present whenever sedation–analgesia is administered. It is recommended that an individual with advanced life support skills be immediately available (within 5 min) for moderate sedation and within the procedure room for deep sedation.[2]

CONCERNS IN SPECIFIC LOCATIONS

A. Magnetic Resonance Imaging (MRI)

The MRI suite is a hazardous location because of the presence of a very strong static magnetic field, high-frequency electromagnetic (radiofrequency) waves, and a time-varied (pulsed) magnetic field.

Secondary dangers of these energy sources include high-level acoustic noise, systemic and localized heating, and accidental projectiles.

There may be significant challenges to anaesthetic administration and monitoring capabilities due to static and dynamic magnetic fields as well as radiofrequency energy emissions. Direct patient observation may be compromised by noise, darkened environment, obstructed line of sight, and other characteristics unique to this environment (*e.g.* distractions). Unlike a conventional operating room, the MRI environment frequently requires the anaesthesiologist to assume broader responsibility for immediate patient care decisions.

In 2009, the ASA published the "Practice Advisory on the Anaesthetic Care for Magnetic Resonance Imaging" (Figs 14.2 and 14.3).[11]

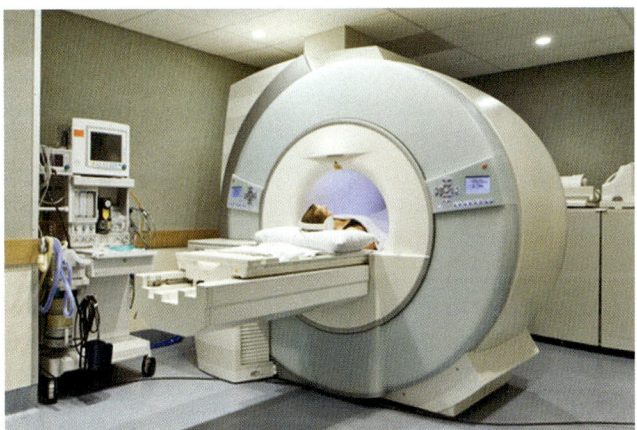

Fig. 14.2. MRI suite

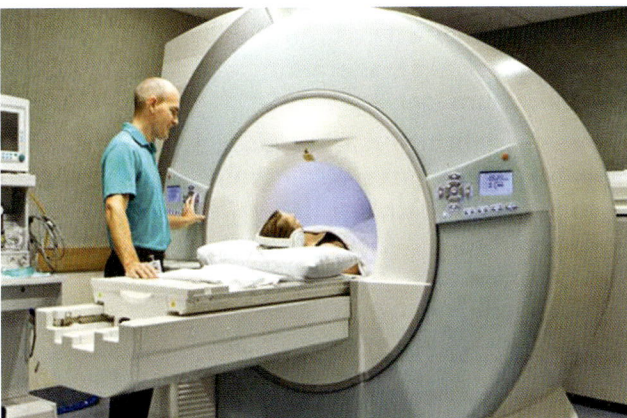

Fig. 14.3. MRI suite with MRI in progress

- There is agreement that the safety, preparation and care of the patients who receive MRIs are a shared responsibility between the anaesthesiologists, radiologists, MRI technologists, and nursing staff. Most of the ASA Closed Claims (70%) from radiology involved anaesthesia in the MRI scanner. Like other remote locations, the majority of the claims were for oversedation. Additional claims resulted from burns from non-MRI compatible electrodes.[12]

- Anaesthetic care providers, ancillary support personnel and patients should not bring ferromagnetic items into the Zone III (region in which free access by unscreened non-MR personnel or ferromagnetic objects or equipment can result in serious injury or death) or Zone IV (MRI scanner magnet room) of the MRI. These items include stethoscopes, pens, watches, wallets, hair clips, name tags, pagers, cell phones, credit cards and batteries.[11]

- Members of the patient care team should not have spinal cord stimulators or implanted objects. Patients need to be screened for aneurysm clips, surgical clips, prosthetic heart valves, intravenous infusion pumps, coronary arterial stents, and implanted dental magnet keepers. There are reports of hemorrhage associated with exposure to iron fillings and image artifacts, burns, swelling and puffiness occurring with eyeliner tattoos. Increased temperatures have been documented in patients with deep brain stimulators, neuro- and spinal cord stimulators. Displacement of leads, pulse generators, or other components of deep brain stimulators and middle ear prostheses may occur. The MRI scanning may interfere with pacemakers and cardioverter-defibrillators resulting in "pacing artifacts, reed switch closures, generator movement or displacement, alterations of pacing rate, and temperature increase.[11]

- Patients with high-risk include those with "neonatal status or prematurity, intensive care or critical care status, impaired respiratory function, haemodynamic instability with vasoactive infusion requirement and comorbidities, such as obesity and peripheral vascular disease."

- In patients with acute or severe renal insufficiency, "the anaesthesiologist should not administer gadolinium because of the increased risk of nephrogenic systemic fibrosis".[11]

- The most desirable situation is to have an MRI-safe/conditional anaesthesia machine available. Metals, such as stainless steel, nickel and titanium as well as plastic, are all suitable for the MRI environment.

- The ASA task force advisory statement indicates that the anaesthesiologists should make sure that all monitors used in zone IV are safe/conditional for the scan.[11] A monitor should be available to view vital signs from zone III when the anaesthesia care provider is not in zone IV. If not, then inhalation anaesthetics may be administered from an anaesthesia machine inside zone III via an elongated circuit through a wave guide. If total intravenous anaesthesia is used, it should be administered by using either MRI-safe/conditional pumps in Zone IV or traditional (MRI-unsafe) pumps in zone III with intravenous tubing passed through a wave guide.[11]

- Equipment-related risks may result from physiologic and invasive monitoring equipment, intubation, oxygenation and ventilation equipment, as well as intravenous infusion pumps. There are case reports of infusion pumps being drawn into the scanner and striking a patient.[13] A death was reported when a non-MRI-compatible oxygen cylinder was drawn into the magnet.[14] "Care should be taken in positioning ECG and other monitors to eliminate burns, even with non-ferromagnetic leads".[11]

- Pulse oximetry probes should be available in multiples sizes. In general, the equipment and drugs for anaesthetic care in the MRI suite should be similar to what is available in the operating room.

- The type of anaesthesia required will depend on the study requirements. General anaesthesia may be needed in younger children who may be uncooperative even under sedation where motion artifact and the need for breath-holding may necessitate use of general anaesthesia. The duration of the procedure, along with patient positioning may play a role in the practitioner's decision to use either an LMA or endotracheal tube.

- If an emergency does occur, a preplanned strategy is advised. The patient should be removed from the zone IV of the MRI suite to a previously designated "safe" location. A call for help should be initiated.

- Cardiopulmonary resuscitation should begin immediately, if needed. The safe location should have in place a defibrillator, vital signs monitor, and a code cart that includes resuscitation drugs, airway equipment, oxygen, and suction.[11]

- Anaesthesiologists should become familiar with projectile emergencies, fire response and "quenching" which can occur as a result of intentional shutdown of the MRI scanner. When a fire does occur, the ASA Practice Advisory for the prevention of and management of operating room fires should be followed.[14] For projectile emergencies, team members should follow their institutions protocol.

B. Computed Tomography Suite

Paediatric patients or those patients undergoing biopsies or percutaneous drainage performed under CT guidance may require the care of an anaesthesiologist. The equipment space issues remain with minimal room for the anaesthesia equipment and personnel. Like the MRI, there can be limited access to the patient. The obvious advantage is that without the strong MRI field, there are few compatibility problems with equipment. The CT scans tend to be much quicker. Paediatric patients, for example, may receive sedation which is titrated to effect for short non-invasive scans. Because of the high levels of ionizing radiation, anaesthesia personnel should monitor the patient through a radiation-shielded window and stop the scan before entering MRI suite, if emergency care must be provided.[15]

COMMON MEDICATIONS USED IN PAEDIATRIC SEDATION (Table 14.1)

Chloral Hydrate and Pentobarbital

Historically, chloral hydrate and pentobarbital have been the hypnotics of choice for paediatric sedation.[16–18] Both medications have no analgesic properties. They are useful for non-painful procedures as sole agents and with adjuvant analgesics for interventional procedures. Rates of successful sedation with chloral hydrate and pentobarbital range from 85 to 98%.[19,20] Both pentobarbital and chloral hydrate are medications which have almost 100 years of clinical experience. Because of their extended half-life (nearly 24 h), they have been associated with prolonged recovery times and sedation-related morbidity. Adverse events with these medications include oxygen desaturation, nausea, vomiting, hyperactivity, respiratory depression, and failure to adequately sedate.[17,21] Chloral hydrate is only available as an oral sedative. Pentobarbital, on the other hand, can be administered intravenously, intramuscularly or orally. Children less than 1 year of age respond well to these two medications when given in the oral form.

Midazolam

Midazolam is a short-acting benzodiazepine with sedative, anxiolytic, muscle relaxant, and amnestic effects with rapid onset and short duration of action. It is administered orally, intravenously, intramuscularly, as well as intranasally. Midazolam is usually administered to provide anxiolysis, with accompanying mild sedation. This state usually suffices for short diagnostic procedures, especially in children who are tired, sleepy, or close to their regular nap time. Adverse effects with midazolam include respiratory depression and hypotension, with rare effects including headache, nausea, emesis, cough, and/or hiccups. Contraindications include acute

Table 14.1	Sedative medications for paediatric use				
S. no.	**Sedative**	**Route**	**Dose**	**Maximum dose**	**Comments**
1.	Chroral hydrate	Oral/rectal	30–50 mg/kg	100 mg/kg	45–60 min before procedure
2.	Midazolam	IV	0.025–0.05 mg/kg	6 mg/kg (in children < 6 years	Over 2–3 mins, 5–10 mins prior to procedure. Reduce dose by 50% when combined with opioids
3.	Ketamine	IVIM Oral	1–2 mg/kg 2–5 mg/kg 6–10 mg/kg	2 mg/kg in children 1 month to 12 years 13 mg/kg	Adjusted according to response
4.	Dexmedetomidine	(Approved for adult use)	2–3 mg/kg over 10 min	3 µg/kg	1–2 mg/kg/hr as an infusion for sedation maintenance
5.	Propofol	IV	1–2 mg/kg	4 mg/kg by IV infusion	Over 1–5 min

narrow-angle glaucoma, uncontrolled pain, existing central nervous system depression, and shock.[22]

Dexmedetomidine

Dexmedetomidine is a highly selective alpha-2 adrenoceptor agonist approved for use in intubated and non-intubated adults. Dexmedetomidine is not approved for paediatric use by the FDA. It is, however, used for paediatric sedation in several settings such as diagnostic radiologic imaging studies and intensive care units.

Dexmedetomidine offers the advantage of providing sedation and analgesia with little respiratory depression and in most a tolerable decrease in blood pressure and heart rate.[23] The half-life of dexmedetomidine is shorter than that of pentobarbital and chloral hydrate making it easier to titrate, quicker to recover from, and potentially associated with fewer prolonged sedation-related adverse events. There is literature to support that dexmedetomidine has some analgesic properties.[24–26] It may be useful for select interventional radiology procedures that require sedation and minimal analgesia. It can be particularly effective when supplemented with a local anaesthetic during the procedure. Although there are no absolute contraindications to dexmedetomidine, the concurrent use of digoxin is often considered a relative contraindication, as it has been associated with extreme bradycardia in children and cardiac arrest in adults.[27,28]

Ketamine

Ketamine is a rapid-acting dissociative agent that is administered via intravenous, intramuscular, oral, rectal, nasal, epidural, or intrathecal routes. Ketamine can produce a rapid onset of deep sedation and analgesia with minimal respiratory depression and cardiovascular side effects.[29,30] Ketamine is unique because it provides deep sedation and profound analgesia while still maintaining airway muscle activity and upper airway patency.[31] Large doses of ketamine can produce a state of general anaesthesia. When given in small bolus doses, ketamine provides analgesia for an average of 30 min. As an infusion, ketamine can produce a continuous state of analgesia which may be titrated up and down in response to (or in anticipation of) the painful stimulus. It is especially useful for patients who will undergo an exceptionally painful procedure, those on long-term treatment with opioids, or those who have a high tolerance to opiates. Ketamine provides an effective alternative to narcotics in these patients.

The use of ketamine for paediatric sedation and analgesia has been described in various non-operating room settings. Most of the experience with ketamine in children is drawn from emergency medicine and, lately, from interventional radiology.

Hallucinations, delusions, nightmares, and emergence delirium are commonly described as potential side effects of ketamine; commonly noted in adults;[31,32] presence in the paediatric population controversial.[33,34] In adults, the concomitant administration of benzodiazepines (midazolam or diazepam) decreases the incidence of these events. Again, the utility of benzodiazepines in reducing these events in children is yet to be proven.[35–37] Some reports indicate that the addition of benzodiazepines leads to an increased incidence of oxygen desaturation events.[38] Under age 5, there is no definitive evidence that benzodiazepine administration will reduce the hallucinations, delusions, and excitatory behaviour that can occur with ketamine. Children over age 5 may benefit from concomitant benzodiazepine administration.

Propofol

Propofol is an intravenous anaesthetic approved for use in the induction and maintenance of general anaesthesia in children and adults. It has a rapid onset of action, distributed extensively and rapidly cleared from the body. Emergence from anaesthesia occurs quickly. Common adverse events include apnoea (children and adults). Other common adverse events in adults include bradycardia, arrhythmias, blood pressure problems, decreased cardiac output, burning/stinging at the site of injection, hyperlipidemia, respiratory acidosis, rash, and pruritus.

Propofol is also used in monitored anaesthesia care for deep sedation in intensive care units and areas outside the operating room, including radiology and nuclear medicine suites. There has been an increasing interest by non-anaesthesiologists in using propofol as a sedation agent.[39,40] Propofol is commonly administered first via a slowly titrated load to achieve the targeted depth of sedation which is then maintained with a continuous infusion at doses of

100 µg/kg/min upwards.[41] Propofol administration requires that the sedation provider be proficient and expert in the identification and management of airway compromise: even at low-dosing ranges, the cross-sectional area of the airway at the level of the tongue and epiglottis narrows, and patients can manifest signs of obstruction.[42,43]

Narcotic

The choice of narcotic depends on the duration of the procedure and the extent of analgesia required. Morphine and fentanyl are the more popular narcotics. Morphine requires approximately 10 min to take effect and has a duration of action of approximately 2 hours. Fentanyl works quicker, has 100 times the potency of morphine, and can produce analgesia in minutes. It generally needs to be re-dosed at least every 30–60 min depending on the procedure. Narcotics should be administered prior to (i.e. in anticipation of) the painful stimulus so that adequate analgesia is present at the time of the stimulus. Respiratory depression is the most common adverse event. In addition, rapid administration of fentanyl may result in rigid chest syndrome. Naloxone is the opioid antagonist indicated for the reversal of opioid-induced respiratory depression. Naloxone, as well as other drugs and equipment for resuscitation, should be readily available in the radiology/nuclear medicine suites.

Combination Therapy

Additional medications increase the risk of adverse events, so the sedation physician or anaesthesiologist should be aware of the possible adverse events that may result from the medications administered. Drugs with long durations of action must be allowed to manifest their pharmacologic actions and peak effects before additional doses are considered. The practitioner must know whether the previous dose of any drug has taken full effect before administering additional medications.[3] If the mechanisms of action of concomitant medications are similar, synergistic effects may be potentiated, and the risk of adverse events is magnified. Respiratory depression is a common pathway of adverse events and may result unexpectedly and quickly. Practitioners must also be cognizant that drug interactions may occur.

SUMMARY

Anaesthesia in remote locations is associated typically with small dark rooms, bulky and sometimes outdated equipment and personnel that are not always familiar with emergency equipment and procedures. It is the role of the anaesthesiologist to ensure that well-equipped anaesthesia machines, standard monitoring (electrocardiogram, oxygen saturation and non-invasive blood pressure), trained personnel and an anaesthetic plan are in place. Since analysis of closed claims suggests that administration of anaesthesia and sedation at remote locations is associated with a significant risk of adverse effects, it is imperative that the anaesthesiologist be particularly attentive to patients when visual and auditory clues of impending cardiorespiratory events may be hindered.[12] There is substantial evidence that the use of continuous monitoring of respiration by capnography is extremely important in patients receiving both general anaesthesia and sedation. Transportation of the patients, especially if significant distance must be travelled to reach the recovery location should consist of an oxygen cylinder, a patient monitor, emergency drugs and a portable suction device if available. Post anaesthesia care for the patient who has undergone a procedure in a remote location should be similar to that for postsurgical patients. The practicing anaesthesiologist should remain familiar with the ASA practice guidelines, advisories and standards as they relate to anaesthesia in remote locations.

REFERENCES

1. American Academy of Pediatrics; American Academy of Pediatric Dentistry, Cote´ CJ, Wilson S; Work Group on Sedation. Guidelines for monitoring and management of pediatric patients during and after sedation for diagnostic and therapeutic procedures: an update. Pediatrics 2006; 118:2587–2602.

2. American Society of Anaesthesiologists Task Force on Sedation and Analgesia. Practice guidelines for sedation and analgesia by non-anesthesiologists. Anesthesiology 2002;96(4):1004–1017.

3. Cote CJ, Wilson S. Guidelines for monitoring and management of pediatric patients during and after sedation for diagnostic and therapeutic procedures: an update. Pediatrics 2006;118(6):2587–2602.

4. Kaplan RF, Cravero JP, Yaster M, Cote C. Chap. 48. Sedation for diagnostic and therapeutic procedures outside the operating room. In: Cote CJ, Lerman J, Todres ID (Eds).

A Practice of Anaesthesia for Infants and Children. Philadelphia: Saunders/Elsevier; 2009.

5. Joint Commission for Accreditation of Hospitals (JCAHO). Operative or other high-risk procedures and/or the administration of moderate or deep sedation or anaesthesia. The Comprehensive accreditation manual for Hospitals: official handbook. Oakbrook Terrace: JCAHO; 2007;p.PC-41.

6. Mason KP, Sanborn P, Zurakowski D, et al. Superiority of pentobarbital versus chloral hydrate for sedation in infants during imaging. Radiology 2004;230(2):537–542.

7. Cravero JP, Beach ML, Blike GT, Gallagher SM, Hertzog JH. The incidence and nature of adverse events during pediatric sedation/anaesthesia with propofol for procedures outside the operating room: a report from the Pediatric Sedation Research Consortium. Anesth Analg 2009;108 (3):795–804.

8. Sanborn PA, Michna E, Zurakowski D, et al. Adverse cardiovascular and respiratory events during sedation of pediatric patients for imaging examinations. Radiology 2005;237(1):288–294.

9. The Royal College of Radiologists. Safe sedation, analgesia and anaesthesia within the radiology department. September 2003 [accessed 30 May 2011]. Available from: http://www.rcr.ac.uk/publications.aspx? pp.ID5310 and PublicationID5186

10. National Institute for Health and Clinical Excellence (NICE) clinical guideline sedation in children and young people. December 2010 [accessed 30 May 2011]. Available from: http://www.nice.org.uk/nicemedia/live/ 13296/52130/52130.pdf

11. Practice Advisory on Anesthetic Care for Magnetic Resonance Imaging: A Report by the American Society of Anesthesiologists Task Force on Anesthetic Care for Magnetic Resonance Imaging. Anesthesiology 2009;110(3): 459–479.

12. Metzner J, Posner KL, Domino KB. The risk and safety of anesthesia at remote locations. The US closed claims analysis. Cur Opin Anesthesia 2009;22:502–508.

13. Wynnychenko TM, Szokol JW, Murphy GS. Infusion pump use in the MRI. Anesth Analg 2000;91:249–250.

14. Landrigan C. Preventable deaths and injuries during magnetic resonance imaging. N Engl J Med 2001;345(13): 1000–1001.

15. Henderson KH, Lu JK, Strauss KJ, et al. Radiation exposure of anesthesiologists. J Clin Anes 1994;6:37–41.

16. American Academy of Pediatrics Committee on Drugs and Committee on Environmental Health: use of chloral hydrate for sedation in children. Pediatrics 1993;92(3): 471–473.

17. Greenberg SB, Faerber EN, Aspinall CL, Adams RC. High-dose chloral hydrate sedation for children undergoing MR imaging: safety and efficacy in relation to age. Am J Roentgenol 1993;161(3):639–641.

18. Greenberg SB, Faerber EN, Aspinall CL. High dose chloral hydrate sedation for children undergoing CT. J Comput Assist Tomogr 1991;15(3):467–469.

19. Napoli KL, Ingall CG, Martin GR. Safety and efficacy of chloral hydrate sedation in children undergoing echocardiography. J Pediatr 1996;129(2):287–291.

20. Thompson JR, Schneider S, Ashwal S, Holden BS, Hinshaw Jr DB, Hasso AN. The choice of sedation for computed tomography in children: a prospective evaluation. Radiology 1982;143(2):475–479.

21. Ronchera-Oms CL, Casillas C, Marti-Bonmati L, et al. Oral chloral hydrate provides effective and safe sedation in paediatric magnetic resonance imaging. J Clin Pharm Ther 1994;19(4):239–243.

22. Macias CG, Chumpitazi CE. Sedation and anesthesia for CT: emerging issues for providing high-quality care. Pediatr Radiol 2011;41(Suppl 2):517–522.

23. Evers AS, Crowder CM, Balser JR. General anesthetics. In: Brunton LL, Laso JS, Parker KL (Eds). Goodman & Gilman's The Pharmacological Basis of Therapeutics, 11th edn. McGraw-Hill Professional 2006;pp.341–368.

24. Bamgbade OA. Dexmedetomidine for perioperative sedation and analgesia in alcohol addiction. Anaesthesia 2006;61(3):299–300.

25. Jackson 3rd KC, Wohlt P, Fine PG. Dexmedetomidine: a novel analgesic with palliative medicine potential. J Pain Palliat Care Pharmacother 2006;20(2):23–27.

26. Rich JM. Dexmedetomidine as a sole sedating agent with local anesthesia in a high-risk patient for axillofemoral bypass graft: a case report. AANAJ 2005;73(5):357–360.

27. Berkenbosch JW, Tobias JD. Development of bradycardia during sedation with dexmedetomidine in an infant concurrently receiving digoxin. Pediatr Crit Care Med 2003;4(2):203–205.

28. Precedex (dexmedetomidine hydrochloride) Hospira, Inc. Lake Forest, IL 60045 USA. http://www.precedex. com/wp-content/uploads/Precedex_PI.pdf. Accessed 12 March 2013.

29. Way WL, Trevor AJ. Pharmacology of intravenous nonnarcotic anesthetics. In: Anesthesia, 2nd edn. New York: Churchill Livingstone; 1986;p.813–817.

30. Drummond GB. Comparison of sedation with midazolam and ketamine: effects on airway muscle activity. Br J Anaesth 1996;76(5):663–667.

31. Fine J, Finestone SC. Sensory disturbances following ketamine anesthesia: recurrent hallucinations. Anesth Analg 1973;52(3):428–430.

32. Meyers EF, Charles P. Prolonged adverse reactions to ketamine in children. Anesthesiology 1978;49(1):39–40.

33. Roelofse JA, Joubert JJ, Roelofse PG. A doubleblind randomized comparison of midazolam alone and midazolam combined with ketamine for sedation of pediatric dental patients. J Oral Maxillofac Surg 1996;54(7):838–844; discussion 845–846.

34. Sherwin TS, Green SM, Khan A, Chapman DS, Dannenberg B. Does adjunctive midazolam reduce recovery agitation after ketamine sedation for pediatric procedures? A randomized, double-blind, placebo-controlled trial. Ann Emerg Med 2000;35(3):229–238.

35. Green SM, Johnson NE. Ketamine sedation for pediatric procedures: part 2, review and implications. Ann Emerg Med 1990;19(9):1033–1046.

36. Hollister GR, Burn JM. Side effects of ketamine in pediatric anesthesia. Anesth Analg 1974;53(2):264–267.

37. Wathen JE, Roback MG, Mackenzie T, Bothner JP. Does midazolam alter the clinical effects of intravenous ketamine sedation in children? A double-blind, randomized, controlled, emergency department trial. Ann Emerg Med 2000;36(6):579–588.

38. Sussman DR. A comparative evaluation of ketamine anesthesia in children and adults. Anesthesiology 1974;40(5):459–464.

39. Mallory MD, Baxter AL, Yanosky DJ, Cravero JP. Emergency physician-administered propofol sedation: a report on 25,433 sedations from the pediatric sedation research consortium. Ann Emerg Med 2011;57(5):462–481.

40. Cravero JP, Beach ML, Blike GT, Gallagher SM, Hertzog JH. The incidence and nature of adverse events during pediatric sedation/anesthesia with propofol for procedures outside the operating room: a report from the Pediatric Sedation Research Consortium. Anesth Analg 2009;108(3):795–804.

41. Frankville DD, Spear RM, Dyck JB. The dose of propofol required to prevent children from moving during magnetic resonance imaging. Anesthesiology. 1993;79(5):953–958.

42. Evans RG, Crawford MW, Noseworthy MD, Yoo SJ. Effect of increasing depth of propofol anesthesia on upper airway confi guration in children. Anesthesiology 2003;99(3):596–602.

43. Reber A, Wetzel SG, Schnabel K, Bongartz G, Frei FJ. Effect of combined mouth closure and chin lift on upper airway dimensions during routine magnetic resonance imaging in pediatric patients sedated with propofol. Anesthesiology 1999;90(6):1617–1623.

15

Foetal Surgery

Raminder Sehgal

- ▪ Physiological considerations
- ▪ Anaesthetic considerations
- ▪ Anaesthetic technique
- ▪ Complications associated with foetal surgery
- ▪ Ethical considerations

Foetal surgery is a specialty which offers therapeutic options for foetus with congenital abnormalities which if untreated will result in death or severe disability after birth. The goal is to improve the natural history of these anomalies by their correction before birth. Historically, Barcroft performed the first foetal surgery on a lamb foetus under subarachnoid block.[1] In 1960s and 1970s, foetal surgery was done in animals to simulate human congenital anomalies and by 1980 attempts were made to correct these surgically created anatomic defects. Hydrops foetalis due to Rh sensitization was the first foetal disorder treated successfully in humans [2] and Harrison et al performed the first surgery on a human foetus.[3] The specialty of foetal medicine came on its own following the development of real-time sonography which provided safe and non-invasive visualization of the living foetus. Sonography helped in the diagnosis of abnormal foetal anatomy, guided needle puncture to aspirate amniotic fluid, urine or ascites, helped biopsy of foetal tissues and finally, guided foetal surgery.

Though conceptually simple, foetal surgical procedures are challenging both for the surgeon and the anaesthesiologist. They are also associated with significant morbidity for the foetus as well as the mother. Therefore, it is important to establish an accurate diagnosis, rule out other chromosomal or anatomic abnormalities in the foetus and assure an acceptable risk-benefit ratio for mother as well as the foetus.[4] Though several anomalies are being treated with foetal interventions, only open repair of meningomyelocele and endoscopic laser ablation for twin-to-twin transfusion syndrome are currently supported by randomized clinical trials.[5,6] Common structural malformations treated by foetal surgery are listed in Table 15.1.

PHYSIOLOGICAL CONSIDERATIONS

A thorough understanding of the maternal, foetal and the uteroplacental physiology is necessary for the success of foetal surgery.

Maternal Factors

The physiological changes during pregnancy have direct impact on the anaesthetic management of a woman scheduled for surgery on her foetus. Increase in body weight, enlarged breasts and capillary engorgement of the respiratory tract makes the airway management a challenge. Increased oxygen consumption and decreased functional residual capacity makes the pregnant woman prone to desaturation and, therefore, merits preoxygenation. Decrease in the tone of lower oesophageal sphincter increases the risk of

Table 15.1	Common structural malformations treated by foetal surgery
Anomaly	**Procedure**
■ **Early–mid gestation**	
Twin-twin transfusion syndrome	Foetoscopic laser ablation of placental vessels
	Bipolar umbilical cord cautery
	Radiofrequency ablation of umbilical cord
■ **Mid gestation**	
Congenital diaphragmatic hernia	Foetoscopic tracheal balloon occlusion
Meningomyelocele	Open surgical closure of defect
Bladder outlet obstruction	Bladder decompression
Sacro-coccygeal teratoma	Debulking, ablation of feeding vessels
Congenital high airway obstruction	Tracheal decompression
■ **Late gestation**	
Cystic hygroma	Exit procedure
Airway teratoma	Exit procedure
Congenital cystic adenomatoid malformation	Exit procedure for pulmonary lobectomy

aspiration pneumonitis and mandates aspiration prophylaxis as well as rapid sequence induction. Decrease in oncotic pressure and increased capillary permeability increases the risk of pulmonary oedema especially when tocolytics are administered post-operatively.

Supine hypotension due to aortocaval compression by the gravid uterus is a well-known complication during pregnancy. The risk of this complication is increased in these patients because several conditions requiring foetal surgery are associated with poly-hydramnios. A lateral tilt is a must whether it is an open or a minimally invasive procedure. There is an increased risk of venous thromboembolism, and therefore, VTE prophylaxis is a must in pregnant women undergoing surgery. They are also more sensitive to the effect of local anaesthetics and muscle relaxants. Also, the MAC of volatile anaesthetics is lower in the pregnant women and, therefore, lower doses of these drugs are needed during anaesthesia.

Foetal Factors

Teratogenicity and placental transfer of drugs are the two important foetal considerations while adminis-tering anaesthesia to a pregnant woman. Anaesthetic agents have potentially harmful effects on cell division as well as cell motility and are known to prolong DNA synthesis.[7] Nitrous oxide has been shown to be a weak teratogen in cell cultures and animal studies.[8] However, there is no evidence to link any anaesthetic

agent, opioids, benzodiazepine or muscle relaxant to teratogenicity.[8] There is also some concern regarding impairment of brain development after exposure to anaesthesia early in life, but its effect on learning disabilities has not been proven.[9]

Most anaesthetic agents cross the placenta to produce foetal anaesthesia. The MAC for inhalational anaesthetics is reduced and their uptake by the foetus is much slower than the maternal uptake.[10] This is an important consideration as adequate time (>20 min) should be given to achieve sufficient depth of anaesthesia in the foetus before allowing the surgical procedure. When administered in high concentration for uterine relaxation during open foetal surgery, most inhalational anaesthetics depress the foetal cardio-vascular system and produce foetal acidosis. Opioids and induction agents reduce the heart rate variability but do not produce foetal acidosis unless maternal haemodynamics are depressed. The opioids are metabolised slowly and half-life of fentanyl in very premature infants may be more than 12 hours.[11] Therefore, intraoperative administration of opioids to the foetus may provide postoperative analgesia for several hours. Muscle relaxants do not cross placenta to affect the foetus.

The immaturity of foetal organ systems is another important consideration during foetal surgery. The foetal myocardium is stiffer and has impaired relaxation as compared to the adult myocardium.[12] The cardiac output is more dependent on the heart rate and any stress results in foetal bradycardia. The coagulation factors are produced in the foetus independently and the maternal coagulation factors do not cross the placenta. The mean prothrombin time at 19–23 weeks is 32.5 seconds with an INR of 6.4 and the mean activated partial thromboplastin time is 168.8 seconds.[12] At mid-gestation, the blood volume of the foetus varies between 40 and 60 ml and, therefore, minimal blood loss results in hypovolaemia which should be replaced with blood transfusion.[13] The thin, easily bruised skin predisposes the foetus to fluid and heat loss on prolonged exposure. Hypovolaemia due to fluid or blood loss decreases foetal blood flow to the placenta, decreases foetal oxygenation and may lead to foetal demise. Therefore, evaporative and heat loss should be minimised by limiting the surgical time and by using warm irrigation fluids. Foetal ECHO, oxygenation saturation and ABG should be monitored for foetal safety.[13]

Uteroplacental Factors

The foetus depends on adequate placental blood flow for nutrition and oxygenation. Uterine vasculature is fully dilated during pregnancy and thus uterine blood flow is dependent on uterine perfusion pressure. Factors, like increased uterine tone, maternal hypotension, aortocaval compression and myometrial vasoconstriction, decrease uterine blood flow and may compromise foetal well-being. Thus, maternal hypotension should be corrected early with the help of fluids or vasopressors. Amongst the vasopressors, ephedrine which possesses primarily beta-adrenergic effects and has minimal effect on uterine blood flow has been the drug of choice to treat hypotension during pregnancy. However, it crosses the placenta to cause hypermetabolism.[14] Phenylepherine is better for foetal pH status and has been found to be equally safe and effective for maintenance of blood pressure during pregnancy.[15] Neuraxial block does not alter uterine blood flow as long as the blood pressure is maintained. Volatile anaesthetics decrease uterine tone and cause hypotension but this effect is compensated by uterine vasodilatation during light or moderately deep anaesthesia. With deeper plane of anaesthesia, this compensation is inadequate and may lead to fatal acidosis. Intravenous anaesthetics do not affect the uterine blood flow as much as the volatile anaesthetics. Maternal hypocapnia decreases

and hypercapnia increases uterine blood flow and foetal oxygenation. Other factors which affect uterine blood flow and foetal oxygenation include kinking or compression of umbilical cord and loss of utero-placental integrity.

ANAESTHETIC CONSIDERATIONS

Foetal Pain and Response to Surgical Stimulation

The concept of foetal pain is a controversial subject. Behavioural patterns, foetal endocrine response to stress and circulatory redistribution studies also indicate that preterm baby is sensate.[16] Stress response related to surgical stimulus can be blocked by analgesics but it is not clear if it is related to relief of foetal pain.[12] Anatomical studies demonstrate that brain and spinal cord begins to develop as early as 8 weeks of intrauterine life, while thalamus and subcortical structures which are necessary for consciousness are present at 20 weeks of gestation.[16] The somatosensory evoked potentials appear around 29 weeks post-conception and EEG pattern denoting wakefulness is seen at 30 weeks. This indicates that the foetus is capable of feeling pain by 30 weeks gestation. In fact, the pain felt by the foetus may even be greater than that of a term neonate or an adult due to immaturity of descending inhibitory fibres.[16] Therefore, foetus undergoing any surgical intervention should be provided adequate analgesia and anaesthesia. Besides relieving pain, foetal anaesthesia serves other purposes including inhibiting foetal movements, preventing hormonal stress response and possibly long-term neurodevelopment and behaviour responses.[17]

Tocolysis

Pregnant uterus is very sensitive to any manipulation or stimulation. Therefore, foetal surgery, especially when done after 27 weeks gestation can stimulate strong uterine contractions which may precipitate placental separation. The degree of uterine stimulation is directly proportional to the size of uterine incision. Thus, open foetal surgery is more likely to result in preterm labour or postoperative abortion than minimally invasive procedures. An important aspect of anaesthetic management for foetal surgical procedures is prevention of uterine contractions both intra- and postoperatively. Tocolytic therapy is needed

Table 15.2	Tocolytic drugs and their side effects
Drugs	**Side effects**
Volatile anaesthetics (2–3 MAC)	Foetal acidosis after prolonged use
β-adrenergic agents (IV or SC terbutaline, ritodrine)	Maternal tachycardia, hypotension, myocardial ischaemia, decreased fluid tolerance, pulmonary oedema
Magnesium sulphate	Decreased foetal heart rate variability, decreased muscle tone at birth
Glyceryl trinitrate	Maternal hypotension, pulmonary oedema
NSAIDs (indomethicin)	Short-term use (48 h) before 32 weeks gestation, risk of premature closure of ductus arteriosus in the foetus, decreased renal function, oliguria, risk of necrotising enterocolitis and intraventricular haemorrhage
Calcium channel antagonists	Maternal hypotension

to prevent as well as treat preterm labour after these procedures. It is usually not required after intrauterine transfusion or cordocentesis. Volatile anaesthetics act as the primary tocolytics during the intraoperative period. Other drugs used as tocolytics are listed in Table 15.2. However, these drugs are not without side effects. Claim of premature closure of ductus arteriosus following indomethicin usage early in pregnancy have been refuted.[18]

Preanaesthetic Evaluation and Preparation

Anaesthesia for foetal surgery is fundamentally similar to that for any non-obstetric surgery performed during pregnancy except that one has to balance the needs of two surgical patients, namely the mother and the foetus. Other concerns include prevention of preterm labour, maintenance of maternal homeostasis in view of deep anaesthesia, tocolytic therapy, maintenance of foetal homeostasis and providing foetal anaesthesia.

After the initial suspicion of any abnormality on routine ultrasound, the foetus is further evaluated by echocardiography to assess the cardiac status, whole body ultrasound is done to delineate the defect and the severity of hydrops, and the magnetic resonance imaging is done to visualise the detailed anatomy. The maternal evaluation includes detailed history, examination including airway and spine examination and investigations to rule out comorbidities or pregnancy-induced conditions, like pre-eclampsia, which might preclude foetal surgery. The severity of symptoms related to aortocaval compression and gastroesophageal reflux is also assessed to plan the anaesthetic technique. In addition, both parents undergo a psychosocial evaluation and meet a multidisciplinary team of doctors to discuss the procedure and its associated risks.

ANAESTHETIC TECHNIQUE

It is important for the anaesthesiologist to know about the foetal lesion and the surgical approach for its correction to chart out the anaesthesia plan. Foetal surgical interventions can be divided into three types of procedures. In the *open procedures,* a hysterotomy is performed, the foetus is exteriorized for surgery and postoperatively it is placed back into the uterus to grow till delivery. *Minimally invasive procedures* are performed via percutaneous needle punctures or small trocars placed into the uterus. The timing of open surgical procedures and minimally invasive interventions varies but are commonly performed during mid-gestation (21–27 weeks). The third group of procedures are called *ex utero intrapartum treatment (EXIT) procedures.* These procedures are performed at or near term and end with the delivery of the baby. A hysterotomy is performed and the surgery is done on the foetus before clamping of cord while the foetus is getting oxygenated by placental transfer of oxygen.

Anaesthesia for Open Surgical Procedures

Common congenital lesions operated upon by open technique include severe meningomyelocoele, sacral teratoma, cystic lung lesions and bladder outlet obstruction. On the morning of surgery, an ultrasound examination is performed to assure the maternal and foetal well-being. The fasting status of the mother is assured and aspiration prophylaxis is administered. Tocolysis is commenced by administering indomethacin 50 mg as rectal suppository. The availability of adequate crossmatched blood for the mother and type O, Rh-negative, cytomegalovirus-negative, leucocyte-depleted packed red cells for the foetus in small aliquots of 50 ml is also confirmed.

The operating room is warmed to 26°C and the mother is positioned on a wedge for left uterine displacement. After placing standard monitors and achieving intravenous access, a lumbar epidural catheter is inserted for postoperative pain relief and its position is confirmed with a test dose. The mother is preoxygenated and rapid sequence induction is performed with sodium thiopentone (5 mg/kg), succinylcholine (2 mg/kg) and fentanyl (1–2 mg/kg). After tracheal intubation, anaesthesia is maintained with 0.5 MAC of volatile anaesthetic in oxygen and vecuronium bromide is administered for muscle relaxation. Desflurane is the preferred volatile anaesthetic as its low solubility allows rapid emergence from deep anaesthesia. Ultrasound mapping of the placenta and the foetus is done to plan the surgical access. An anteriorly attached placenta increases the risk of bleeding, requires greater manipulation of the uterus and predisposes the foetus to hypoxia.[10] The anaesthesiologist uses this time to place an orogastric tube and urinary catheter. An arterial catheter and a second wide bore intravenous cannula are inserted to monitor and treat haemodynamic instability.

Before commencement of surgery, the concentration of volatile anaesthetic is increased to 2 or 3 MAC to relax the uterus and it is then titrated to the desired effect. Additional relaxation is provided by tocolytics, like nitroglycerine given in small intravenous boluses of 50 to 100 µg or by continuous intravenous infusion at the rate of 0.5–1 µg/kg/minute.[19] Low dose desflurane supplemented by intravenous propofol and remifentanil has also been used to provide adequate uterine relaxation with less need for foetal resuscitation.[20] Total intraoperative fluids are usually limited to 500 ml of crystalloid to avoid the risk of postoperative pulmonary oedema. The maternal blood pressure is maintained within 10% of the baseline with titrated intravenous ephedrine (5–10 mg) or phenylephrine (1–2 µg/kg). The placental mapping is done to optimize surgical approach and the uterine incision is made with a uterine stapling device which seals the amniotic membranes and the myometrium. The foetal part to be operated upon is delivered through the incision and intramuscular

injections of fentanyl (20 µg/kg), vecuronium (0.2 mg/kg) and atropine (20 µg/kg) are administered to the foetus. Throughout the procedure, foetal oxygenation is maintained via the placenta. The uterine cavity is continuously infused with pressurised, warm lactated Ringer's solution to make up for the lost amniotic fluid and prevent umbilical cord kinking. If required, foetal intravenous access is secured and sterile tubing is handed to the anaesthesiologist over the drapes. In addition to direct observation, foetal monitoring is done by ultrasound, pulse oximetry and foetal echocardiography. The foetal saturation of oxygen varies between 40 and 70%.[21] A decrease in foetal oxygen saturation or foetal bradycardia is indicator of foetal distress which usually occurs due to hypoperfusion or umbilical cord kinking. It necessitates administration of blood, fluid or adrenaline to the foetus. Foetal temperature, hematocrit, acid-base status monitoring and Doppler assessment of the umbilical cord blood flow are also recommended.

At the time of uterine closure, tocolysis is provided by magnesium sulphate (6 g bolus followed by infusion at the rate of 3 g/h). The volatile anaesthetic concentration is decreased and the epidural catheter is dosed with bupivacaine (15–20 ml of 0.25% solution) and morphine (0.05 mg/kg) to supplement anaesthesia and provide postoperative analgesia. Neuromuscular monitoring of the mother is recommended before reversal as magnesium sulphate can potentiate the effect of vecuronium. While reversing the neuromuscular block, it should be kept in mind that anticholinesterase agents can trigger uterine contractions which are not desirable in these patients.[22] For the same reason, shivering, nausea and vomiting upon awakening should be treated aggressively.

Postoperatively, the mother is observed in an obstetric intensive care unit and the uterine activity and foetal heart rate are monitored. Important postoperative considerations include premature labour, pulmonary oedema, amniotic fluid leak and foetal demise. Tocolysis is continued with magnesium sulphate for 2–3 days which is later replaced by oral nifedipine or subcutaneous terbutaline till delivery of the baby. Adequate pain control with patient controlled epidural analgesia is crucial to the success of foetal surgery. The DVT prophylaxis is continued and mother is advised bed-rest for remainder of her pregnancy.

Anaesthesia for Minimally Invasive and Percutaneous Procedures

Minimally invasive procedures involve percutaneous access to the foetus for surgery on the placenta, membranes or the foetus. Varied ultrasound-guided procedures are with needle or radiofrequency probes or multiple trocars for laparoscopy (fetoscopy) or for robot-assisted repair of meningomyelocele.[12] Common lesions treated by fetoscopic surgery include tracheal balloon occlusion for congenital diaphragmatic hernia, laser atrial septostomy, resection of urethral valves, radiofrequency ablation of non-viable twin and laser photocoagulation of vessel in twin to twin transfusion syndrome. This approach has the advantage of reduced length of hospital stay, fewer complications and reduced need for postoperative tocolysis. The anaesthetic technique for these procedures varies from local infiltration of the abdominal wall for procedures, like intrauterine blood transfusion, cordocentesis or amniocentesis, to regional anaesthesia for multiple needle punctures or minilaparotomy, to general anaesthesia when procedure requires uterine exteriorization. Other considerations for the choice of anaesthesia include uterine activity, location of placenta and umbilical cord, position of the foetus, location of foetal lesion and chance of conversion to an open procedure. Local infiltration does not assure foetal immobility and it is usually achieved with direct administration of opioids and muscle relaxant to the foetus. Continuous infusion of remifentanil has also been used for maternal sedation and foetal immobility.[23] Balanced anaesthesia can be used for these procedures instead of deep inhalational technique used for open surgical procedures. An arterial catheter, orogastric tube, additional intravenous line or postoperative epidural analgesia are usually not required for minimally invasive procedures.

Anaesthesia for Ex Utero Intrapartum Treatment (EXIT) Procedures

EXIT procedures are a modification of open foetal procedures which are performed later in pregnancy and end with delivery of the baby. The technique was initially developed to remove tracheal clips placed during an open tracheal occlusion procedure to promote lung growth in congenital diaphragmatic hernia.[18] Presently, its indications have expanded to include cases where an obstructed airway (congenital high airway obstruction syndrome or CHAOS, laryngeal web or laryngeal cyst) or difficulty in securing the airway (cystic hygroma) is anticipated after birth, or when large thoracic or mediastinal masses require emergent excision to promote ventilation. It is also indicated in cases with associated cardiac lesion requiring immediate extracorporeal membrane oxygenation (ECMO) cannulation.[4] ECMO also shortens the time on placental support thereby preventing major maternal haemorrhage.[24] The essential components of the procedure include maintenance of uteroplacental blood flow and foetal oxygenation throughout the procedure until a definite airway has been established or the thoracic mass is excised. The uterus is opened with staplers as for open procedures. For airway procedures, only the foetal head and shoulders are delivered and for the thoracic mass excision, baby is delivered and kept on mother's abdomen for surgery. Care is taken to keep the umbilical cord moist with warm fluids. The procedure is done under general anaesthesia and sufficient time is allowed for uterine relaxation before commencement of the procedure. Foetal anaesthesia is supplemented with an opioid and neuromuscular blocker. Foetal anaesthesia is important as any spontaneous breath before airway intubation will induce transitional-pattern circulation and cause impairment of placental support.[25] Respiratory depression in the postoperative period is not an issue as all fetuses are intubated and ventilated at the end of an EXIT procedure. When general anaesthesia is not possible, a central neuraxial block supplemented with nitroglycerine can be used.[8] An intravenous line is always established in the foetus for fluid or blood resuscitation and foetal monitoring is established with pulse oximeter placed on the exposed hand. Maternal monitoring and epidural catheter placement is done as for open foetal procedures. After delivery of the baby, the inhalational anaesthetic is reduced or stopped and oxytocics are given to prevent uterine atony and blood loss. Ideally, a second anaesthesiologist should be present to take care of the baby and a second operation theatre is kept ready in case the baby needs further surgery. EXIT procedures provide maternal, foetal and uteroplacental stability and these procedures usually last for a short duration. However, continuous placental circulation maintained up to 1h has also been reported.[26]

COMPLICATIONS ASSOCIATED WITH FOETAL SURGERY

Maternal outcome after foetal procedures is generally good but as the maternal physiology is manipulated to facilitate surgery on the foetus, these procedures can expose the mother to several risks. Complications, like haemorrhage, scar dehiscence and wound infection, can occur after open surgical procedures. Cardiac dysfunction and haemodynamic disturbances which occur from prolonged exposure to high concentrations of volatile anaesthetics may compromise uterine and foetal blood flow. Preterm labour, premature rupture of membranes, preterm delivery and placental abruption have also been reported following foetal surgery.[27] Good postoperative analgesia minimizes the risk of preterm labour. Placental abruption may present with blood in the amniotic fluid, new onset maternal hypotension and foetal bradycardia or desaturation. The mother has to be explained the need for caesarean section in the future pregnancies. Uterine rupture in a subsequent pregnancy is a possibility as the baby is delivered by a classic caesarean incision for an EXIT procedure.

Intraoperative and postoperative pulmonary oedema is a dreaded complication which occurs in 25% of mothers presenting for foetal surgery, regardless of open or fetoscopic approach.[4] The mechanism of pulmonary oedema is not fully understood but it is mostly related to the tocolytic therapy especially with beta-sympathomimetics ritodrine and terbutaline. Prolonged therapy (>48 h) with magnesium sulphate decreases the maternal serum oncotic pressure and increased capillary permeability. Pulmonary oedema following nitroglycerine therapy is prolonged and difficult to treat. Another factor specific to the fetoscopic surgery is the significant amount of fluid absorbed into the maternal circulation to produce fluid overload.

The foetus is also at risk following surgery. Foetal distress can occur due to kinking and compression of the cord, increased uterine tone and maternal hypotension or hypoxia. Other foetal risks include bradycardia, hypoxia, hypothermia, central nervous system injuries, haemorrhage, heart failure and death.[28] Foetus may need resuscitation with left uterine displacement, administering vasopressors to the mother and administering atropine, adrenaline or blood to the foetus.[12] Increase in foetal heart rate and decrease in stroke volume have been observed during surgery on foetuses with normal cardiovascular system.[29] It is probably due to the combined effect of anaesthesia, surgery and tocolytic agents.

ETHICAL CONSIDERATIONS

Foetal surgery is a specialised field where the foetus is considered a primary patient with the mother acting as its operation theatre. As the access to the foetus is through the mother, it raises several ethical issues concerning informed consent, balancing the risk-benefit of the procedure and the duties of the physician to the pregnant woman and her foetus.[30] The consent of the mother is of utmost importance. Her life should never be put at risk and her choice should be respected. Moreover, all foetal therapeutic interventions are not of proven efficacy. Even procedures, like foetal blood transfusion for cells destroyed by Rh sensitised mother's immune system, which have proven efficacy, can cause severe foetal morbidity. Therefore, procedures on the foetus should only be undertaken, if there is a realistic chance of saving the foetus without any irreversible disability.

CONCLUSION

Foetal surgery has opened up a new and exciting field where foetus is the primary patient in his own right who can benefit from early correction of a congenital abnormality. It offers a third alternative to treat these abnormalities other than therapeutic abortion and neonatal death or severe sequelae after birth. Foetal surgery for congenital abnormalities is performed with the idea that result will be better than if surgery is performed after birth. However, these procedures should only be performed when there is a reasonable probability of foetal benefit and minimal risk to the mother. Research in this field is limited by ethical and practical reasons. A good communication between the surgeon and the anaesthesiologist, both intra- and postoperatively, is mandatory for the success of these procedures.

REFERENCES

1. Jancelewicz T, Harrison MR. A history of fetal surgery. Clin Perinatol 2009;36:227–236.

2. Liley AW. Intrauterine transfusion of the foetus in haemolytic disease. Br Med J 1963;2:1107–1109.

3. Harrison MR, Golbus MS, Filly RA. Management of the fetus with a correctable congenital defect. JAMA 1981;246:774–777.

4. Partridge EA, Flake AW. Maternal-fetal surgery for structural malformations. Best Practice and Research Clinical Obstetrics and Gynaecology 2012;26:669–682.

5. Adzick NS, Thom Ea, Spong CY, Brock 3rd JW, Burrows PK, Johnson MP, et al. A randomized trial of prenatal versus postnatal repair of myelomeningocele. N Engl J Med 2011;364:993–1004.

6. Senat MV, Deprest J, Boulvain M, Paupe A, Winer N, Ville Y. Endoscopic laser surgery versus serial amnio-reduction for severe twin-to-twin transfusion syndrome. N Engl J Med 2004;351:136–144.

7. Stephanova E, Topouzove-hristove T, Haarosova R, Moskova V. Halothane-induced alterations in cellular structure and proliferation of A549 cells. Tissue Cell 2008; 40:397–404.

8. Van de Velde M, De Buck F. Fetal and maternal analgesia/ anesthesia for fetal procedures. Fetal Diagn Ther 2012; 31:201–209.

9. Sprung J, Flick RP, Wilder RT, et al. Anesthesia for caesarean delivery and learning disabilities in a popu-lation-based birth cohort. Anesthesiology 2009;111: 302–310.

10. Myers LB, Cohen D, Galinkin J, Gaiser R, Kurth CD. Anaesthesia for fetal surgery. Paediatr Anaesth 2002; 12:569–578.

11. Okamoto M, Walewski JL, Artusio JF, WF Riker Jr. Neuromuscular pharmacology in rat neonates: develop-ment of responsiveness to prototypic blocking and reversal drugs. Anesth Analg 1992;75:361–371.

12. Tran K, Cohen DE. Anesthesia for fetal surgery. In: Davis PJ, Cladis FP, Motoyama EK (Eds). Smith's Anesthesia for Infants and Children, 8th edn. Elsevier Mosby: Philadelphia. 2011;589–604.

13. Galinkin JL, Kurth CD. Anesthesia for fetal surgery. ASA Refresher Course 2002;30:111–119.

14. Ngan Kee WD, Khaw KS, Tan PE, Ng FF, Karmakar MK. Placental transfer and foetal metabolic effects of pheny-lephrine and ephedrine during spinal anesthesia for cesarean delivery. Anesthesiology 2009;111:506–512.

15. Lee A, Ngan Kee WD, Gin T. A quantitative systematic review of randomized controlled trials of ephedrine versus phenylephrine for the management of hypotension during spinal anesthesia for caesarean delivery. Anesth Analg 2002;94:920–926.

16. Brusseau R, Myers L. Developing consciousness: Fetal anesthesia and analgesia. Seminars in Anesthesia, Perioperative Medicine and Pain 2006;25:189–195.

17. Lee SJ, Ralston HJP, Drey EA, Partridge JC, Rosen MA. Fetal Pain. A systematic review of the evidence. JAMA 2005;294(8):947–954.

18. Cauldwell CB. Anesthesia for fetal surgery. Anesthesiol Clin North America 2002;20:211–226.

19. Sviggum HP, Kodali BS. Maternal anesthesia for fetal surgery. Clin Perinatol 2013;40:413–427.

20. Ngamprasertwong P, Michelfelder EC, Arbabi S, Choi YS, Statile C, Ding L, Boat a, Eghtesady P, Holland K, Sadhasivam S. Anesthetic techniques for fetal surgery: Effects of maternal anesthesia on intraoperative fetal outcomes in the sheep model. Anesthesiology 2013;118: 796–808.

21. Johnson N, Johnson VA, Fisher J, et al. Fetal monitoring with pulse oximetry. Br J Obstet Gynaecol 1991;98:36–41.

22. Ramirez MV. Anesthesia for fetal surgery. Rev Colomb Anestesiol 2012;40:268–272.

23. Van de Velde M, Van Schoubroeck D, Lewi LE, et al. Remifentanil for fetal immobilization and maternal sedation during fetoscopic surgery: a randomized, double-blind comparison with diazepam. Anesth Analg 2005;101: 251–258.

24. DeBuck F, Van de Velde M. Anesthesia for fetal surgery. Curr Opin Anesthesiol 2008;21:293-297.

25. Zadra N, Giusti F. Ex utero intrapartum surgery (EXIT): indications and anaesthetic management. Best Practice & Research Clinical Anaesthesiology 2004;18(2):259–271.

26. Boris P, Cox PBW, Gogarten W, Struwper D, Marcus MAE. Foetal surgery, anaesthesiological considerations. Curr Opin Anaesthesiol 2004;17:235–240.

27. Golombeck K, Ball RH, Lee H, Farrell JA, Farmer DL, Jacobs VR, Rosen MA, Filly RA, Harrison MR. Maternal morbidity after maternal-fetal surgery. Am J Obstet Gynecol 2006;194:834–839.

28. Rosen MA. Anesthesia for fetal surgery and other intrauterine procedures. In: Chestnut DH, Tsen LC, Polley LS, Wong CA (Eds). Chestnut's Obstetric Anesthesia: Principles and Practice, 4th edn. Mosby Elsevier 2009; 7:123–140.

29. Rychik J, Tian Z, Cohen MS, Ewing SG, Cohen D, Howell LJ, Wilson RD, Johnson MP, Hedrick HL, Flake AW, Crombleholme TM, Adzick NS, et al. Acute cardio-vascular effects of fetal surgery in the human. Circulation 2004;110:1549–1556.

30. Noble R, Rodeck CH. Ethical considerations of feta surgery. Best Practice & Research Clinical Obstetrics and Gynaecology 2008;22(1):219–231.

16

Dental Procedures in Children: Challenges and Concerns

Namita Kalra, Amit Khatri

- Primary concern in children undergoing dental procedures
- Indications and contraindications for general anaesthesia
  - Circumstances and conditions suitable for general anaesthesia
  - Circumstances and conditions not suitable for general anaesthesia
- Children with medical problems
- Ethical considerations
- Treatment planning in children presenting for various dental procedures

INTRODUCTION

Paediatric dental patients are mostly overcome by anxiety and fear of unknown. It is extremely difficult to overcome their anxiety which results in uncooperative behaviour. Paediatric dentists are, therefore, trained to understand the psychology of the growing child and follow behaviour management techniques and methods. The different methods of pain control vary from simple behaviour management to full intubational general anaesthesia in a hospital set up.[1]

In 1929, American Society for the Advancement of Anesthesia and Sedation in Dentistry was founded by a group of dedicated dentists under the leadership of Dr M Hillel Feldman. Anaesthesia techniques were initially developed specifically for dentistry and blossomed in the middle of the 20th century. Drs Morgan Allison, Adrian Hubbell, and Leonard Monheim were among the first pioneers to become noted for advancing the training of dentists in the practice of general anaesthesia for dentistry. Around this same time, other dentists, including Drs Niels Jorgensen, Ed Driscoll, and Norman Trieger developed what was then a new technique, termed "conscious sedation." Conscious sedation used subanaesthetic doses of general anaesthetic drugs, along with good local anaesthesia, to provide a comfortable and safe form of anaesthesia. These new anaesthesia concepts and ideas led to the establishment of the American Dental Society of Anesthesiology (ADSA) in 1953.[2]

PRIMARY CONCERN IN CHILDREN UNDERGOING DENTAL PROCEDURES

The commonest problem encountered in children presenting for any dental procedure which results in a very uncooperative child is anxiety. Therefore, the primary concern remains methods to recognize and alleviate anxiety during a primary visit itself.

Commonly employed method and technique to allay anxiety are as follows:

- Child friendly operator.
- Soothing subtle music with facility for music in head rest of child.
- Friendly talk with familiarization of the environment and methods.

Some established strategies for behaviuor management include:

- Audiovisual distraction
- Systematic desensitization

- Positive reinforcement
- Voice control

In normal healthy children, failure of behaviour management technique takes place only rarely. The majority of paediatric dental procedures are performed on an out-patient basis. In normal children, local anaesthesia, with or without sedation is sufficient to accomplish most procedures. However, when extensive dental care is required, and/or the child is severely retarded, or has serious behavioural problem, or is medically compromised, special monitoring and deep sedation or general anaesthesia may be required.

The armamentarium for pain and anxiety management includes:

- Non-pharmacologic
  - Behaviour management skills
  - Hypnosis
- Pharmacologic
  - **Pre-procedural enteral sedation:** Techniques of sedation requiring drug administration by oral or rectal route. This term is synonymous with premedication.
  - **Peri-procedural sedation:** This involves induction of general anaesthesia and can be thus either inhalational (relative analgesia and N20 sedation) or parenteral.
  - Local anaesthesia
  - General anaesthesia

Optimum techniques or combinations of the above pharmacological procedures are most advantageous with lower risk to patients. At the same time, it will suffice in achieving treatment goals namely, sedation with local anaesthesia.

Pharmocological management is indicated for children who cannot be managed with traditional behaviour management technique and local anaesthesia.

Decision between Sedation and General Anaesthesia[1]

There are no set rules for deciding whether dental treatment should be provided under conscious sedation or general anaesthesia and patient need to be assessed individually. No child should be taken under general anaesthesia without consideration for potential risk. The decision whether a paediatric patient should be treated under conscious sedation or general anaesthesia depends on the following factors:

- Age of child
- Degree of surgical trauma involved
- Anxiety level
- Complexity of operative procedure involved
- Medical status of child

American Society of Anaesthesiologists (ASA) Classification provide an excellent guide to the type of sedation or anaesthesia appropriate to individual patient's medical and behavioural problem (Box 16.1).

Box 16.1: American Society of Anesthesiologists— classification

- **ASA I:** A normal healthy patient.
- **ASA II:** A patient with mild systemic disease.
- **ASA III:** A patient with severe systemic disease.
- **ASA IV:** A patient with severe systemic disease that is a constant threat to life.
- **ASA V:** A moribund patient who is not expected to survive without the operation.
- **ASA VI:** A declared brain-dead patient whose organs are being removed for donor purposes.
- **E:** Emergency operation of any variety (used to modify one of the above classifications, i.e. ASA III-E).

ASA Physical Status Classification System is reprinted with permission of the American Society of Anaesthesiologists, 520 N. Northwest Highway, Park Ridge, IL 60068-2573.

INDICATIONS AND CONTRAINDICATIONS FOR GENERAL ANAESTHESIA

Indications

1. Patients with certain physical, mental, or medically compromising conditions, e.g. Down's syndrome, severe mental retardation, renal failure, cerebral palsy.
2. Patients to whom local anaesthesia is ineffective due to acute infections, anatomic variations and allergy to local anaesthetic components.
3. Extremely uncooperative, fearful, anxious or uncommunicative child/adolescent who requires immediate dental care.
4. Patients with extensive orofacial and dental trauma (e.g. from accidents)
5. Patients with dental needs who otherwise would not obtain necessary dental care, e.g. children in

Table 16.1	Reasons for administration of general anaesthesia	
Reason		**%**
▪ Medically compromised/handicapped		39.14
▪ Uncooperative/lacking cooperative ability		23.40
▪ Coming from far/inability for repeated visits		37.40

rural areas which are inaccessible to dental treatment.

6. Patients requiring dental care for whom the use of general anaesthesia may protect the developing psyche.

Reasons for administration of general anaesthesia: The common reasons for administrations were evaluated by Tharian and Tandon,[3] and the results were grouped as shown in Table 16.1.

Contraindications

1. Cooperative child with extensive dental treatment.
2. Medical contraindications to general anaesthesia, e.g. enlarged tonsils, acute infections.
3. Cooperative child with minimal dental treatment needs.

Circumstances and Conditions Suitable for General Anaesthesia[4,5]

1. Severe pulpitis requiring immediate relief.
2. Acute soft tissue swelling requiring removal of the infected tooth/teeth.
3. Surgical drainage of an acute infected swelling.
4. Single or multiple extractions in a young child unsuitable for conscious sedation.
5. Symptomatic teeth in more than one quadrant.
6. Moderately traumatic or complex extractions, e.g. ankylosed or infraoccluded primary molars, extraction of broken down permanent molars.
7. Teeth requiring surgical removal or exposure.
8. Biopsy of a hard or soft tissue lesion.
9. Debridement and suturing of orofacial wounds.
10. Established allergy to local anaesthesia.
11. Postoperative haemorrhage requiring packing and suturing.
12. Examination under GA, including radiographs, for a special needs child where clinical evidence exists that there is a dental problem which warrants treatment.

13. Severe pulpitis and acute infection are by far the most common conditions treated under GA.

Circumstances and Conditions not Suitable for General Anaesthesia

1. Carious, asymptomatic teeth with no clinical or radiographic signs of sepsis.
2. Orthodontic extraction of sound permanent premolar teeth in a healthy child.
3. Patient/carer preference, except where other techniques have already been tried.
   Extenuating circumstances that override the above limitations are: Physical, emotional, learning impairment or a combination of two or more of these.
4. Children who have attempted treatment using LA alone or LA combined with conscious sedation and have been unable to co-operate.

CHILDREN WITH MEDICAL PROBLEMS

These should be managed in collaboration with the child's paediatrician. When appropriate the dental surgeon should seek advice from a physician which should be provided in writing. This advice should cover any special problems related to preoperative, intraoperative and postoperative care of the child.[6,7] The American Society of Anaesthesiologists (ASA) Physical Status classification is a useful guide to suitability for day care GA.[8] A child with a severe underlying medical condition in categories ASA III or ASA IV should be admitted to a paediatric ward and clinical care shared with a paediatric team.

ETHICAL CONSIDERATIONS

Consent of surrogates (such as parents, legal guardians and courts) should be taken for any general anaesthesia procedure.

Factors affecting consent:

1. Considering the patients best interest in mind.
2. Parental influences, like moral attitude, past experiences, beliefs and inability to make decisions, may prevent caregivers from giving consent. They will then start insisting on many forms of therapy that may not be beneficial and increase the child's suffering.
3. Dentist should give proper information of the procedure and the need for the procedures.
4. Parent motivation.

Informed Consent

Fully discloses the benefits, therapeutic and non-therapeutic alternatives and potential complications of the procedure. It must provide:

- Adequate information of procedure
- Should be in clear language/understandable

Assent

American Association of Paediatric Dentistry 2008[9] suggests physicians to seek "permission" from parents and to seek "assent" from the child whenever possible. This is done because the American Association of Pediatric Dentistry in encouraging the development of healthy, involved, fully decisional adults through helpful encounters with paediatricians and others.

TREATMENT PLANNING IN CHILDREN PRESENTING FOR VARIOUS DENTAL PROCEDURES

Comprehensive planning aims at ensuring that all the treatment required is carried out under a single GA. The practice of extracting the most grossly carious and/or symptomatic teeth and leaving restorable teeth for future visits as an outpatient using LA with or without sedation is to be depreciated. This has been shown to result in a high rate of repeat GA.[10] The inability of the child to accept treatment using LA is an important factor in determining the need for GA.

Radiographs

A comprehensive treatment plan is not possible without recent radiographs. An exception to this is when removal of carious primary incisor teeth is planned, where radiographs are of limited diagnostic value.

Extractions

If an urgent GA is indicated, unrestorable asymptomatic teeth should be removed in addition to those causing pain or sepsis.[11,12]

Balancing and Compensating Extractions

Guidelines exist for the planning of extraction patterns in paediatric dentistry, and these should be followed.[12]

Extraction of a Permanent Molar

If a permanent molar is to be considered for extraction under GA, the orthodontic implications should be considered, and the need for loss of further permanent molars discussed with the child and parents.

Restorative Treatment Options

Restorative care provided under GA can be more durable than that provided under other circumstances, particularly in very young children.[13–15] The most predictably successful restoration should be provided. A temporary/provisional restoration may be indicated by other circumstances (e.g. imminent exfoliation).

Preventive Counselling

Parents of children who require the treatment of extensive disease under GA need further preventive advice.[16,17] The SIGN guideline "Preventing Dental Caries in Children at High Caries Risk" provides an important source of preventive advice.[18]

Clinical Effectiveness

A primary tooth restored under GA should be expected to exfoliate naturally without failure. Preformed metal crowns are the most predictable and durable restorations for pulp therapy for primary teeth should be provided with caution under GA, given the clinical failure rates of the medicaments available. Exceptional circumstances (e.g. haemangioma/lymphangioma in supporting tissues) may be a contraindication to extraction.[19]

In the paediatric dentistry, anaesthesia falls into three main categories:[1]

1. Outpatient/short-case dental chair anaesthesia with a laryngeal mask.
2. Outpatient/day-stay intubation anaesthesia
3. Inpatient/hospital-stay intubation anaesthesia

Outpatient/short-case dental chair anaesthesia with a laryngeal mask: This is used for ASA class I or class II patients requiring short, 2–10 min, procedures with rapid induction and early recovery, e.g. dental extraction.

Outpatient/day-stay intubation anaesthesia: This is used for ASA class I or class II patients who require dental treatment that last more than 10 min, e.g. removal of impacted teeth and supernumerary teeth, minor oral maxillofacial procedures, e.g. mucocele.

Inpatient/hospital–stay intubation anaesthesia: This is used for ASA class III patients. These patients have a medical problem that constitutes a significant risk, and are advised by the anaesthesiologist that they be treated in a hospital operating theatre.

CONCLUSION

1. Most paediatric patients can be treated using behaviour management under local anaesthesia.
2. Paediatric dentist/anaesthetist who want to use sedation technique with child patient should receive training in sedation.
3. It is also essential that whole dental team is trained in sedation and general anaesthesia
4. All techniques requiring sedation and anaesthesia, appropriate monitoring equipment should be available.

REFERENCES

1. Richard Welbury, Monty Duggal and Marie Therese Hosey. Paediatric Dentistry (3rd edn), Oxford University Press.
2. Ganzberg S, Rashid RG, Davidian E. Contribution of Dentist Anesthesiologists to Dental Anesthesiology Research. Anesthesia Progress 2011;58(1):14–21. doi:10.2344/0003–3006-58.1.14.
3. Sowjanya V, Tandon S, Tharian E. Physiological response to dental anxiety in children. J Indian Soc Pedod Prev Dent 1995;13(1):13–17.
4. Blain KM, Hill FJ. The use of inhalation sedation and local anaesthesia as an alternative to general anaesthesia for dental extractions in children. Br Dent J 1998;184(12): 608–611.
5. Shaw A. Inhalation sedation can be used for many children referred for general anaesthesia. Br Dent J 1998; 184(12): 601.
6. Landes DP, Clayton-Smith AJ. The role of pre-general anaesthetic assessment for patients referred by general dental practitioners to in the Community Dental Service. Community Dent Health 1996;13(3):169–171.
7. Harrison MG, Roberts GJ. Comprehensive dental treatment of healthy and chronically sick children under intubation general anaesthesia during a 5-year period. Br Dent J 1998 ;184(10):503–506.
8. American Society of Anesthesiologists. ASA Physical Status Classification System.http://www.asahq.org/clinical/physicalstatus.htm.
9. American Academy of Pediatric Dentistry special issue: reference manual 2007–2008. Pediatr Dent 2007;29(7suppl): 66–68,121–122.
10. Harrison M, Nutting L. Repeat general anaesthesia for paediatric dentistry. Br Dent J 2000;189(1):37–39.
11. Camilleri C, Roberts G, Ashley P, Scheer B. Analysis of paediatric dental care under general anaesthesia and levels of dental disease in two hospitals. Br Dent J 2004;196(4): 219–223.
12. Guideline for first permanent molar extraction.http://www.rcseng.ac.uk/fds/clinical _guidelines/documents/guideline_molar_e.
13. O'Sullivan EA, Curzon ME. The efficacy of comprehensive dental care for children under general anesthesia. Br Dent J 1991;171(2):56–58.
14. Eidelman E, Faibis S, Peretz B. A comparison of restorations for children with early childhood caries treated under general anesthesia or conscious sedation. Pediatr Dent 2000;22(1):33–37.
15. Tate AR, Ng MW, Needleman HL, Acs G. Failure rates of restorative procedures following dental rehabilitation under general anesthesia. Pediatr Dent 2002;24(1): 69–71.
16. Hood CA, Hunter ML, Kingdon A. Demographic characteristics, oral health knowledge and practices of mothers of children aged 5 years and under referred for extraction of teeth under general anaesthesia. Int J Paediatr Dent 1998;8(2):131–136.
17. Almeida AG, Roseman MM, Sheff M, Huntington N, Hughes CV. Future caries susceptibility in children with early childhood caries following treatment under general anesthesia. Pediatr Dent 2000;22(4):302–306.
18. Preventing dental caries in children at high caries risk. Scottish Intercollegiate Guidelines Network. 2000.
19. Randall RC, Vrijhoef MM, Wilson NH. Efficacy of preformed metal crowns vs. amalgam restorations in primary molars: a systematic review. J Am Dent Assoc 2000;131(3): 337–343.

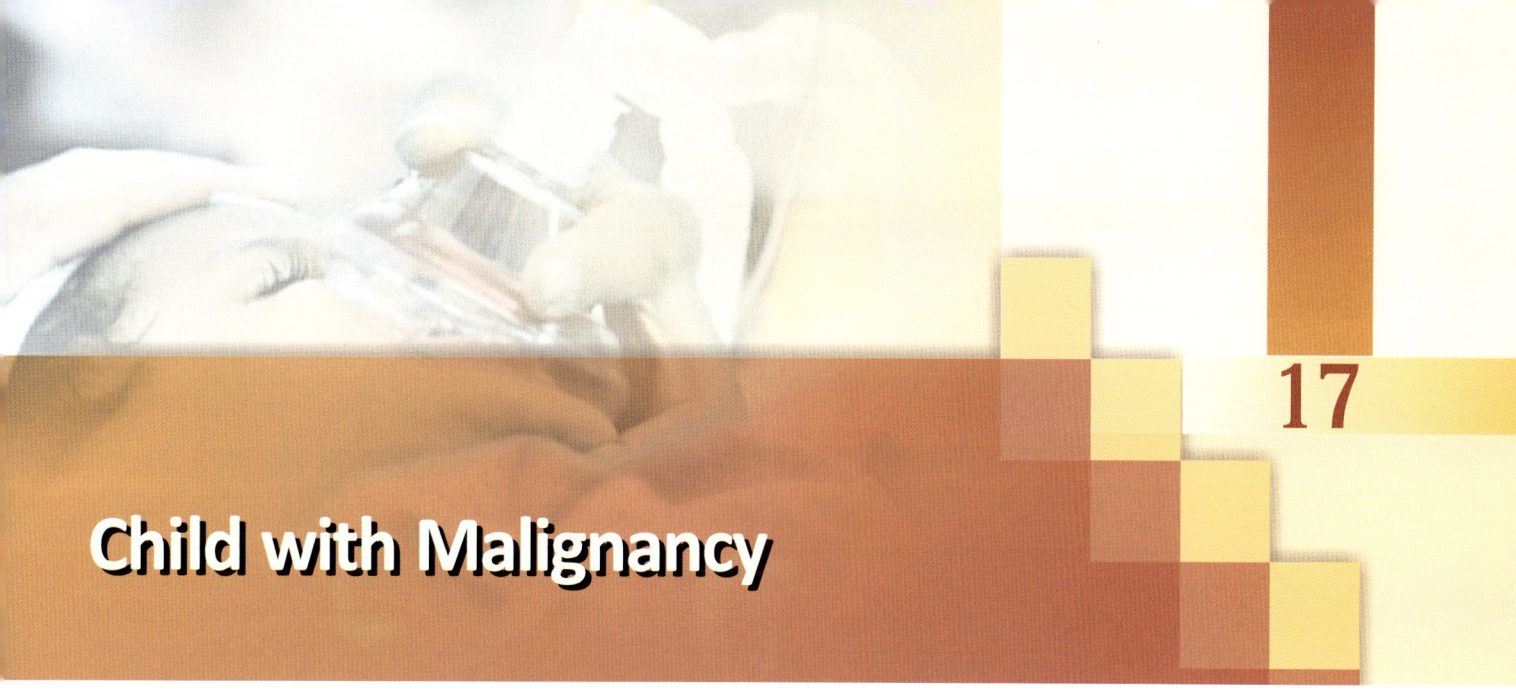

Child with Malignancy

Poonam Motiani

- Incidence and mortality
- Causes of childhood cancer
- Overview of common paediatric malignancies
- Role of anaesthetist
- Reasons for surgery
- Toxicity of therapy
  - Effects of chemotherapy
  - Effects of radiotherapy
- Anaesthesia for short procedures in remote locations
- Alternate site anaesthesia concerns
- Anaesthesia for radiotherapy
  - Fundamentals of external beam radiotherapy
  - Anaesthetic management of paediatric radiotherapy treatment

INCIDENCE AND MORTALITY

Worldwide, childhood cancer has an incidence of about 175,000 per year, and a mortality rate of approximately 96,000 per year.[1]

In the United States, cancer is the second commonest cause of death among children aged 1 to 14 years, exceeded only by accidents.[2] In developed countries, childhood cancer has a 20% mortality as compared to 80–90% in the world's poorest countries.[3]

CAUSES OF CHILDHOOD CANCER

- Identified **familial and genetic factors** (5–15%)
- Known **environmental exposures** and exogenous factors (<5–10%)[4–8] including:

- **External agents:**
  - Physical carcinogens:
    - Ionizing radiation (X-ray)
    - Non-ionizing radiation (electromagnetic fields, UV)
  - Biological carcinogens:
    - Infections from viruses (Epstein-Barr virus: *Burkitt's lymphoma and Hodgkin's disease;*
    - Hepatitis B: *Liver carcinoma*
    - HHV8 and HIV: *Kaposi's sarcoma*)
  - Chemical carcinogens:
    - Tobacco: mothers who smoke during pregnancy
    - Pesticides, asbestos—parental occupation
    - Aflatoxin, arsenic—food and drinking water contaminants
    - Drugs and medication—pregnant women treatment (diethylstilbesterol: *Cell adenocarcinoma of the vagina or cervix*)
  - Dietary constituents
- **Internal agents:**
  - Inherited factors
    - Predisposition to particular familial diseases
    - Genetically determined features
- **Unknown 75–90%**[9,10]

In most cases, cancers involve multiple risk factors and variables.

OVERVIEW OF COMMON PAEDIATRIC MALIGNANCIES

The most common cancers in children are childhood leukaemia (34%), brain tumours (23%), and lymphomas (12%).[11] Considerable improvements in treatment have led to a dramatic improvement in survival rates.

- **Leukaemia:** One-third of all childhood cancers.
  - Peak incidence: 2–3 years of age.
  - **Factors contributing to improved outcomes include** increased intensity of treatment and effective use of multi-agent chemotherapy regimens.
- **Brain and CNS tumours:** Second most common group of cancers.
  - Forty-three percent—astrocytomas.
  - **Mainstay of treatment:** Surgery, chemotherapy and radiotherapy.
- **Lymphoma:** 10–20% of all cancers.
  - Incidence: Two-fold in boys; increases with age
  - 0–10 years: Non-Hodgkin's lymphoma more common.
  - 10–14 years: Hodgkin's lymphoma more common.
  - **Mainstay of treatment:** Chemotherapy but radiotherapy and surgical resection may also be used.
- **Embryonal tumours:** Comprise 15% of childhood cancers
  - Arise due to proliferation of tissue normally only seen in the developing embryo. They include: medulloblastoma, neuroblastoma, retinoblastoma, nephroblastoma (Wilms' tumour), and hepatoblastoma.
- **Other tumours:** Less common
  - Include bone cancers, soft tissue sarcomas and germ cell and gonadal tumours.

ROLE OF ANAESTHETIST

The anaesthesiologist forms a key part of the multidisciplinary team caring for the child with malignancy. Anaesthesia will be required at all stages of their care including diagnosis, treatment, tumour surveillance and pain management. This will include anaesthesia for major and minor surgical procedures, anaesthesia for short painful procedures (lumbar puncture, bone marrow aspiration, and trephine biopsy) or to facilitate radiotherapy. Knowledge of the physiological effects of the malignant process and its treatment are vital for any anaesthesiologist involved in the care of such patients.

REASONS FOR SURGERY

Surgery can be required for multiple reasons:
- **As part of diagnosis:** Surgical intervention (biopsy or sampling of involved tissues), may be required to define the exact type of cancer, the true nature of the tumour (malignant or benign), and to determine, if the tumour has spread to other organs or areas in the body.
- **In support of treatment:** Surgery may be needed to prepare patients for treatments that require chemotherapy or drugs by providing a route of access (placement of a central venous line or port-a-cath to administer these agents), or to address complications of treatment, such as infections or obstructions.
- **As a primary component of treatment:** Sometimes surgery is the best option in the treatment of a child's tumour, or it may be part of a multi-modality approach (in combination with chemotherapy, radiotherapy, immunotherapy, etc.) to the global treatment of a cancerous tumour.

Open surgical removal of the tumours occurring in any of the sites, such as abdomen, thorax, chest wall, HFN (head, face, neck), brain and extremities, is the option which has been practiced traditionally and even in the present era. Nevertheless with the advances in science and technology and with ever increasing usage and expertise of laparoscopy in children, paediatric oncologic surgeons are now skilled in minimally invasive as well as open surgical procedures. The benefits of a minimally invasive approach include cosmetic appearance, reduced hospital stay, faster recovery, no/minimal bowel adhesions, much less pain and discomfort, reduced analgesic requirement, minimal postoperative disability, shorter length of postoperative ileus and rapid wound healing.[12,13]

Absolute contraindications to MIS in paediatric surgical oncology include an associated coagulation disorder, respiratory compromise and an infective focus, especially in the anterior abdominal wall.

Relative contraindications include extensive previous surgery and ablative MIS when tumour is very huge as it may lead to tumour spillage.

Judicious conversion to open surgery should not be considered as a complication. The conversion rate for paediatric surgical MIS procedures is usually between 7 and 10%.[14] **Complications** of minimal invasive surgery include atelectasis [15] and trocar site herniation.[16]

TOXICITY OF THERAPY

It is important to recognise that children with cancer can develop organ dysfunction at any time for a number of different reasons. The previously uncomplicated anaesthetic is not always a safe predictor. A detailed anaesthetic assessment and appropriate ordering of investigations, paying particular attention to the anatomical and physiological effects of the cancer is vital for all paediatric oncology patients.

Effects of Chemotherapy

Combination therapy results in potential toxicity to nearly every organ system (Table 17.1). Of concern are the detrimental effects chemotherapy and radiotherapy have on the airway and cardiopulmonary systems. Sub-clinical but relevant cardiomyopathy is common and can be unmasked during the perioperative period. A careful assessment of all systems should be made before giving an anaesthetic.

Cardiac Toxicity

Anthracycline based chemotherapeutic agents, including doxorubicin, daunorubicin, fluorouracil and cyclophosphamide are frequently used to treat leukaemias and lymphomas. Recognised cardiotoxic effects of these agents include myocardial depression and ischaemia, hypotension, hypertension, myocarditis, endomyocardial fibrosis and conduction defects leading to supraventricular tachycardia and heart block. It is thought cardiotoxicity is caused by the generation of free radicals, which interfere with mitochondrial function. Specific risk factors predisposing patients to cardiotoxicity include cumulative drug dose given, total dose given on any day of treatment, rate and route of administration, drug combination and dosing schedule.

Cardiotoxicity can manifest early or late. Children receiving cardiotoxic chemotherapy should have surveillance echocardiography during and after treatment.

Pulmonary Toxicity

Chemotherapeutic agents cause a broad-spectrum of pulmonary complications. These can manifest early (Table 17.2) or late in the treatment process. Amongst late manifestations, pulmonary fibrosis predominates.

Bleomycin results in toxicity in up to 10% of patients receiving it. Bleomycin causes a spectrum of lung disease including bleomycin-induced pneumonitis (BIP). BIP can progress to pulmonary fibrosis and treatment involves the cessation of therapy and commencing steroids. Evidence suggests that delivery of high inspired oxygen concentrations (FiO_2) during or after bleomycin therapy may promote pulmonary toxicity because bleomycin-induced lung injury is mediated via oxidant pathways. This is of particular relevance to the anaesthetist as intraoperative inspired oxygen concentrations should be as low as safely possible during and after bleomycin therapy.

S.No.	Chemotherapy	Complications
Table 17.1	**Toxicity of various chemotherapeutic agents**	
1	Vincristine	Myelosuppression, SIADH, peripheral neuropathy, mucositis
2	Anthracyclines	Myelosuppression, cardiomyopathy, arrhythmias
3	Cyclophosphamide	Myelosuppression, cardiomyopathy, arrhythmias, haemorrhagic cystitis
4	Ifosfamide	Myelosuppression, Fanconi's syndrome, renal failure
5	Cisplatin	Seizures, hypomagnesaemia, renal failure
6	Nitrosureas	Pneumonitis, renal failure
7	Bleomycin	Allergic reactions, pulmonary fibrosis, Reynaud's
8	Methotrexate	Myelosuppression, mucositis, pneumonitis, renal failure

Table 17.2	Pulmonary toxicity of chemotherapeutic agents
Agent	**Complication (early)**
Methotrexate, bleomycin, paclitaxel	Interstitial pneumonitis
Bleomycin, interleukin -2	Acute non-cardiogenic pulmonary oedema
Vinblastine, methotrexate	Bronchospasm
Pleural effusion	Methotrexate

Haematological Toxicity

Myelosuppression is the most common dose limiting effect of cancer chemotherapy and manifests as anaemia, neutropenia and thrombocytopenia. It must also be considered that myelosuppression is a common direct effect of cancer in children and may be present even in the pre-treatment phase. Haematological abnormalities commonly encountered are often multifactorial in origin. Anaemia is common at the diagnosis of many paediatric malignancies and occurs in up to 80% of children presenting with ALL. The ability of the child to cope with the physiological complications of such anaemia may be compromised in the presence of chemotherapy-induced cardiac dysfunction.

- **Neutropenia** is usual on presentation in patients with ALL. Leucopenia is the most common haematological toxicity of cancer therapy and often leads to cessation or dose limitation of therapy.

- *Specific considerations for the anaesthetist in the neutropenic patient:*
  - Careful adherence to aseptic technique during invasive procedures
  - Avoidance of per rectum medications
  - Appropriate perioperative isolation of the patient
  - Awareness of the increased risk of mucositis and its associated potential airway complications.

- **Thrombocytopenia** is a common side effect of myelosuppression. Clinically significant bleeding frequently occurs and is the commonest cause of premature death in children with leukaemia. Of relevance to the anaesthetist is the variance of local protocol regarding acceptable platelet counts for invasive procedures. Typically, the platelet count should be above $50 \times 10^9/L$ for lumbar puncture and $20 \times 10^9/L$ for bone marrow trephine.

Gastrointestinal Toxicity

GI system side effects from chemotherapeutic agents are common and often treatment limiting. They include:

- Nausea and vomiting
- Diarrhoea
- Mucositis
- Enterocolitis
- Stomatitis

These may co-exist and lead to anorexia, malnutrition and subsequent alterations in electrolytes, vitamins and serum proteins. Specific anaesthetic considerations include the risk of delayed gastric emptying and aspiration. This is confounded by the concurrent use of opiate pain relief. The presence of dehydration, acute renal failure (ARF) and electrolyte imbalance should be considered.

Renal Toxicity

Cisplatin, carboplatin and ifosfamide are the agents most commonly associated with ARF in children. Cisplatin produces a dose-dependent and cumulative nephrotoxicity. High dose methotrexate therapy is associated with severe renal impairment in 2% of children. The use of amphotericin B, cyclosporin A, acyclovir, immunoglobulin and some antibiotics may contribute to the development of ARF.

Neurotoxicity

The platinum-based chemotherapeutic agents (e.g. cisplatin, carboplatin) are associated with increased incidence of neurotoxicity. Other implicated agents include: methotrexate, vincristine and cyclosporin. Serious neurotoxicity is especially associated with ifosfamide and systemic or intrathecal methotrexate.

Effects of Radiotherapy

Radiotherapy leads to the cell death of both tumour cells and healthy tissues by causing damage to cellular DNA. Healthy or 'normal' tissues have a greater capacity to repair the ionizing effects of radiation but require time to do so and thus the total radiotherapy dose is divided into a series of fractions to be given over days or weeks. Conformal radiotherapy represents a major advance in treatment and helps to minimize damage to surrounding tissues. Despite this, children's developing tissues are particularly susceptible to radiotherapy. The susceptibility of normal tissues to damage from radiation depends on multiple factors including total and fractional dose received, sensitivity of tissues to radiation, volume of tissue irradiated, time course of treatment and the presence concurrent chemotherapy.

Airway Issues

The airway is at particular risk following high-dose radiotherapy to the neck and oral cavity. Mucositis is a common complication.

Chronic radiotherapy effects predisposing to airway difficulty:

- Fibrosis and stiffness of soft tissue resulting in limited mouth opening and neck extension
- Airway mucosal fibrosis
- Subglottic oedema
- Supra- and subglottic narrowing or stenosis
- Hypoplasia of jaw and xerostomia

Cardiopulmonary Issues

Radiation-induced heart disease can affect all components of the heart. The risk is increased with concomitant vincristine or doxorubicin therapy. Radiation-induced pericardial disease can develop in 2 months to years following therapy.

Effects of radiation-induced heart disease:

- Pericarditis
- Pericardial effusion
- Endocardial fibrosis
- Valvular fibrosis
- Conduction defects
- Coronary artery disease

Radiation-induced pneumonitis is common due to the susceptibility of lung tissue to damage. Severity of disease is related to the total volume of lung exposed to radiation, the total radiation dose, and the size of the individual fractions of dose given. Previous chemotherapy, previous radiotherapy and withdrawal of steroids are recognised risk factors for radiation-induced pneumonitis.

Toxic effects of chemotherapy and chest irradiation typically lead to a restrictive defect on pulmonary function tests. The results of these tests and the severity of such restriction should be reviewed prior to embarking upon anaesthesia.

Airway complications and mucositis: Airway tumours are uncommon in children. Airway concerns relate mostly to the toxic effects of treatment. The presence of an anterior mediastinal mass (AMM) must always be considered. Enlarged tonsils and adenoids secondary to leukaemic infiltration can cause obstructive sleep apnoea. Infiltration of retropharyngeal lymph nodes can present as stridor in severe cases and cervical lymphadenopathy can cause airway compromise.

Mucositis is characterised by ulcerative, erythematous and extremely painful lesions. It may cause supraglottic oedema and airway bleeding secondary to tissue friability and this may cause a previously routine airway to become difficult. It is prevalent and dose-limiting during high dose chemotherapy, haemopoietic stem cell transplantation (HSCT) and radiation therapy to the head and neck. It can emerge 7–10 days after the start of chemotherapy and persist for 1–2 weeks. It is most acute 2–4 weeks after radiotherapy treatment.

Tumour Lysis Syndrome

This potentially fatal syndrome most frequently occurs in patients presenting with a large tumour load especially in acute leukaemias or those with high-grade lymphomas. The syndrome results from the sudden release of intracellular components into the circulation following the rapid death of large numbers of malignant cells. This leads to a rapidly rising potassium and progressive renal impairment from urate nephropathy and phosphate precipitation. The increase in serum phosphate production may be accompanied by hypocalcaemic seizures. Further complications include severe metabolic acidosis, cardiac arrhythmias, and sudden death. Emergency management includes control of hyperkalaemia, correction of hypocalcaemia and hyperhydration to prevent urate nephropathy. These patients should be managed on an intensive care unit as many will require a period of haemofiltration. Those at high risk of tumour lysis syndrome should have preventative measures initiated prior to chemotherapy or anaesthetic intervention. Such measures include: hyperhydration, administration of allopurinol and alkalination of the urine. The recombinant urate oxidase enzyme rasburicase has proved effective in prophylaxis of high-risk paediatric patients. Of specific importance to the anaesthetist is the fact that steroids have potent anti-cancer properties and have been shown to inadvertently precipitate tumour lysis syndrome. Steroids, such as dexamethasone, as an antiemetic, should be used cautiously under anaesthesia.

Pain and Psychological Impact of Disease

Many children report that the single most painful experience of their treatment for paediatric cancer was a painful medical procedure (lumbar puncture or bone marrow aspiration) or surgery. A general anaesthetic was the only variable that provided a reduction in pain scores. General anaesthesia should be provided, if deemed appropriate and safe. Severe pain in children often requires short- or long-term opioid use, which can lead to tolerance. A multimodal approach to analgesia in children is of great benefit. This includes the use of regional techniques where possible. However, the increased risks in this subset of patients (especially epidural haematoma) must be considered. The anaesthetist must be aware of the psychological effects that both the diagnosis and treatment of paediatric cancer has on patient and family. It is the anaesthetist's duty to help reduce the emotional stress of multiple painful procedures and surgeries by providing a calm, non-threatening environment pre-operatively and by effective management of post-operative complications, especially pain and nausea and vomiting.

ANAESTHESIA FOR SHORT PROCEDURES IN REMOTE LOCATIONS

- Modern chemotherapy involves the use of intrathecal cytotoxics with regular bone marrow aspirates and trephines to follow the response to treatment. Anaesthesia for these short procedures often takes place in remote locations, such as day case oncology units, radiology/imaging suites.
- External beam radiation therapy (EBRT) has become one of the cornerstones in the management of paediatric oncology cases. Children over five years of age may tolerate radiotherapy without a general anaesthetic, if they have suitable preparation. However, in younger children anaesthesia is usually required. Anaesthesia for these short procedures is required in remote locations, such as radiotherapy suites.

ALTERNATE SITE ANAESTHESIA CONCERNS

The provision of anaesthesia for patients undergoing short procedures in remote locations may present a deceptively simple challenge to the anaesthesiologist. These cases are often very short in duration, there is essentially no blood loss or fluid shift. How then can we explain the discomfort that anaesthesia providers experience when faced with these cases?

This is because:

1. Locations outside the OR (radiology dept, radiotherapy suite, etc.) tend to be ill-equipped for anaesthesia and resuscitation. The anaesthesiologist is usually unfamiliar with the surroundings; location of drugs and instruments, the room is usually scarcely lit and full of equipment with difficult access to the patient, typical example being magnetic resonance imaging (MRI) suite.
2. The personnel in these locations, although well trained in their field, are unfamiliar with anaesthesia. Assistance with intravenous lines, difficult airways, additional personnel support, extra drugs, or equipment or anaesthetic emergencies may be delayed/completely unavailable.
3. Cardiorespiratory stability is another challenge, particularly in children with weakened physical state (due to chemotherapeutic drugs, infections, sepsis, parenteral nutrition, exhaustion and loss of weight) and without a protected airway. Though the procedure is usually brief, the patient must remain motionless and sometimes prone.
4. However, the greatest source of concern seems to be the physical distance that must be maintained from the patients. While many alternate-site anaesthetizing locations force the anaesthesiologist to be at a considerable distance from the patient, perhaps even in a different room (CT scanner, MRI suite), the EBRT (external beam radiotherapy) area is unique in that there is no means of directly viewing the patient or the patient monitors. Instead, one relies solely upon the use of closed circuit television monitoring (Fig. 17.1).
5. Other considerations in the EBRT suite include the possibility of the child being required to wear a face mould, if irradiation is to be delivered to the head or cervical spine; and prone position.

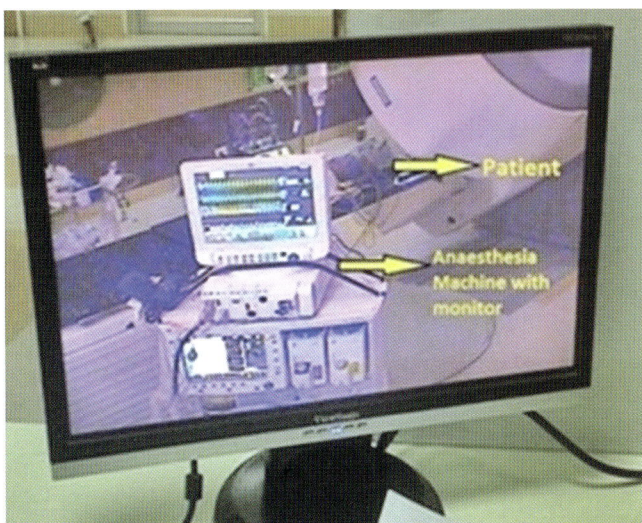

Fig. 17.1 Closed circuit television monitoring outside a radiation oncology suite in DSCI

ANAESTHESIA FOR RADIOTHERAPY

Fundamentals of External Beam Radiotherapy (EBRT)

A basic understanding of radiotherapy department is essential for the anaesthesiologist. The most obvious piece of equipment in the radiotherapy suite is the linear accelerator.

Linear Accelerator (Fig. 17.2)

In this machine, electrons are accelerated to very high energy states and forced to collide with tungsten to release energy in the form of X-rays[17] which is focused to degrade the genetic material within the tumour cells. The energy absorbed by the tissues is measured in terms of gray (Gy). 1Gy is equivalent to 100 rad units.[18]

Simulation

When a child is accepted for radiotherapy, he/she first undergoes a treatment planning session, know as **simulation** in a simulation suite. The **simulator** (simulation machine) provides radiographs of the treatment fields and aids the radiotherapy team in planning radiation doses and points of entry. It is, however, incapable of delivering therapeutic doses of radiation. Further, it offers a trial to see if the child will be cooperative and immobile during the treatment. Since therapeutic radiation is not used, the anaesthesia team can remain in the room wearing lead shields or safely observe the patient through a panel of leaded glass from an adjacent room, also called the **console**. Depending upon the sites to be treated, plaster immobilization casts of the head[19] (Fig. 17.3) or/and blocks, radio-opaque shields to shield radio-sensitive organs, e.g. kidneys and eyes from the ionizing radiation may be required (Fig. 17.4).

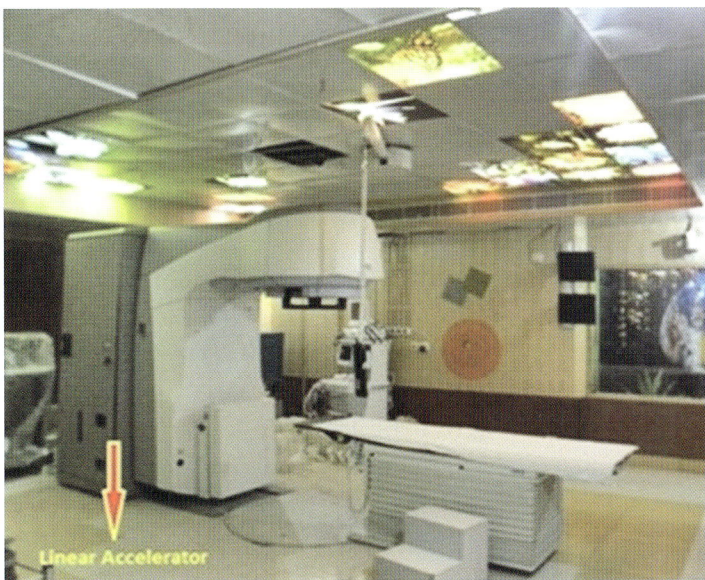

Fig. 17.2. View of a radiation oncology suite at DSCI

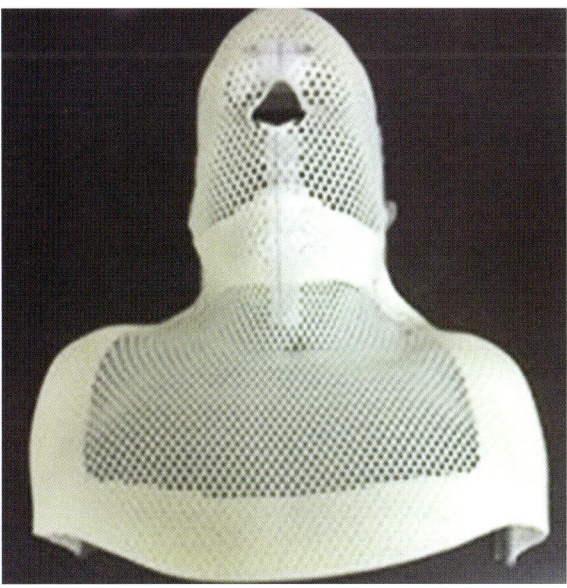

Fig. 17.3. Plaster immobilization cast

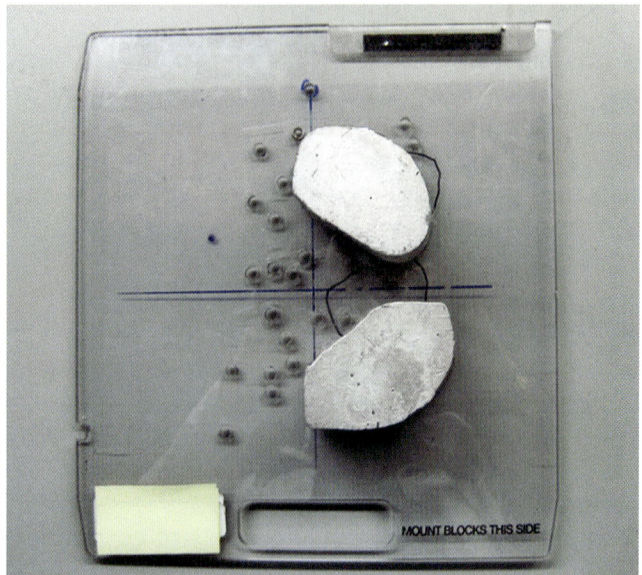

Fig. 17.4. Blocks used to shield radiosensitive organs

Simulation phase is followed by treatment with doses varying from 25 to 80 Gy divided into 30 equal portions, five days/weeks over a 6-week period. Depending upon the number of fields, the entire process is completed in 5 to 20 minutes.

Anaesthetic Management of Paediatric Radiotherapy Treatment

- Anaesthetic technique
- Airway management
- Equipment and monitoring
- Personnel
- Non-pharmacological methods of anxiolysis.

Anaesthetic Technique

For daily radiation therapy, the anaesthetic should provide immobility and amnesia whilst limiting the side effects and disruption to the child's routine.

Historically, a variety of anaesthetic techniques and drugs have been used to facilitate paediatric radiation therapy, including inhalation anaesthesia;[20] IM and IV methohexital;[21,22] oral, IM and IV ketamine;[21,23] IV thiopental;[24] IV meperidine; IV midazolam; and oral chloral hydrate.[25]

Many institutions now advocate the use of an intravenous over an inhalational technique advantages being rapid speed of onset and recovery, diminished movement and no requirement for scavenging of anaesthetic gases. A few of these children have an intravascular port present. Alternatively, intravenous access via a peripheral vein can be obtained Monday morning, left in throughout the week, and removed on Friday.[26] EMLA can greatly facilitate the process.

- Propofol has been cited as being an excellent *stand-alone* drug for use in EBRT without the need for benzodiazepine premedication. Its merits include rapid and predictable induction, easily titratable depth, maintenance of spontaneous ventilation with minimal need for airway manipulation, and rapid recovery,[25,27] particularly important in the context of repetitive daily anaesthesia. With a centrally accessed port, the likelihood of burning during propofol administration is highly unlikely. Propofol-based total intravenous anaesthesia (TIVA) is induced by administering successive boluses of 1 mg/kg followed by an infusion @ 100–250 µg/kg/min.

- Alternatively, after benzodiazepine pretreatment (0.05 mg/kg IV midazolam), an initial propofol dose in the range of 0.5–0.8 mg/kg has been shown to provide adequate sedation for EBRT while still allowing for spontaneous respiration and airway control.[28] This is followed by a continuous propofol infusion in the range from 7.4[29] to 10[30] mg/kg/hr throughout the treatment phase. Thus propofol, combined with midazolam, provides excellent therapeutic conditions throughout the entire course of treatment.

- For patients with a history of agitation on emergence from propofol, painful conditions (e.g. recent postoperative status), allergy or intolerance to propofol, propofol may be supplemented with benzodiazepines, opioids and/or ketamine.

- More recently, the infusion of the α-2 agonist dexmedetomidine has been described.[31]

- Ketamine is another drug that is also used successfully, following midazolam pretreatment.[32] Tachyphylaxis may develop with repeated doses of ketamine. By the fifth or sixth week of therapy, the child may require twice the dosage to obtain the same effect as seen during the first or second week.

- Rarely, general anaesthesia may be required. However, a muscle relaxant may not be necessary (the exception, is retinoblastoma, which requires paralysis of the extraocular muscles). The subglottic swelling that may develop with repeated daily intubations can be obviated by the use of a supra-glottic airway, such as the LMA. The emetic effects of radiotherapy, chemotherapy and stress can result in vomiting. Ondansetron 0.1 mg/kg is the agent of choice for most practitioners.

Airway Management

Supplemental oxygen is provided by face mask. The airway position is manipulated by chin lift and placement of a chest roll, as dictated by the clinical situation.

When the prone position is required, the airway is managed identically, but oxygen tubing alone or nasal prongs are used instead of the face mask. In rare cases, when upper airway obstruction cannot be controlled by these measures, placement of an oral airway or LMA is required.

Equipment and Monitoring

Remote monitoring of the patient receiving radiotherapy typically uses two cameras, each with independent control to provide visual monitoring[27] of the patient to observe for consistent breathing and absence of other movements. The other camera is focused upon the monitors, which typically include continuous ECG, NIBP, HR, pulse oximetry and end-tidal CO_2. If the patient is receiving general anaesthesia, the field of vision can be widened to include the ventilator and anaesthesia machine as well. A microphone is also present to transmit the pulse oximeter tone.

Personnel

Appropriately experienced and recovery staff as well as full paediatric resuscitation equipment must be available at all times.

Anaesthetics are administered by an anaesthesiologist. During the treatment period, the EBRT room is evacuated. Any reasonable request by the anaesthesiologist to reenter the room at any time should be honoured by the radiation therapist.

Nonpharmacological Methods of Anxiolysis

Some practitioners use interactive intervention concepts including cognitive distraction, behavioural rehearsal and psychosocial methods either in lieu of or as a supplement to pharmacologic sedation. However, a busy EBRT service might not be able to devote the necessary time and patience to foster the atmosphere necessary for such methods.

Radiation therapy in alternate sites includes:

- Brachytherapy or the intracavity implantation of radiotherapeutic material (e.g. intrauterine isotopes).
- Surgeons, radiation oncologists, and anaesthesiologists work as a team to provide intraoperative radiation therapy (IORT). This is especially useful for tumours which cannot be fully resected or have a high probability of local recurrence. In these cases after surgical exposure and debulking of the tumour, the wound is covered and the patient transported to the EBRT suite to receive high dose external beam radiation directly to the exposed tissue. The child is then returned to the OR for surgical closure. These cases, typically performed under general anaesthesia, require a great degree of coordination between all specialties including careful attention to maintaining a sterile field as well as continued provision of anaesthesia and analgesia with cardiovascular stability. Further, monitoring, airway, and PALS supplies should accompany the patient during the transit phase.[33]
- Stereotactic radiosurgery is used to treat conditions as diverse as malignancies, arteriovenous malformations, acoustic neuromas, and trigeminal neuralgia. In contrast to EBRT derived from a linear accelerator, only a single session of radiotherapy is needed to treat the disease. Anaesthetic management is much like what has been described for traditional EBRT.

CONCLUSION

Alternate-site anaesthesiology has become more routine over the last decade. While some clinicians still feel uncomfortable emerging from the "protection" of the OR, others have embraced the chance to expand their practice beyond its traditional borders. EBRT offers the anaesthesiologist both a physical layout and a patient population that can be challenging initially but ultimately extremely rewarding.

REFERENCES

1. Stiller CA, Draper GJ. The epidemiology of cancer in children. In: Voute AP, Barrett A, Steverns MCG, Caron HN (Eds). Cancer in Children, Clinical Management. Oxford University Press, 2005.

2. US Mortality Data, 2006. National Center for Health Statistics. Centers for Disease Control and Prevention, 2009.

3. Children and Cancer, in Children's Health and the Environment, a WHO Training Package for the Health Sector, World Health Organization. In turn citing: Scott CH. Childhood cancer epidemiology in low-income countries". Cancer 2007;112(3):461–472.

4. Belpomme D. The multitude and diversity of environmental carcinogens. Environ Res 2007;105(3):414–429. Epub 2007 Aug 9.

5. Bunin GR. Nongenetic causes of childhood cancers: evidence from international variation, time trends, and risk factor studies. Toxicol Appl Pharmacol 2004;199(2): 91–103.

6. Kheifets L, Shimkhada R. Childhood leukemia and EMF: review of the epidemiologic evidence. Bioelectromagnetics 2005;Suppl 7:S51–59.

7. Moore SW, et al. The epidemiology of neonatal tumours. Pediatr Surg Int 2003;19:509–519.

8. Schüz J. Implications from epidemiologic studies on magnetic fields and the risk of childhood leukemia on protection guidelines. Health Phys 2007;92(6):642–648.

9. Birch JM. Genes and cancer. Arch Dis Child 1999;80: 1–3.

10. Lichtenstein P, et al. N Engl J Med 2000;13;343(2):78–85.

11. Kaatsch P, Sikora E, Pawelec G. "Epidemiology of childhood cancer". Cancer Treatment Reviews 2010;36(4): 277–285.

12. Tagge EP. Minimal access cancer management in children. In: Greene FL, Heniford BT (Eds). Minimally Invasive Cancer Management. Springer: USA, 2001;335–346.

13. Ehrlich PF, Newman KD, Haase GM, Lobe TE, Wiener ES, Holcomb GW. Lessons learned from a failed multi-institutional randomized controlled study. J Pediatr Surg 2002;37:431–436.

14. Meng M, Miller T, Cha I, Stoller MA. Cytology of morcellated renal specimens: Significance in diagnosis and dissemination. J Urol 2003;169:45–48.

15. Holcomb GW 3rd, Tomita SS, Haase GM, Dillon PW, Newman KD, Applebaum H, et al. Minimally invasive surgery in children with cancer. Cancer 1995;76:121–128.

16. Waldhaussen JH. Incisional hernia in a 5-mm trocar site following pediatric laparoscopy. J Laparoendosc Surg 1996;6:S89–90.

17. DeVita V, Hellman S, Rosenberg S. Principles and Practice of Anesthesiology, 4th edn, Philadelphia, Lippincott Raven Publishers, 1993.

18. Johns HE, Cunningham JR. The Physics of Radiology, Thomas, Springfield, Ill, USA, 1983.

19. Glauber DT, Audenaert SM. Anesthesia for children undergoing craniospinal radiotherapy. Anesthesiology 1987;67(5): 801–803.

20. Brett CM, Wara WM, Hamilton WK. Anesthesia for infants during radiotherapy: an insufflations technique. Anesthesiology 1986;64:402–405.

21. Jeffries G. Radiotherapy and children's anaesthesia. Anaesthesia 1988;43:416–417.

22. Metriyakool K. Methohexital as alternative to propofol for intravenous anesthesia in children undergoing daily radiation treatment: a case report. Anesthesiology 1998; 88:821–822.

23. Shewale S, Saxena A, Trikha A, et al. Oral ketamine for radiotherapy in children with cancer. Indian J Pediatr 2000;67:263–266.

24. Menache L, Eifel PJ, Kennamer DL, et al. Twice-daily anesthesia in infants receiving hyperfractionated irradiation. Int J Radiat Oncol Biol Phys 1990;18:625–629.

25. Seiler G, De Vol E, Khafaga Y, et al. Evaluation of the safety and efficacy of repeated sedations for the radiotherapy of young children with cancer: a prospective study of 1033 consecutive sedations. International Journal of Radiation Oncology Biology Physics 2001;49(3):771–783.

26. Rodarte A. Heparin-lock for repeated anesthesia in pediatric radiation therapy. Anesthesiology 1982;56(4): 316–317.

27. Keidan I, Perel A, Shabtai EL, Pfeffer RM. Children undergoing repeated exposures for radiation therapy do not develop tolerance to propofol: clinical and bispectral index data. Anesthesiology 2004;100:251–254.

28. Weiss M, Frei M, Buehrer S, Feurer R, Goitein G, Timmermann B. Deep propofol sedation for vacuum-assisted bite-block immobilization in children undergoing proton radiation therapy of cranial tumors. Paediatric Anesthesia 2007;17(9):867–873.

29. Scheiber G, Ribeiro FC, Karpienski H, Strehl K. Deep sedation with propofol in preschool children undergoing radiation therapy. Paediatric Anesthesia 1996;6(3):209–213.

30. Buehrer S, Immoos S, Frei M, et al. Evaluation of propofol for repeated prolonged deep sedation in children undergoing proton radiation therapy. British Journal of Anesthesia 2007;99(4):556–560.

31. Shukry M, Ramadhyani. Dexmedetomidine as the primary sedative agent for brain radiation therapy in a 21-month old child. Paediatric Anesthesia 2005;15(3):241–242.

32. Sherwin TS, Green SM, Khan A, Chapman DS, Dannenberg B. Does adjunctive midazolam reduce recovery agitation after ketamine sedation for pediatric procedures? A randomized, double-blind, placebo-controlled trial. Annals of Emergency Medicine 2000; 35(3):229–238.

33. De Cosmo G, Gualtieri E, Bonomo V, Rosica C, Primieri P, Villani A. Intraoperative radiotherapy: anesthesiologic problems during transport of patients. Minerva Anesiologica 1991;57(6):373–377.

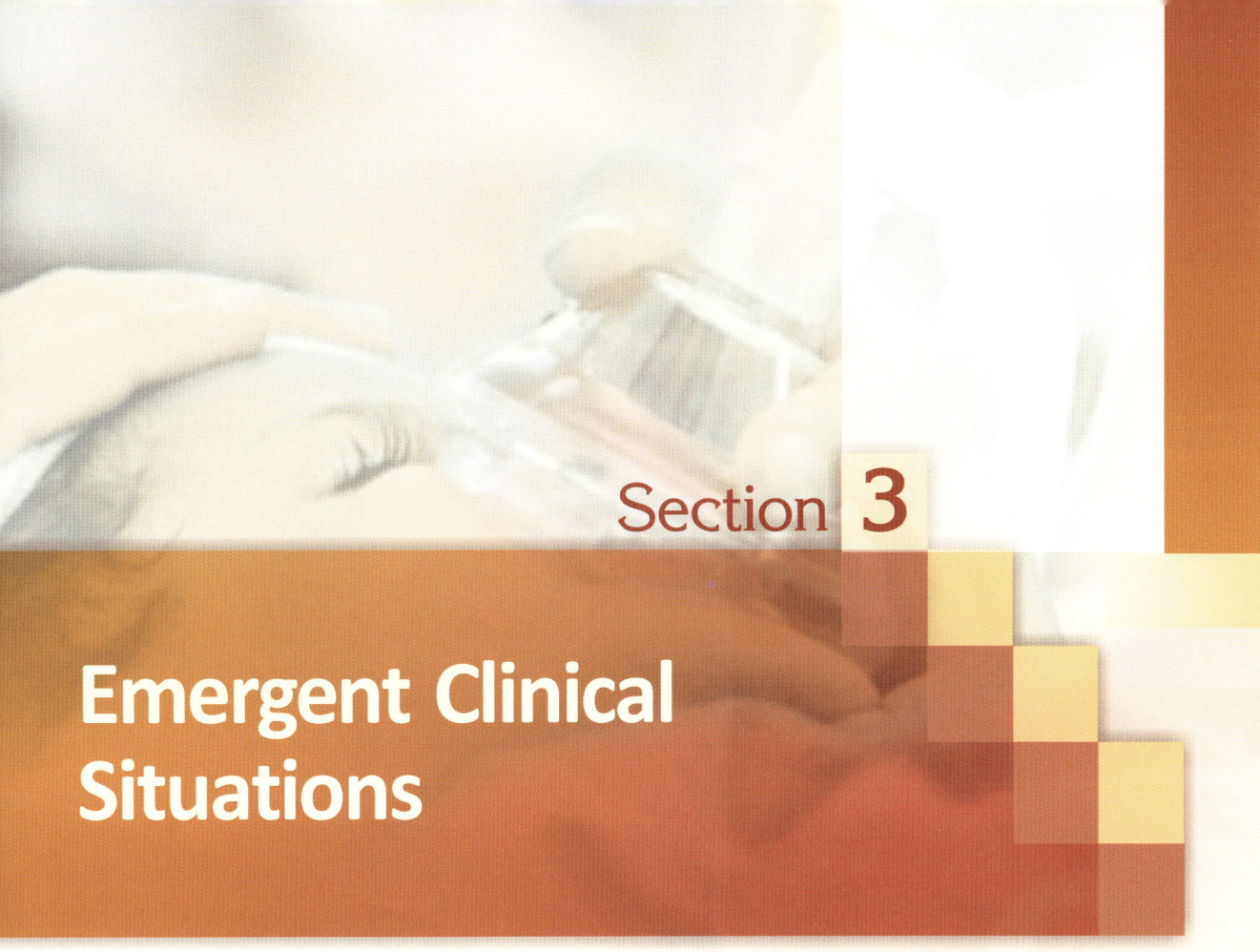

Section 3

Emergent Clinical Situations

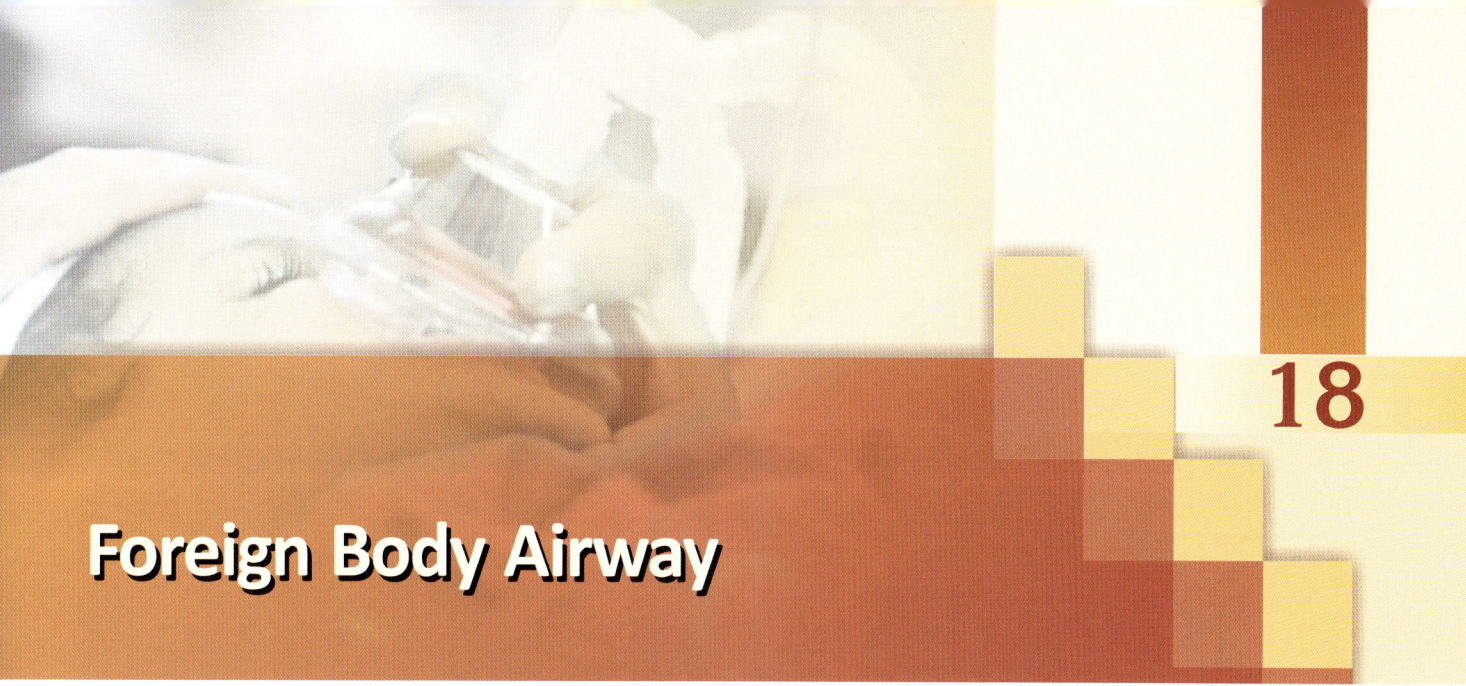

Foreign Body Airway

Dilip Pawar

- ■ Pathophysiology
- ■ Equipment
- ■ Anaesthetic techniques
  - ● Preoperative preparation
  - ● Premedication
  - ● Induction and maintenance of anaesthesia

Foreign body in the tracheobronchial tree is a leading cause of death in children less than a year.[1] It's a challenge to the skill of the anaesthetist and endoscopist.

PATHOPHYSIOLOGY

When a foreign body (FB) is lodged in any part of airway there is always a compromise in gaseous exchange of varying degree.[2] As the foreign body offers resistance to movement of air across it (depending on the degree of airway compromise), there will be obstruction to air entry or exit beyond the FB. This will lead to a distension of the lung (something like an auto-PEEP) distal to the obstruction, which gradually increases to involve a larger part of the lobe. Hyperinflation of lung field or emphysema beyond the foreign body is the earliest and most common lung pathology seen on X-ray chest (Figs 18.1A and B). It is deceptive when the foreign body is non-radio-opaque and/or area of emphysema is small and likely to be missed.

When the obstruction persists and along with it the lung expansion, gradually it might lead to barotrauma and pneumothorax. In case of complete obstruction of the bronchus, it can lead to collapse of the lung (Fig. 18.1C). In long-standing cases,when superadded with infection can lead to lung consolidation (Fig. 18.1D). These complications are rarely seen nowadays.

The foreign bodies can be described as reactive or non-reactive depending on their ability to initiate inflammatory process in the tissue. Common reactive FBs are vegetable FBs, like groundnut, betel, leaf, grass, or animal FBs, like fish, leather or meat. These get swollen after inhalation and initiate an inflammatory reaction on the tracheobronchial mucosa,

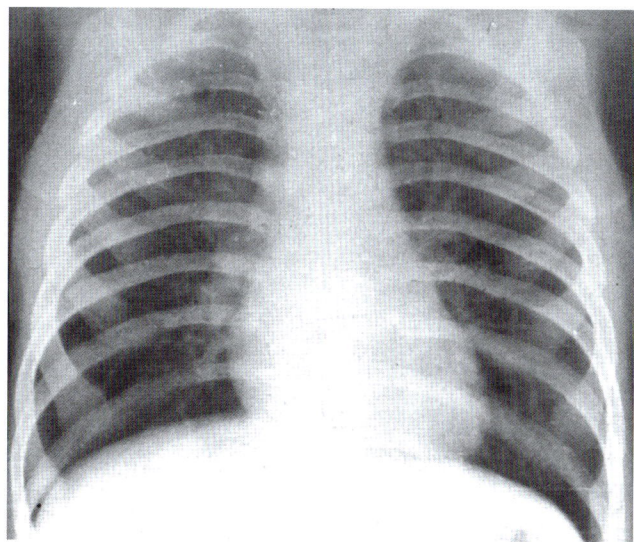

Fig. 18.1A. X-ray chest showing hyperinflated zone of lung beyond obstruction—right lower lobe, likely to miss unless seen carefully

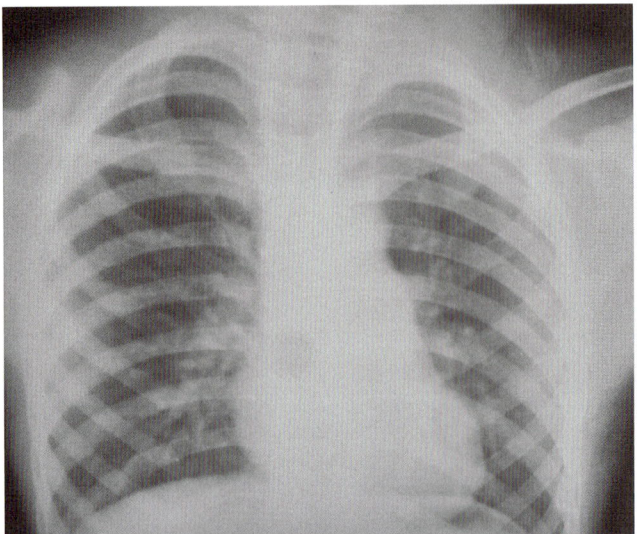

Fig. 18.1B. X-ray chest showing hyperinflated zone of lung beyond obstruction—whole of right lung with distinct widening of rib space and gross emphysema

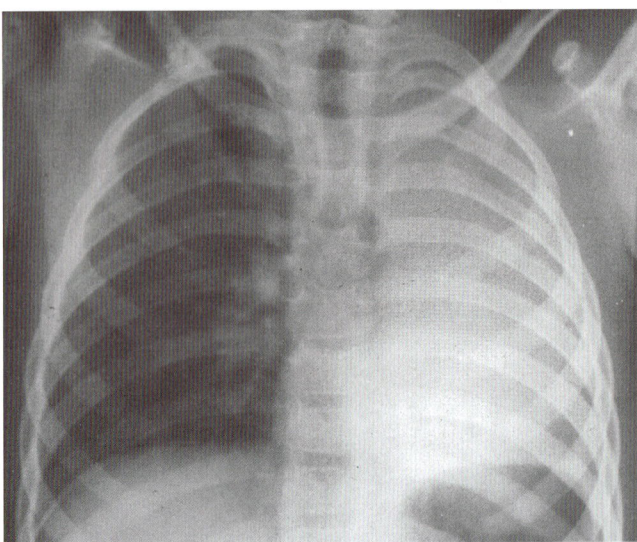

Fig. 18.1C. X-ray chest showing hyperinflated zone of lung beyond obstruction—atelectasis

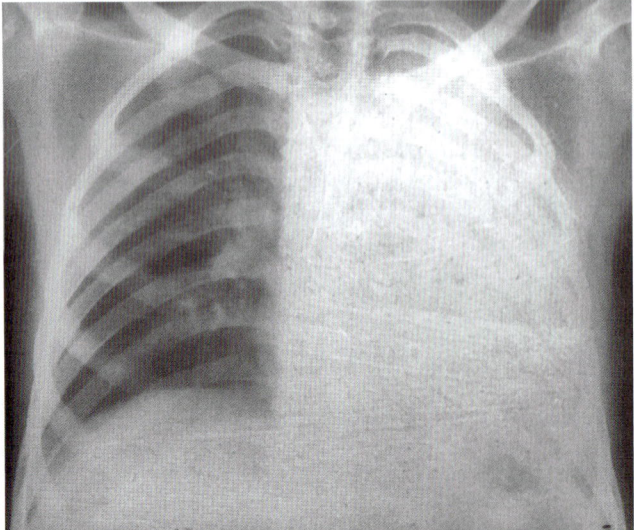

Fig. 18.1D. X-ray chest showing hyperinflated zone of lung beyond obstruction—consolidation

airway. On long-standing cases, however, granulation tissue may grow around it. The sharp object like, a pin, might pierce through the airway to reach mediastinum or even pericardium.[5]

Depending on the degree of lung pathology, there is direct effect on degree of derangement of gaseous exchange. Indirectly ventilation perfusion mismatch in these pathological lung areas will further contribute to the hypoxia and hypercarbia.

EQUIPMENT

Equipment used for removal of FB consists of (Fig. 18.2):
1. A rigid bronchoscope
2. A telescope
3. An alligator forceps
4. Optically guided FB removal forceps
5. Light source

Technique

Bronchoscope is inserted into the larynx and trachea under laryngoscopy assistance to minimize time of intubation and trauma (Fig. 18.3). The bronchoscope has side ports, one for ventilation, where a 15 mm adaptor or a 'T' piece adaptor fits directly, the other port for the light source. There is another port on the side of main port for multiple uses, like biopsy, suctioning, etc. This port needs to be closed when not

which gradually becomes oedematous and might lead to growth of granulomatous tissue. They easily get fragmented during retrieval.[3]

The non-reactive FBs are plastic, aluminium, steel, hairpin, nail, glass beads, even bullet,[4] etc. It is unbelievable the ingenuity of the tiny tots what all they can inhale. In our set up whistle tip of the plastic toys are the most common FBs. These FBs, do not initiate inflammatory response and can move in the

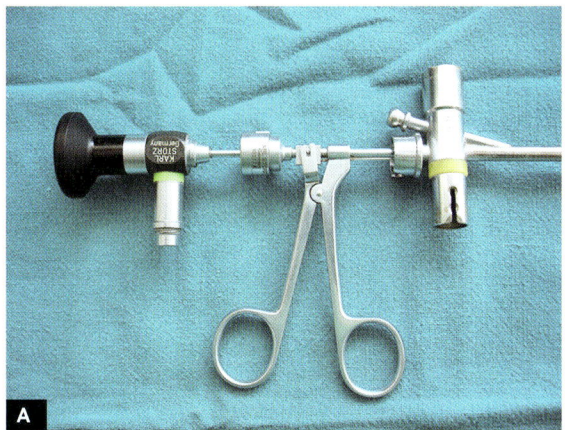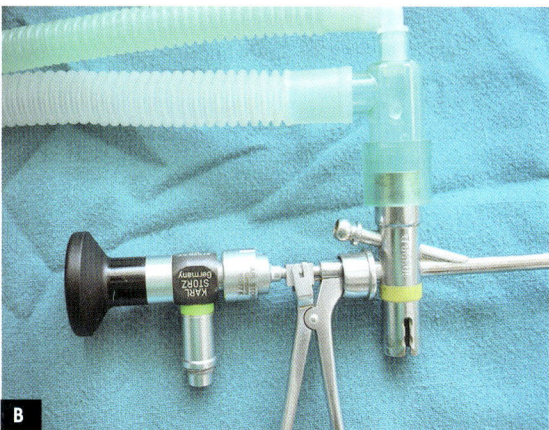

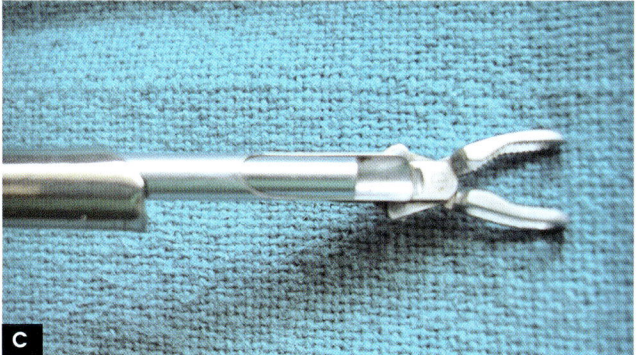

Fig. 18.2. Rigid bronchoscope: (A) Mounted with forceps and telescope; (B) T-piece; (C) The optical-guided forceps tip

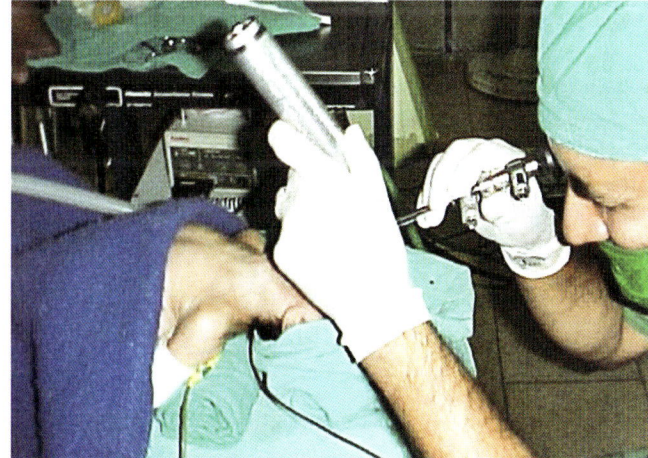

Fig. 18.3. Patient position with roll under shoulder and no head ring

in use. The main viewing port takes the telescope. The telescope is based on the Hopkins rod principle and gives magnified view of the airway.

Once the FB is sited and the tissue debris, blood, mucous cleaned FB is ready for removal. Telescope is withdrawn and mounted in the FB removal forceps,

before its insertion into the bronchoscope. With optical guidance, the forceps removes FB. As and when alligator forceps is used it becomes almost a blind procedure, as distal end may not be visible clearly.

After removal of FB, a check bronchoscopy is always done. The bronchoscope with telescope and FB removal forceps, increase airway resistance, tremendously (>200%).

The posture of the patient for rigid bronchoscopy is odd. A roll under the shoulder and head hanging with or without a ring, this position further impairs respiration (Fig. 18.3).

For sharp FBs, like glass piece, a razor blade, pin, fish bone, etc. it is better to go for open thoracotomy and removal by bronchotomy to avoid further injury to airway during retrieval.[6,7]

ANAESTHETIC TECHNIQUES

Preoperative Preparation

In our country, it is uncommon for these patients to come early to hospital. It could be because of lack of awareness amongst guardians as well as general practitioners. They come late after some complications have set in, often in critical condition needing resuscitation.

These cases should always be considered emergency even if it is an old FB or the patients' condition is stable as they have a potential to deteriorate any time. The preparation depends on the child's presenting condition. Often they need fluid resuscitation as they might have lost fluid due to heavy breathing and less of fluid intake. They might also need oxygenation and their breathing assisted.

Premedication

Any sedative premedication is avoided. Atropine used to be administered routinely earlier prophylactically to avoid bradycardia. As it is well known that most common cause of bradycardia during bronchoscopy is hypoxia, nowadays it is kept ready and used only to treat persistent bradycardia even after correction of hypoxia.

Induction and Maintenance of Anaesthesia

If lung pathology is minimal, both inhalational induction with halothane/sevoflurane or intravenous induction with thiopantone or propofol are practiced depending on the individual preference and institutional practice.[8] Sick patients are usually induced with inhalational agents. Lignocaine spray prior to endoscopy decreases the need of anaesthetic drugs.[9]

Standard monitoring with, ECG, NIBP, SpO$_2$, EtCO$_2$ are used. It should be noted that EtCO$_2$ could be fallacious because of the leak around the system.

During the maintenance phase, there is a difference in clinical practice, some leave them on spontaneous breathing others control the ventilation. Our understanding on the subject is primarily based on case reports, retrospective studies of case series, individual practices, surgeons and institutional preferences and not based on any hard-core evidence.[8] In all the series of cases where patients have been managed on spontaneous breathing, children's respiration needed assistance. Ours is the first prospective study comparing spontaneous and controlled breathing.[2] We observed that children on spontaneous breathing needed respiratory assistance, whereas in the controlled group, it was possible to manage even depth of anaesthesia throughout the procedure.

It is rightly so, because:

1. They have various degrees of lung pathology and abnormal gaseous exchange.
2. The equipment used offers a great resistance to the airway and there is little space outside the scope for breathing.
3. The posture during endoscopy further embarrasses breathing.
4. Anaesthetic drugs further depress respiration.

Spontaneously breathing patients need respiratory assistance, especially after the effect of anaesthesia but it might be difficult to synchronise assistance, as their rate of breathing is high. It might be difficult to maintain even depth of anaesthesia with inhalational agents as there is leak in the breathing system. Some authors use ketamine, propofol, remifentanil infusion on spontaneously breathing children.[10-12] These children also need respiratory assistance.

Older children, whose tracheal diameter bronchoscope ratio is higher and have minimal lung pathology, may be managed on spontaneous breathing successfully. Some other situations where leaving the patient on spontaneous breathing will be beneficial are; (a) any moving or tracheal FB, (b) evidence of airway injury and pneumomediastinum.

Controlled ventilation can be achieved by IPPV through 'T' piece or Jet ventilation.[13,14] Atracurium is the relaxant of choice in these patients when paralysed. However, if the surgeon is good, a single dose of suxamethonium might be too long. The fear of positive pressure ventilation pushing the FB distally is an unfounded myth, never been reported and probably a theoretical fear.

During retrieval, there is always possibility of dislodgement of FB. It depends on the skill of the endoscopist and availability of proper equipment rather than the technique of anaesthesia.[13]

The most dangerous situation during removal of FB is, where a vegetable FB occluding one main stem bronchi gets dislodged and gets into the healthy main stem bronchi during retrieval (Fig. 18.4). The FB should be dislodged and pushed to the original site of lodgment for any resuscitation to be effective.

Because of multiple insertion of bronchoscope, there is always possibility of various degree of trauma to larynx, subglottic region and trachea. That may lead to simple persistence cough and laryngeal oedema. IV lignocaine 1.5 mg/kg is helpful in reducing the

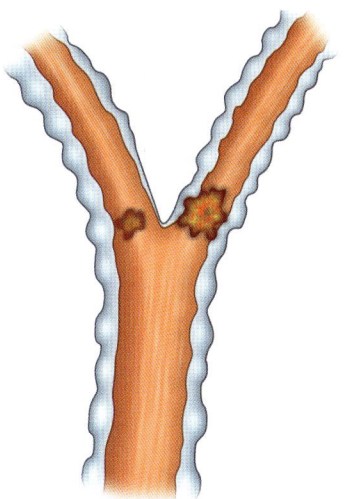

Fig. 18.4. Red-granulation tissue, gray-foreign body. Most dangerous situation when FB gets fragmented during removal from right main stem bronchus gets lodged on the left main stem bronchus, thereby occluding both the bronchi

irritable cough. Some prefer to administer hydro-cortisone. These drugs may be administered 10–20 min before the end of procedure.

In the recovery, they should be monitored for SpO_2. Agitation and crying should be avoided, which might further increase the airway oedema. If the larynx has been sprayed with lignocaine feeding should be delayed to avoid gastric aspiration at least for one hour after spray.

The most common postoperative complication is persistent cough. Hypoxic injury, hypoxia, laryngeal oedema, and subglottic oedema are not so commonly seen complications.[15]

CONCLUSION

There is no fit solution for all the cases of foreign body tracheobronchial tree. Every child presenting with foreign body offers different pathophysiology and challenges, individual treatment option for a particular patient offers optimum care. Competent anaesthetist, a skilled surgeon assisted by a team and availability of right equipments are the key to successful outcome.

REFERENCES

1. Haynes SR, Bonner S. Anaesthesia for thoracic surgery in children. Pediatr Anesth 2000;10:237–251.
2. Soodan A, Pawar D, Subramanium R. Anesthesia for removal of inhaled foreign bodies in children. Pediat Anesth 2004;14:947–952.
3. Sih T, Bunnag C, Ballali S, Lauriello M, Bellussi L. Nuts and seed: a natural yet dangerous foreign body. Int J Pediatr Otorhinolaryngol 2012;14(76 Suppl 1):S49–52.
4. Arora MKA. Rare foreign body (bullet) in the bronchus of a child. Pediatr Anesth 2007;17:703–704.
5. Sondekoppam RV, Kajal K, Jain K, Bhatia N. Open safety pin causing fatal pneumopericardium: the effect of positive-pressure ventilation. Pediatr Anesth 2012;22:589–591.
6. Ma G, Yang J, Liu S. Anesthetic management of bronchial rupture following extraction of a fishbone from the bronchus after 5 months. Paediatr Anaesth 2014;24:544–546.
7. Hoff SR, Chang KW. The proximal bronchoplasty retrieval technique for removal of embedded distal airway foreign bodies. Int J Pediatr Otorhinolaryngol 2014;78:148–151.
8. Pawar D. Authors' reply Pediatr Anesth 2005;15:533–534.
9. Moustafa MA. Nebulizedlidocaine alone or combined with fentanyl as a premedication to general anesthesia in spontaneously breathing pediatric patients undergoing rigid bronchoscopy. Pediatr Anesth 2013;23:429–434.
10. Landy C, Massoure PL, Gauthier J, Eve O, Kaiser E. Interest of ketamine for the management of a large foreign body in the trachea. Pediatr Anesth 2012;22:608–609.
11. Teksan L, Baris S, Karakaya D, Dilek A. A dose study of remifentanil in combination with propofol during tracheobronchial foreign body removal in children. J Clin Anesth 2013;25:198–201.
12. Chai J, Wu XY, Han N, Wang LY, Chen WM. A retrospective study of anesthesia during rigid bronchoscopy for airway foreign body removal in children: propofol and sevoflurane with spontaneous ventilation. Pediatr Anesth 2014;24:1031–1036.
13. Pawar DK. Dislodgement of bronchial foreign body during retrieval in children. Pediatr Anesth 2000;10:333–335.
14. Baraka A. Oxygen enrichment of entrained room air during Venturi jet ventilation of children undergoing bronchoscopy. Pediatr Anesth 1996;6:383–385.
15. Tomaske M, Gerber AC, Weiss M. Anesthesia and periinterventional morbidity of rigid bronchoscopy for tracheobronchial foreign body diagnosis and removal. Pediatr Anesth 2006;16:123–129.

19

Child with Trauma

- Role of anaesthesiologist in paediatric trauma management
- Resuscitation
- Unique features of paediatric trauma
- Anaesthetic management
  - Preoperative assessment and management
  - Airway management
  - Fluid management
  - Monitoring
  - Postoperative management
- Traumatic brain injury
- Spinal injuries
- Thoracic trauma
- Abdominal trauma

Trauma is a leading cause of morbidity and mortality in children all over the world. In United States, 45% of total mortality in paediatric patients is due to trauma.[1] The injury mechanisms in children vary with age.[2] Child abuse is common in infants, whereas the predominant mechanism in toddlers is fall from height. Older children and adolescents most frequently suffer from road traffic accidents (RTAs) and sports injuries. The children are pedestrians in more than 50% and cyclists in 20% of RTAs.[3] In India, the highest incidence of trauma has been seen in school going age-group (6–12 years), with male children getting injured more than females.[4] Fall from height is the commonest cause followed by RTAs, burns, sports-related injuries and assaults, etc.

ROLE OF ANAESTHESIOLOGIST IN PAEDIATRIC TRAUMA MANAGEMENT

The anaesthesiologists have a significant role at various stages of management of injured children:

1. Initial resuscitation and stabilization in emergency department
2. Anaesthetic management during surgical procedures
3. Intensive care management of critically injured children
4. Providing sedation and monitoring for patients undergoing imaging procedures, such as computed tomography (CT) scan or magnetic resonance imaging (MRI)
5. Providing analgesia to acutely injured children

RESUSCITATION

The basic principles of trauma care remain same for the adults and the children. The common structured approach has components of rapid primary survey, resuscitation of vital functions, detailed secondary survey, and finally, the initiation of definitive care.[5] During the primary survey, life-threatening conditions are identified and managed simultaneously. It involves the ABCDE sequence, which stands for airway management with cervical spine protection; breathing and ventilation; circulation with haemorrhage control; disability in terms of neurologic status; and exposure/environmental control.

Ensuring a patent airway is the first priority in the management of an injured child. Possibility of cervical spine injuries, head injury and full stomach should always be considered.[2] Manual in-line immobilization must be applied at the time of airway manipulations in patients with uncleared cervical spine. Intubation may be required either for airway protection, e.g. in unconscious patients, those having severe maxillo-facial trauma, those at risk of aspiration or airway obstruction; or for ventilation and oxygenation, e.g. in cases of inadequate or no respiratory efforts, suspected raised intracranial pressure, Glasgow Coma Scale (GCS) <8, or massive blood loss.[5] Details of airway management will be discussed under 'Anaesthetic Management'.

Breathing and ventilatory pattern should be assessed. It is important to know normal respiratory rate at different ages. The respiratory rate of an infant is 30–40 breaths/min, whereas that of an older child is 15–20 breaths/min. Normal spontaneous tidal volume for infants and children is 6–8 ml/kg and slightly larger volumes of 7–10 ml/kg are required during assisted ventilation.

Hypoxia is the commonest cause of cardiac arrest in children. Children have high oxygen consumption, low functional residual capacity and increased chest wall compliance. These factors predispose them to airway collapse and hypoxia. Urgent intervention is required for management of tension pneumothorax, open pneumothorax, haemothorax, or flail chest.[2]

The important elements in evaluation of circulation include assessment of pulse, arterial pressure, level of consciousness, skin colour, capillary refill and urine output.[2] Children can maintain their systolic blood pressure even in shock state due to their better physiologic reserves than adults. Therefore, hypovolemia in early stages is recognized by tachycardia and poor skin perfusion. However, tachycardia may also occur due to pain and fear. The mean normal systolic blood pressure of children is 90 mm Hg plus twice the age in years, whereas 70 mm Hg plus twice the age in years is considered the lower limit of normal range.[5] Blood pressure remains normal with loss of less than 30% blood volume and becomes low normal with 30–45% blood volume loss. Hypotension indicates loss of more than 45% blood volume. It may be associated with tachycardia changing to brady-cardia. Appropriate fluid resuscitation should be started early without waiting for the hypotension to develop. If percutaneous access is unsuccessful after two attempts, intraosseous placement of a bone marrow needle in the marrow cavity of proximal tibia or distal femur in an uninjured extremity should be considered. Besides replacing intravascular volume, definitive control of bleeding is essential.

For assessment of disability, a brief neurological examination is conducted to determine conscious level and pupillary size and reaction. The responses for assessing GCS in children above 5 years of age remain similar to adult GCS. However, for smaller children, the responses need to be modified for age (Table 19.1).[6] Following the neurological examination, the patient is completely undressed for a thorough physical examination and assessment. At the same time, care should be taken to prevent hypothermia by covering the patient with blankets, infusing warm fluids and maintaining warm environment.

Despite identical assessment and management priorities for adult as well as paediatric trauma patients, one needs to keep in mind certain unique physical characteristics of paediatric patients.

UNIQUE FEATURES OF PAEDIATRIC TRAUMA

- Due to smaller body size of children, trauma results in application of greater force per unit body area.
- Children have less fat and connective tissue. Moreover, multiple organs are located in smaller area. This results in higher incidence of multiple injuries.
- Young children have larger head in relation to the body, resulting in more frequent brain injuries.
- Bones are incompletely calcified, more pliable and have multiple active growth centres. Therefore, internal organs may be damaged without overlying bony fractures.
- Due to higher body surface area in comparison to body volume, children can develop hypothermia more quickly.
- Very small children are psychologically unstable.
- Injury can adversely affect subsequent growth and development of the child. Injuries involving growth centres may result in abnormal development of that bone. Sometimes, even minor injuries in children may result in prolonged cerebral dysfunction, difficulty in psychological adjustment and organ system disability.

Table 19.1	Child's Glasgow Coma Scale[6]	
	Age >5 years	**Age <5 years**
Eye opening		
4	Spontaneous	Spontaneous
3	To voice	To voice
2	To pain	To pain
1	None	None
Verbal		
5	Orientated	Alert, babbles, coos, words or sentences—normal for age
4	Confused	Less than usual ability, irritable cry
3	Inappropriate words	Cries to pain
2	Incomprehensible sounds	Moans to pain
1	No response to pain	No response to pain
Motor		
6	Obeys commands	Normal spontaneous movements
5	Localizes to supraorbital pain	Withdraws to touch
4	Withdraws from nail bed pain	Withdraws from nail bed pain
3	Flexion to supraorbital pain	Flexion to supraorbital pain
2	Extension to supraorbital pain	Extension to supraorbital pain
1	No response to supraorbital pain	No response to supraorbital pain

ANAESTHETIC MANAGEMENT

Injured children may need to be anaesthetized for emergency procedures, e.g. craniotomy and laparotomy; or semielective procedures after initial stabilization, e.g. fixation of long bone fractures.

Preoperative Assessment and Management

In procedures being performed after initial stabilization, thorough history and examination is conducted. However, in emergency procedures, only brief history can be taken.[1] The mnemonic AMPLE helps to remember the important points in quick history taking (A=Allergies; M=Medications; P=Past medical history; L=Last meal time, last tetanus immunization; E=Events related to injury). For clinical examination, only a quick assessment of airway, breathing and circulation is possible in these circumstances.

The operating room should be adequately prepared to successfully manage paediatric trauma patients. Besides checking and preparing equipment and medications according to the child's age; infusion pumps, fluid warmers and rapid infusion devices also should be kept ready. Ambient temperature should be raised to 26°C for infants and small children.[7]

Essential investigations in haemodynamically unstable patients include haemoglobin/haematocrit and typing and crossmatching of blood. Coagulation profile becomes important in critically injured children due to association of coagulopathy with trauma, specifically head injury.[8] Serial arterial blood gas analysis provides vital information about oxygenation and acid-base status in these patients. X-ray chest is very useful in patients with thoracic injuries.

Airway Management

The airway management in children is more challenging than in adults and, therefore, it is preferable to have an experienced person to handle it. The oral cavity is small with a large tongue and delicate gums. There is a possibility of enlarged tonsils or adenoids, or loose deciduous teeth. The larynx is short, high and anterior; and the epiglottis is long and floppy. These features result in potentially difficult laryngoscopy, and possibility of endobronchial intubation. Nasotracheal intubation or even use of nasal airway can result in bleeding. The size of the endotracheal tube should be chosen considering the fact that the airway is narrowest at the cricoid cartilage.

The larger size of a small child's head causes passive flexion of the cervical spine, predisposing to airway obstruction. To optimize the airway, the plane of the face should be kept parallel to the plane of the stretcher and cervical spine should be maintained in neutral alignment.[5] This can be achieved by keeping a 1-inch thick padding under the infant's torso. Jaw thrust manoeuvre with manual in-line spinal immobilization is used to open the airway. Oxygen is administered to all trauma patients.

Oral airway may be used in unconscious child; however, the technique used in adults, i.e. inserting the airway backward and then rotating it by 180° is not recommended in children due to risk of soft tissue trauma leading to haemorrhage. It should be gently inserted either directly into the oropharynx or with the help of a tongue depressor.[5]

Orotracheal intubation under direct vision with immobilization and protection of cervical spine remains the best method to establish airway and ventilate lungs of a child. Earlier, it was recommended to use uncuffed endotracheal tubes in small children; however, recent evidence suggests that cuffed tubes with improved cuff designs may be used safely.[9] It is recommended to measure cuff pressures, with 30 mm Hg being the upper safe limit.[10]

All patients should be preoxygenated. As infants and young children have a more pronounced vagal response to endotracheal intubation, atropine administration in a dose of 0.01–0.02 mg/kg is recommended in infants, children aged 1–5 years receiving succinylcholine and adolescents receiving second dose of succinylcholine.[12,13] The choice of sedatives (induction agents) and paralytics used for RSI and their doses depend on the child's level of consciousness and vital signs. Etomidate, thiopental and propofol are commonly used induction agents in children. These agents are also the preferred agents in cases of head injury due to their beneficial effects on intracranial pressure.[14–16] However, etomidate is preferred in patients with shock due to greater haemodynamic stability achieved with this drug.[17,18] For neuromuscular blockade, succinylcholine remains the preferred agent due to its rapid onset and short duration of action. Rocuronium is a safe alternative in conditions where succinylcholine is contraindicated, i.e. children with crush injury, burns more than 24 hours old, history of neuromuscular disease or renal insufficiency.[17]

In cases of failed laryngoscopy and intubation, alternative devices, e.g. laryngeal mask airway or videolaryngoscope may be used. Cricothyroidotomy may be required, if it is not possible to oxygenate a patient with bag-mask ventilation, orotracheal intubation or other devices.

Fluid Management

As children have small blood volume, delay in appropriate fluid resuscitation may result in rapid development of significant hypovolemia. For fluid resuscitation, isotonic crystalloids remain the fluid of choice. Hypotonic fluids may result in development of cerebral oedema. Also hyperglycaemia is associated with poor neurological outcome in head-injured patients. Therefore, dextrose-containing fluids are not recommended for trauma patients.[19,20] However, it is also important to avoid hypoglycaemia.[21]

To replace the intravascular volume lost, a bolus of 20 ml/kg warm isotonic crystalloid is infused. Two more such boluses may be repeated which should be followed by packed red cells bolus 10 ml/kg, if there is no clinical improvement.[5,22] Once blood transfusion has been started, administration of other blood products, e.g. fresh frozen plasma (FFP) and platelets should be considered.[5] In case of excessive bleeding, various massive transfusion protocols have been used.[23–25] The optimal approach for multiple transfusions in paediatric patients is currently unknown.[26] However, it has been suggested that implementation of multiple transfusion protocols, allowing for rapid provision of balanced blood products, is feasible.[25]

Normalization of heart rate and adequate urine output are the simple and commonly used end points of fluid resuscitation in children.[1] Other indicators of adequate organ perfusion include clearing of sensorium, return of peripheral pulses and normal skin colour, increased warmth of extremities, increased systolic blood pressure and pulse pressure more than 20 mm Hg.[5]

Monitoring

The standard monitoring while anaesthetizing paediatric patients includes ECG, non-invasive blood pressure, pulse oximetry, capnography and temperature monitoring. Temperature monitoring is specifically important in injured children as hypothermia may exacerbate coagulopathy, make injuries refractory to treatment and also adversely affect central nervous system function. Adequate urine output with normalization of urine specific gravity is a very good indicator of adequacy of volume resuscitation.[5] However, age of the patient must be considered while using this monitor as normal urine output varies with age. It is 2 ml/kg/hr for infants, 1.5 ml/kg/hr for younger children and 1 ml/kg/hr for older children. Patients with head injury may also require invasive arterial pressure, intracranial pressure and neurophysiologic monitoring.[1]

Postoperative Management

It may be required to continue resuscitation and monitoring in the immediate postoperative period. Critically injured children may need to be shifted to intensive care unit (ICU). Some of them may even require mechanical ventilation. Some patients, especially with polytrauma, may also need to undergo imaging after emergency surgery. The anaesthesiologist must be very careful during transport of these patients. One must ensure adequate oxygenation, haemodynamic stability and monitoring before and during the transport. All resuscitation equipment and drugs must be carried along with. In ICU, the patient should be handed over to the ICU team with detailed history, preoperative examination findings and perioperative course verbally conveyed as well as documented in the records. All this is essential for patient safety and continuity of care.[1]

Pain should be adequately treated in postoperative period. This can be achieved by either oral or rectal acetaminophen (paracetamol), ibuprofen, or opioids, e.g. fentanyl or morphine, if pain is more severe. Regional anaesthetic techniques can also be used to provide good postoperative analgesia.

TRAUMATIC BRAIN INJURY

Primary injury to brain occurs at the time of initial trauma due to acceleration, deceleration or rotational forces. This may result in skull fracture; contusion of brain; epidural, subdural or intraparenchymal haematoma; or diffuse axonal injury. Secondary injury may occur due to inflammatory and excitotoxic processes resulting in further oedema, raised intracranial pressure (ICP) and reduced cerebral perfusion pressure (CPP).[27,28] Hypoxemia and hypotension are the two major factors that can result in or exacerbate secondary injury.

In children, cerebral oedema is usually more severe and diffuse than in adults.[29] Anatomical differences, such as unstable neck, large head, and a more compliant skull in infants, may result in greater consequences from acceleration–deceleration injuries. There is little space to accommodate oedema in the skull. The developing brain has incomplete axonal myelination, high water content and inflammatory mediators which may result in more severe oedema in children than in adults.[30]

Guidelines for acute management of severe traumatic brain injury were first published in 2003 by the Society of Critical Care Medicine[31] and then were modified in 2012.[32] The primary goals of anaesthetic management in paediatric patients with TBI include provision of adequate anaesthesia and analgesia, optimization of surgical conditions, control of ICP, maintenance of adequate CPP and avoidance of factors causing secondary injury, i.e. hypoxaemia, hypotension, hypercarbia, hypocarbia, hyperglycaemia and hypoglycaemia.[33]

In respiratory care, PaO_2 $\geq$60 mm Hg and normocarbia should be maintained. Severe hyperventilation to $PaCO_2$ <30 mm Hg should be avoided in the initial 48 hours after injury. If it is used to manage refractory intracranial hypertension, advanced neuromonitoring in the form of jugular venous oxygen saturation or brain tissue oxygen tension measurement is recommended to monitor oxygen delivery.[32]

Haemodynamic support with avoidance of hypotension is extremely important as even a single episode of hypotension can worsen the outcome. Cerebral perfusion pressure should be maintained at 40–50 mm Hg depending on the patient's age, with infants at the lower end and adolescents at the upper end of this range.[32] Intraoperatively normovolemia should be maintained. Normal saline remains the fluid of choice. Glucose containing fluids should not be administered unless serum glucose is $\leq$70 mg/dl.

Intracranial hypertension must be avoided and ICP $\geq$20 mm Hg must be treated so as to avoid further secondary injury. The patient's head should remain in neutral and midline position to avoid jugular venous obstruction and the head of bed should be elevated at 15–30° to lower ICP. Mannitol 0.25–1.0 g/kg helps to treat raised ICP. According to recent evidence, 3% hypertonic saline should be considered for treatment of severe paediatric TBI with intracranial hypertension.[32] For acute use, it can be given in a dose of 6.5 to 10 ml/kg; whereas during ICU management, it can be administered as a continuous infusion of 0.1 to 1.0 ml/kg/hr. The minimum dose needed to maintain ICP<20 mm Hg should be used, with serum osmolarity maintained below 360 mOsm/L.

There is no class I evidence of improved outcome with induced hypothermia. The use of corticosteroids is not recommended due to lack of any beneficial effect and potential for harmful effects due to suppression of pituitary adrenal axis and increased incidence of pneumonia.[32] Haemoglobin should be maintained at 7–10 g/dl. Coagulation abnormalities should be treated with blood products. Infants and small children are a higher risk of developing post-traumatic seizures when compared to adults. Seizure activity may contribute to secondary brain injury by increasing cerebral oxygen consumption and ICP, enhanced neurotransmitter release and haemodynamic fluctuations. Therefore, anticonvulsants should be administered during first week after severe TBI to reduce the incidence of early post-traumatic seizures.

SPINAL INJURIES

Spinal cord injuries (SCI) are less common in children than in adults. This is because a child's spine is more mobile and elastic; and softer cartilaginous vertebrae are less likely to fracture with minor trauma.[34] Subluxations and dislocations are common.[2] The location of spinal injuries also differs with children usually having high cervical injuries at C2 and C3 vertebrae due to underdeveloped neck musculature and disproportionately large head.[35]

It may be difficult to rule out spinal cord injury radiographically in paediatric population as in up to 50% cases there may be spinal cord injury without radiographic abnormality (SCIWORA).[36] CT scans may be more useful to detect such injuries.

As in adults, cervical spine injury must be assumed to be present in all paediatric trauma patients until it has been excluded. Care should be taken to immobilize the spine, especially during airway management.

Succinylcholine administration is contraindicated in patients with spinal cord injury due to hyperkalemic response. However, hyperkalemia does not occur during initial 24 hours after injury. Therefore,

succinylcholine can be used for acute airway management in these patients.[37]

While managing a child with SCI, one must avoid worsening the initial insult. Hypoxia and hypotension must be avoided and spinal cord perfusion pressure must be maintained.

Earlier high dose methylprednisolone treatment was recommended for spinal cord injury patients presenting within eight hours of injury. However, recent guidelines issued by The Congress of Neurological Surgeons (CNS) and the American Association of Neurological Surgeons (AANS) in 2013 state that high dose methylprednisolone should not be used for management of acute SCI in view of lack of medical evidence showing benefits of steroids and evidence of harmful side effects associated with their use.[38]

THORACIC TRAUMA

The common thoracic injuries include pneumothorax, haemothorax and pulmonary contusion. Rarely, cardiac, aortic, tracheobronchial tree and diaphragmatic injuries may also occur.[2] The chest wall in children is very compliant. The risk of rib fractures is reduced; however, energy may be transferred to internal structures.[2] Thus children may suffer severe blunt trauma to the chest without rib fractures.[35] Hence presence of rib fractures is a marker of severe trauma and mandates careful examination to exclude possible injuries to underlying organs, i.e. lungs, liver and spleen.[39]

Pneumothorax, haemothorax and haemopneumothorax are managed with pleural decompression by chest tube insertion in the fifth intercostal space, just anterior to mid-axillary line. In case of tension pneumothorax, immediate needle decompression just over the top of third rib in midclavicular line is done followed by chest tube placement in fifth intercostal space. Chest tube must be inserted before beginning mechanical ventilation in children having clinically significant pneumothorax. Use of nitrous oxide should be avoided in patients at risk for developing pneumothorax.

ABDOMINAL TRAUMA

Abdominal trauma is the leading cause of unrecognized fatal injury in children.[2] They are very vulnerable to suffering injury to intra-abdominal organs as superiorly compliant chest wall allows transmission of forces to liver and spleen; whereas inferiorly, the pelvis fails to protect the bladder. The most commonly injured abdominal organ is spleen followed by liver, kidney, intestine and pancreas.

Abdominal distension can cause respiratory compromise and gastric tube should be inserted in these patients before induction of anaesthesia. Splenic and hepatic injuries can result in significant bleeding which may require massive transfusion.

SUMMARY

Trauma is a major cause of morbidity and mortality in children all over the world. The anaesthesiologists play an important role at various stages in management of injured children which include initial resuscitation; providing analgesia and sedation; anaesthetic management during surgical procedures and intensive care management of critically injured children. The basic principles of trauma care remain same for the adults and the children. However, the unique physical characteristics of children make them very different from adults. The implications of these differences must always be considered while managing these patients.

During initial resuscitation, ABCDE approach is followed, which stands for airway management with cervical spine protection; breathing and ventilation; circulation with haemorrhage control; disability in terms of neurologic status; and exposure/environmental control. All trauma patients should be considered as full stomach and rapid sequence intubation (RSI) is the gold standard for their airway management. However, in case of failure, alternative devices, e.g. laryngeal mask airway or technique, i.e. cricothyroidotomy may be life saving. Children have small blood volume and, therefore, appropriate fluid therapy must be started early. For fluid resuscitation, warm isotonic crystalloids remain the fluid of choice. Normalization of heart rate and urine output more than 1 ml/kg/h are the simplest and commonly used end points of fluid resuscitation in children.

In children with traumatic brain injury, the primary goals of anaesthetic management include provision of adequate anaesthesia and analgesia, optimization of surgical conditions, control of intracranial pressure, maintenance of adequate cerebral perfusion pressure and avoidance of factors causing secondary brain injury, i.e. hypoxaemia, hypotension, hypercarbia, hypocarbia, hyperglycaemia and hypoglycaemia.

Cervical spine injury must be assumed to be present in all paediatric trauma patients until it has been excluded. Care should be taken to immobilize the spine, especially during airway management. In patients with spinal cord injury, one must avoid worsening the initial insult by preventing hypoxia and hypotension and maintaining spinal cord perfusion pressure.

Due to very compliant chest wall, children may suffer severe blunt trauma to the chest without rib fractures.

REFERENCES

1. Ivashkov Y, Bhananker SM. Perioperative management of pediatric trauma patients. Int J Crit Illn Inj Sci 2012;2: 143–148.
2. Cullen PM. Paediatric trauma. Contin Educ Anaesth Crit Care Pain 2012;12:157–161.
3. Cooper A, Barlow B, Davidson L, Relethford J, O'Meara J, Mottley L. Epidemiology of pediatric trauma: importance of population-based statistics. J Pediatr Surg 1992; 27(2):149–153.
4. Sharma M, Lahoti BK, Khandelwal G, Mathur RK, Sharma SS, Laddha A. Epidemiological trends of pediatric trauma: A single-center study of 791 patients. J Indian Assoc Pediatr Surg 2011;16(3):88–92.
5. Advanced Trauma Life Support for doctors. 9th edn. Chicago: American College of Surgeons, 2012.
6. Kirkham FJ, Newton CRJC, Whitehouse W. Paediatric coma scales. Dev Med Child Neurol 2008;50(4):267–274.
7. Varon AJ, Smith CE (Eds). Essentials of trauma anesthesia. Cambridge: Cambridge University Press; 2012.
8. Hymel KP, Abshire TC, Luckey DW, Jenny C. Coagulopathy in pediatric abusive head trauma. Pediatrics 1997;99:371–375.
9. Crankshaw D, McViety J, Entwistle M. A review of cuffed vs uncuffed endotracheal tubes in children. Ped Anesth Crit Care J 2014;2(2):70–73.
10. Tollefsen WW, Chapman J, Frakes M, Gallagher M, Shear M, Thomas SH. Endotracheal tube cuff pressures in pediatric patients intubated before aeromedical transport. Pediatr Emerg Care 2010;26:361–363.
11. Sagarin MJ, Chiang V, Sakles JC, Barton ED, Wolfe RE, Vissers RJ, et al. Rapid sequence intubation for pediatric emergency airway management. Pediatr Emerg Care 2002;18(6):417–423.
12. Gerardi MJ, Sacchetti AD, Cantor RM, Santamaria JP, Gausche M, Lucid W, et al. Rapid-sequence intubation of the pediatric patient. Pediatric Emergency Medicine Committee of the American College of Emergency Physicians. Ann Emerg Med 1996;28(1):55–74.

13. Rapid sequence intubation. In: Hazinski MF, Zaritsky AL, Nadkarni VM, Hickey RW, Schexnayder SM, Berg RA (Eds). Pediatric Advanced Life Support Provider Manual. Dallas, Texas: American Heart Association; 2002; pp. 359–378.

14. Dearden M, McDowall D. Comparison of etomidate and althesin in the reduction of increased intracranial pressure after head injury. Br J Anaesth 1985;57:361–368.

15. Eisenberg HM, Frankowski RF, Contant CF, Marshall LF, Walker MD. High dose barbiturate control of elevated intracranial pressure in patients with severe head injury. J Neurosurg 1988;69(1):15–23.

16. Kelly DF, Goodale DB, Williams J, Herr DL, Chappell ET, Rosner MJ, et al. Propofol in the treatment of moderate and severe head injury: a randomized, prospective double blind pilot trial. J Neurosurg 1999;90(6):1042–1052.

17. Zelicof-Paul A, Smith-Lockridge A, Schnadower D, Tyler S, Levin S, Roskind C, et al. Controversies in rapid sequence intubation in children. Curr Opin Pediatr 2005; 17:355–362.

18. Guldner G, Schultz J, Sexton P, Fortner C, Richmond M. Etomidate for rapid-sequence intubation in young children: hemodynamic effects and adverse events. Acad Emerg Med 2003;10(2):134–139.

19. Kaieda R, Todd MM, Cook LN, Warner DS. Acute effects of changing plasma osmolality and colloid oncotic pressure on the formation of brain edema after cryogenic injury. Neurosurgery 1989;24:671–678.

20. Cochran A, Scaife ER, Hansen KW, Downey EC. Hyperglycemia and outcomes from pediatric traumatic brain injury. J Trauma 2003;55:1035–1038.

21. Udani V, Munot P, Ursekar M, Gupta S. Neonatal hypoglycemic brain. Injury a common cause of infantile onset remote symptomatic epilepsy. Indian Pediatr 2009;46: 127–132.

22. Browne GJ, Cocks AJ, McCaskill ME. Current trends in the management of major paediatric trauma. Emerg Med (Fremantle) 2001;13:418–425.

23. Paterson NA. Validation of a theoretically derived model for the management of massive blood loss in pediatric patients—A case report. Paediatr Anaesth 2009;19:535–540.

24. Chidester SJ, Williams N, Wang W, Groner JI. A pediatric massive transfusion protocol. J Trauma Acute Care Surg 2012;73(5):1273–1277.

25. Hendrickson JE, Shaz BH, Pereira G, Parker PM, Jessup P, Atwell F, et al. Implementation of a pediatric trauma massive transfusion protocol: one institution's experience. Transfusion 2012;52:1228–1236.

26. Diab YA, Edward CC, Wong ECC, Luban NLC. Massive transfusion in children and neonates. Br J Haematol 2013; 161:15–26.

27. Werner C, Engelhard K. Pathophysiology of traumatic brain injury. Br J Anaesth 2007;99:4–9.

28. Chesnut RM, Marshall LF, Klauber MR, Blunt BA, Baldwin N, Eisenberg HM, et al. The role of secondary brain injury in determining outcome from severe head injury. J Trauma 1993;34:216–22.

29. Lang DA, Teasdale GM, Macpherson P, Lawrence A. Diffuse brain swelling after head injury: more often malignant in adults than children? J Neurosurg 1994;80: 675–680.

30. Kochanek PM. Pediatric traumatic brain injury: quo vadis? Dev Neurosci 2006;28:244–255.

31. Carney NA, Chesnut R, Kochanek PM. American Association for Surgery of Trauma; Child Neurology Society; International Society for Pediatric Neurosurgery; et al. Guidelines for the acute medical management of severe traumatic brain injury in infants, children, and adolescents. Pediatr Crit Care Med 2003;4:S1–S75.

32. Kochanek PM, Carney N, Adelson PD, Ashwal S, Bell MJ, Bratton S, et al. Guidelines for the acute medical management of severe traumatic brain injury in infants, children, and adolescents—second edition. Pediatr Crit Care Med 2012;13(Suppl 1):S1–82.

33. Bhalla T, Dewhirst E, Sawardekar A, Dairo O, Tobias JD. Perioperative management of the pediatric patient with traumatic brain injury. Pediatr Anesth 2012;22:627–640.

34. Kewalramani LS, Kraus JF, Sterling HM. Acute spinal cord lesions in a pediatric population: Epidemiologic and clinical features. Paraplegia 1980;18:206–19.

35. Ross AK, Pediatric trauma Anesthesia management. Anesthesiol Clin North Am 2001;19:309–337.

36. Cantor RM, Learning JM. Evaluation and management of pediatric major trauma. Emerg Med Clin North Am 1998; 16:229–256.

37. Dutton RP, McCunn M, Grissom TE. Anesthesia for trauma. In: Miller RD (ed). Miller's Anesthesia 7th edn. Philadelphia, Churchill Livingstone 2010;2277–2311.

38. Hurlbert RJ, Hadley MN, Walters BC, Aarabi B, Dhall SS, Gelb DE, et al. Pharmacological therapy for acute spinal cord injury. Neurosurgery 2013;72(Suppl 2):93–105.

39. Garcia VF, Gotschall CS, Eichelberger MR, Bowman LM. Rib fractures in children: A marker of severe trauma. J Trauma 1990;30(6):695–700.

20

Child with Burns

Rachna Wadhwa

- Assessment
- Pathophysiology
- Pharmacological alterations
- Primary survey and resuscitation
- Perioperative anaesthesia consideration
- Special considerations

INTRODUCTION

Burns represent a unique and common mechanism of thermal injuries in paediatrics. Burn injuries are a frequent cause of morbidity and mortality in paediatrics. In fact it is the second leading cause of accidental death in children aged 1–4 years, exceeded only by motor vehicle accidents.[1] The peak age of accidental burns is also 1–4 years with incidence higher in boys as compared to girls.[2,3] Although the mortality rates have declined over past few decades, still about 265,000 deaths occur every year due to burns (WHO 2014). Burns are associated with intense pain and distress, so, adequate pain relief is mandatory in all victims.

Mortality is attributed to refractory burn shock, inhalational injury associated with airway compromise and sepsis-induced multiorgan failure.[3] Therefore, a holistic approach is required to have good outcome in paediatric burns. Health care workers involved in burns management must have thorough knowledge of associated pathophysiological and pharmacological abnormalities.

Modern age management of thermal injuries should aim at—(a) prevention of thermal injuries, (b) dedicated hospitals/burn centres, (c) improved surgical techniques, (d) safe anaesthesia and pain management, (e) prompt management of associated injuries.

ASSESSMENT

Severity of burn depends on size, depth and location. Different types of mechanisms implicated in burns include thermal, chemical, electrical, ultraviolet and others.

Estimate of skin surface involvement is recorded as percentage of total body surface area (TBSA). Though few clinicians have used clinometric instruments to evaluate percentage of burns, still Lund-Browder estimate is the most common tool in paediatrics (Fig. 20.1).[4,5] It is considered the most accurate of all the methods as it assigns a specific number to each body part depending on age. Wallace rule of nines may be useful for quick estimation in pre-hospital arena where decision to transfer in a burn centre has to be taken immediately.[6]

Palmar method is an alternative way of assessing paediatric burns where size of the patients' palm represents 1% TBSA.[7,8] Modern methods like flexible single use nomogram has been devised to calculate the affected area with precision. It is based on advanced graphics software platform that creates a three-dimensional virtual display.[9,10]

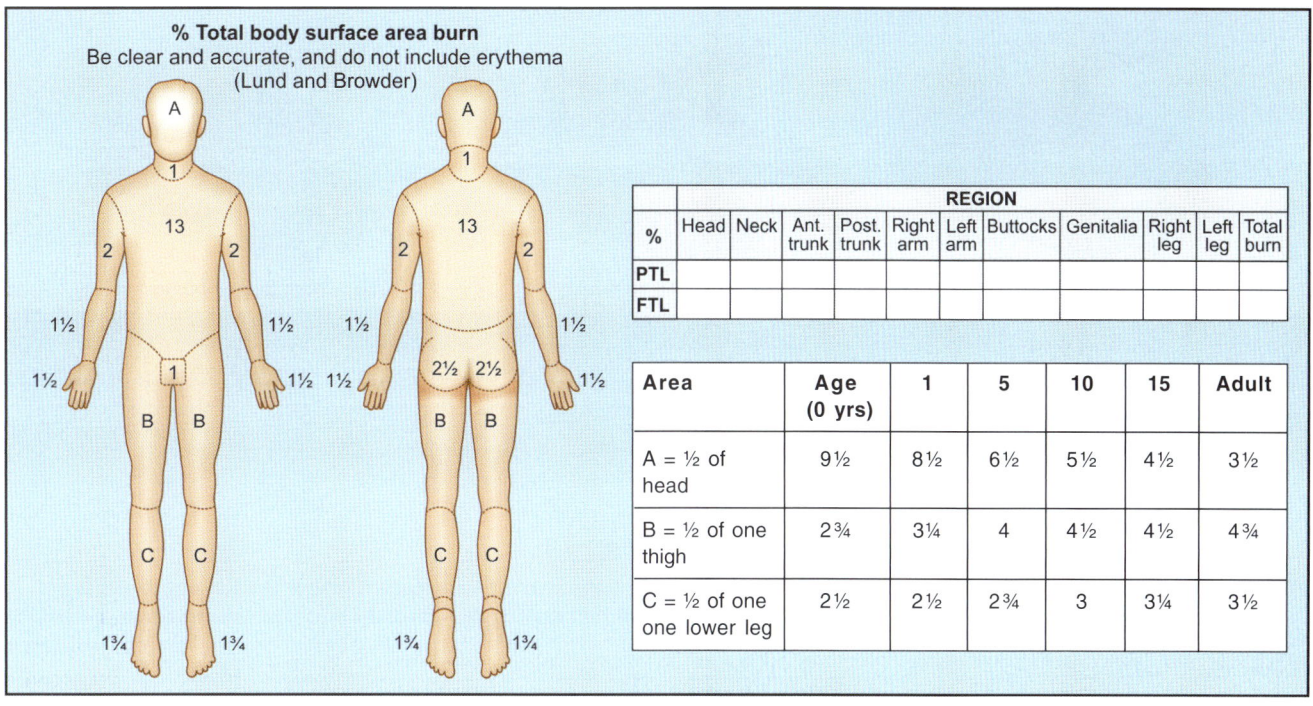

% Total body surface area burn
Be clear and accurate, and do not include erythema
(Lund and Browder)

%	REGION										
	Head	Neck	Ant. trunk	Post. trunk	Right arm	Left arm	Buttocks	Genitalia	Right leg	Left leg	Total burn
PTL											
FTL											

Area	Age (0 yrs)	1	5	10	15	Adult
A = ½ of head	9½	8½	6½	5½	4½	3½
B = ½ of one thigh	2¾	3¼	4	4½	4½	4¾
C = ½ of one one lower leg	2½	2½	2¾	3	3¼	3½

Fig. 20.1. Lund-Browder chart for assessment of total body surface area burned

Depth of burn estimates the actual dermal involvement. The higher the degree, the deeper the burn wound (Table 20.1). The dynamics of dermal injury changes after a period of time and should be observed for their extension to adjacent or deeper tissues.[11]

PATHOPHYSIOLOGY

Skin is an important sense organ that plays crucial role in preventing heat loss, evaporation and infection. Loss of dermal barrier results in hypothermia and predisposition to sepsis. Additionally, several mediators are released from the burned site, thereby, activating intense inflammatory response depending upon degree and percentage of body surface area affected. Cytokines are the key mediators of the systemic effects.[12] Other mediators are complement factors, arachidonic acid metabolites, C-reactive protein and free oxygen radicals. Reactive oxygen species (ROS) production is markedly increased in acute phase of burns, resulting in oxidation of nucleotides, proteins and lipids.[13] The lipid peroxides and endotoxins are implicated in damage to the tissues throughout the body, leading to multiorgan failure. Early debridement of extensive burn tissue may decrease toxic response and hence mortality.

Respiratory System

Inhalational injury and airway obstruction are most common cause for morbidity and mortality in burn patients. Respiratory complications may arise early in cases where victim is confined in a burning environment. The mechanisms implicated are as follows:

Direct Thermal Injury

Direct thermal injury affects upper airways denuding ciliated epithelium and mucosa in proximal bronchi. Massive tissue oedema in laryngeal and tracheal structures above the carina results in acute airway obstruction, especially in children.[14]

Chemical and Toxic Damage

Chemical and toxic damage generally affects the lower airways. Inhalation of nitrogen dioxide and sulphur dioxide released from burning plastic combines with moisture in tracheobronchial tree to form nitric and sulphuric acids thereby damaging the distal airways. Inhalation of toxic fumes results in necrotizing bronchitis, alveolar destruction, oedema, exudation of proteins and development of bronchopneumonitis.[15]

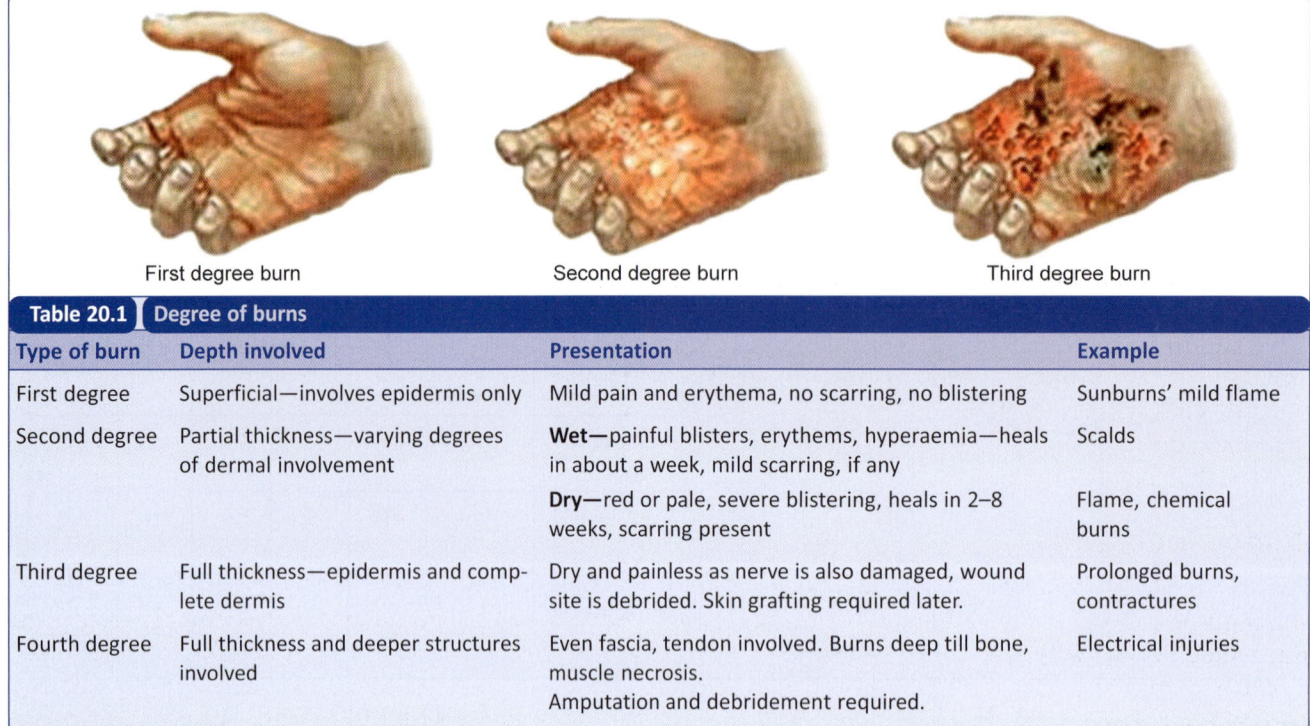

First degree burn   Second degree burn   Third degree burn

Table 20.1	Degree of burns		
Type of burn	**Depth involved**	**Presentation**	**Example**
First degree	Superficial—involves epidermis only	Mild pain and erythema, no scarring, no blistering	Sunburns' mild flame
Second degree	Partial thickness—varying degrees of dermal involvement	**Wet**—painful blisters, erythems, hyperaemia—heals in about a week, mild scarring, if any	Scalds
		Dry—red or pale, severe blistering, heals in 2–8 weeks, scarring present	Flame, chemical burns
Third degree	Full thickness—epidermis and complete dermis	Dry and painless as nerve is also damaged, wound site is debrided. Skin grafting required later.	Prolonged burns, contractures
Fourth degree	Full thickness and deeper structures involved	Even fascia, tendon involved. Burns deep till bone, muscle necrosis. Amputation and debridement required.	Electrical injuries

Carbon Monoxide (CO) and Cyanide (CN) Poisoning

CO is a by product of incomplete organic combustion and its exposure is assumed to be present in all patients who were burned in enclosed areas. Affinity of CO is 240 times that of oxygen, so it displaces O_2 from haemoglobin (Hb) molecule and shifts oxy-Hb curve to left, producing functional anaemia (Table 20.2). Hence, oxygen therapy should be given to all patients of thermal injury. Factually, half-life of COHb in room air is 200 minutes, but it is decreased to around 40 minutes after 100% O_2 therapy. In fact, hyperbaric oxygen has been found to reduce neurological sequelae in adults.[16] Standard pulse-oximetry and arterial blood gas analysis (ABG) cannot give actual insight into CO intoxication, hence assays of COHb levels is recommended. A non-invasive co-oximeter that measures multiple wavelengths can identify COHb and meth-Hb levels.[17] CN binds to ferric ion of cytochrome oxidase, therby limiting aerobic metabolism at mitochondrial level, resulting in decreased ATP production and rapid depletion of energy resources.[18] It produces tissue hypoxia by decreasing extraction of transported oxygen, resulting in high levels of venous oxygen and lactic acidosis not responding to oxygen therapy. Management of cyanide poisoning includes administration of sodium thiosulphate, amyl nitrite, sodium nitrite and cyanocobalamin.[19]

Acute Lung Injury/ Acute Respiratory Distress Syndrome (ALI/ARDS)

Lower airway injury compounded with endobronchial cell destruction and inflammatory changes predispose the patient to ALI and later on ARDS.[20,21] There may be significant ventilation perfusion mismatch and potential for bacterial infection leading to severe bronchopneumonia after sometime. Pulmonary lavage to clear mucous plugs, debris and exudates

Table 20.2	Symptoms of carbon monooxide poisoning
CoHb%	**Clinical signs**
0–10	None
10–20	Headache, flushing and nausea
20–30	Nausea, pulsatile headache and dyspnoea on exertion
30–40	Confusion
40–60	Coma
>60	Convulsions, cherry red appearance coma, death

(Adapted and modified from ATIS student manual.)

may be helpful.[22] Use of aerosolized heparin and mucolytics may reduce cast formation and attenuate risk of respiratory failure.[23] Airway management can be challenging particularly in small children. Though tracheostomy is considered advantageous, still it has many limitations.[24]

Circumferential Chest Burns

They may result in impaired thoracic wall movement and hence reduced compliance. Markedly elevated intra-abdominal and intrathoracic pressures impair venous return with resultant decreased cardiac output. Hence early escharotomies are performed in order to overcome compressive effects of abdomino-thoracic burns.

Cardiovascular System

Paediatric burn patients experience massive fluid shifts due to loss of vascular and endothelial integrity. Burn shock is characterized by significant reduction in cardiac output owing to hypovolemia, decreased cardiac contractility and altered peripheral resistance.[25] This results in hypoperfusion of organ systems and resultant cellular ischaemia. The cardiac output is decreased even before the loss of plasma volume, implicating direct myocardial depression by burns. Cardiac troponin I, marker of non-ischaemic cardiac injury was also found to be elevated in burn patients between 5th and 14th day after injury.[26] Other humoral mediators like, TNFα, interleukins (IL-1β, IL-6) and nuclear factor κβ possess negative inotropic effects and accentuate cardiac depression.[27] Trans-cellular electrolyte shifts and loss of circulating plasma proteins further lead to decreased intravascular volume, generalized oedema and organ hypoperfusion. Children who survive this acute phase develop hyperdynamic state 3–5 days after burn. Hyperdynamic state is characterized by two to three times rise in cardiac output, heart rate and cardiac index. Plasma levels of rennin, aldosterone, catecholamines, vasopressin and ADH are markedly elevated resulting in hypertension and tachycardia. Early burn wound closure may decrease this hypermetabolic response and help in cardiac output reduction.

Renal Function

Acute renal failure (ARF) after burns can be a life-threatening complication.[28] Hypovolaemia, hypo-perfusion, hypoxia, hyperglycaemia, myoglobinuria and haemoglobinuria are all implicated in renal dysfunction. Aggressive fluid resuscitation with the target to maintain urine output within 1 to 1.5 ml/kg/hour minimises the risk of development of ARF.

Mortality rates were quite high in paediatric burns till 1980s because of concomitant ARF, but the concept of early fluid resuscitation has led to decreased incidence of ARF. Delayed intravascular fluid resuscitation may result in ARF and adds on to mortality attributed to burns. Children with burns involving >40% of BSA generally demonstrate renal tubular dysfunction.[29] Free haemoglobin and myoglobin in plasma further adds on to tubular injury. Rhabdo-myolysis, a consequence of electrical burns and crush injury, can also lead to ARF.

Gastrointestinal System

Burns have long been identified as directly associated with gastroduodenal ulcers, like Curlings' ulcer. Now-adays, abdominal compartment syndrome is another matter of concern in fluid therapy. When TBSA affected with burns is high and patient receives 300 ml/kg/day as intravenous fluid, the chances of development of intra-abdominal hypertension is more.[30] This critical volume associated with abdominal compartment syndrome is called Ivy index.[31]

Diversion of blood flow from viscera to vital organs is the hallmark of early post-burn period. Thromboxane is one of the common mediators along with catecholamines and prostanoids implicated in mesenteric vasoconstriction and decreased gut vascularity, although blood flow to adrenals and liver is not affected. A true paralytic ileus persists until the bowel is used. Severe thermal injury-induced gaps in intestinal mucosa favour bacterial translocation and systemic absorption of endotoxins, thereby propagating sepsis.[32,33] Early enteral nutrition decreases gut-related complications, life-threatening bleeding, sepsis and morbidity in thermal injuries.[34] Stress ulcer prophylaxis should be administered to all burn trauma patients to avoid massive bleeding and sepsis.

Metabolism and Thermal Regulation

Classical biphasic pattern is seen after burns with respect to energy expenditure.[35] On initial 1–2 days, energy and oxygen consumption is low, known as *ebb phase*. This is followed by hypermetabolic that is *flow phase*. Release of catecholamines, stress hormones, interleukins, TNFα and prostanoids results in sharply elevated basal energy expenditure, catabolism of skeletal muscle proteins and hyperdynamic circulation.[36] These abnormalities may persist for long after burns. Hence, patients have refractory tachycardia, increased cardiac output and oxygen consumption, hyperpyrexia and increased carbon di oxide production.[37]

Temperature regulation is another important concern in paediatric burns. The infants lose the insulating properties of skin and fail to achieve normothermia. Moreover, hypermetabolic phase and evaporation from open wounds markedly enhance heat loss. This may result in severe hypothermia and predicts poor prognosis. Ambient temperature should be set at 28–33°C, and exposed areas should be covered with sterile sheets to prevent infection and heat loss.

Hepatic Functions

Post-burn hepatic abnormalities also contribute to burn associated morbidity and mortality. In early phases of hypovolemia and hypotension, hepatic blood flow is compromised.[38]

Later on, toxic drug interactions, multiple blood transfusions, hypermetabolism and sepsis may result in hepatocellular dysfunction. Increased serum transaminases, reduced synthesis of proteins and focal hypertrophy are observed in hepatocellular damage. Fatty infiltration of liver and hepatomegaly has also been reported. This may be associated with high amount of carbohydrates used in parentral nutrition.

Haematological Abnormalities

Early post-burn phase is characterized by anaemia owing to red blood cell mass destruction by heat, free radicals and extravascular sequestration.[39] Initially, haemoglobin levels may be normal because of shrunken intravascular volume. Anaemia becomes apparent after fluid resuscitation. Infants and small children have limited circulating blood volume, so blood loss should be precariously managed. Thrombocytopenia is an early manifestation of consumption coagulopathy. It is followed by thrombocytosis, 10–14 days after burns.[40] Sepsis in post-burn period results in persistent thrombocytopenia. Though not so commonly encountered, coagulopathies require aggressive management.

Nervous System

There may be direct trauma to nerve apparatus else neurological dysfunction may be a result of tissue oedema, hypoxia and hypoperfusion. Burn encephalopathy is defined as a complex syndrome associated with variable course of hallucinations, delirium, seizures, coma and behavioural changes.[41] About 30% of pediatric burns face acute post-traumatic stress disorders. Neuropsychiatric disturbances may arise from various factors, like cerebral oedema, stress, severe pain and sleep deficit. Serial monitoring of serum electrolytes is also essential to avoid complications.

Immune System

The immune system is depressed within few hours following burns and directly correlates with percentage of body surface area burnt. The humoral as well as cellular immunity is attenuated, predisposing the patient to infections.[42] Hence, strictly aseptic handling, early wound excision and targeted antibiotic therapy play an important role in improving outcome of the child.

PHARMACOLOGICAL ALTERATIONS

General Considerations

A spectrum of metabolic, fluid and organ–system derangements is associated with burns in children. All medications have to be carefully titrated in view of wide interpatient variability in drug response.[43] If the burns are extensive, the pharmacological alterations are also significant.

Special emphasis is laid upon securing intravenous access, difficult tracheal intubation, monitoring, prevention of heat loss and blood management.

Co-existent hypovolaemia, hypoperfusion and redistribution of blood flow may alter the volume of distribution and clearance of drugs in acute phase of burns.

In addition, uptake of drugs by oral and intramuscular routes becomes unpredictable.

In hypermetabolic phase, the children may require larger than normal doses of all medications. Due to altered synthetic functions of liver, alpha-1 acid glycoprotein concentration is increased as compared to albumin, thereby altering the pharmacologically active free fraction.

Inhalational Agents

Among all anaesthetic agents, inhalational agents have been found to be safest in burn victims.[44] In a haemodynamically stable child, halothane, isoflurane and sevoflurane have been used extensively without any major problems. However, halothane-induced peripheral vasodilatation, increased heat loss, increased operative bleeding and postoperative shivering may preclude its use in hypovolaemic patients. Sevoflurane offers the advantage of rapid induction with minimal airway irritability. However, there is literature reporting emergence delirium after sevoflurane anaesthesia. Paediatric burn patients require frequent dressings and entonox ($O_2/N_2O:50/50$) has also been found effective. Though quite safe and predictable, its long-term use is associated with bone marrow depression.

Intravenous Agents

Ketamine is one of the most commonly used anaesthetic agents in burns from decades. Profound analgesia, predictable onset and recovery time, minimal respiratory and cardiovascular derangements are unique properties of ketamine that makes it suitable for burn patients.[45]

Recently, ketamine combined with dexmedetomidine is considered better alternative for change of dressings in paediatric burns as compared to propofol ketamine combination.[46,47] Propofol sedation is widely accepted for short procedures. But prolonged infusions are discouraged in ICU in fear of fatal complication in paediatrics, i.e. propofol infusion syndrome.[48]

Muscle Relaxants

Burn patient exhibits abnormal response to depolarizing as well as non-depolarizing muscle relaxants (NDMR). It has been postulated that there is proliferation of nicotinic acetylcholine receptors, not only around neuromuscular junction but also on entire muscle membrane.[49,50] The presence of immature receptors in extrajunctional tissues, even at sites away from injury results in variable response to muscle relaxants. Succinylcholine, a depolarizing muscle relaxant, has fast onset of action, and is preferred for rapid sequence induction (RSI) in emergency situations. But its administration may result in dangerous hyperkalemias post-burn. However, succinylcholine may be used in early burns as the hyperkalaemic response has not been observed in first 24 hours.[44] But this response may persist till 18 months, hence avoid succinylcholine and use rocuronium 1.2 mg/kg for RSI in this period.[51] Dose frequency and requirements of NDMR increase during hyperdynamic phase, but reversal agent requirements are unchanged.

Analgesics and Sedatives

High quality pain management is an integral part of burn care. Opioids not only provide excellent analgesia, but also attenuate metabolic demands and anxiety of patients. The most fruitful approach in such patients is frequent assessment of pain and supplement analgesia when relief seems inadequate.[52,53] The attitude towards pain management should be presumptive and preemptive.[54] Morphine, fentanyl, alfentanil are commonly used opioids. Intravenous paracetamol alone or with opioids provides adequate analgesia in children. Dexmedetomidine has also gained wide acceptance in view of its unique properties of sedation, analgesia and minimal respiratory depression.[55]

Regional Anaesthesia

Peripheral nerve blocks prove to be very efficacious for pain relief in limbs, especially for donor sites after skin grafting. Ultrasound guidance has added a new dimension to regional anaesthesia. Continuous nerve blockades have opioids sparing effects and provide pain relief in postoperative period without any side effects.

PRIMARY SURVEY AND RESUSCITATION

The 'ABC' approach of ATLS is followed in initial management of burns.[43,56] The mechanism of injury provides information about smoke inhalation or thermal injury of the upper airway.

Airway

In cases of suspected inhalational injury, progressive airway oedema has to be anticipated and tracheal intubation is performed early. The small diameter of the airways in children is vulnerable to critical narrowing and acute airway obstruction. Small tracheal tubes may be required, cuffed tracheal tubes provide better seal and controlled ventilation.[57] Microcuff tubes, specially designed for paediatrics, provide a greater margin of safety as compared to conventional tubes.

Breathing

Adequate ventilation and oxygenation must be ensured. Smoke inhalation and carbon monoxide poisoning necessitate high inspired oxygen concentrations. Therefore, oxygen must be given to all patients and saturation continuously monitored. Sometimes, there is a need of thoracic and abdominal escharotomy to relieve impairment of thoracic and diaphragmatic excursion.

Circulation

Early goal-directed volume resuscitation is manadatory to achieve better outcome in thermal injuries.[58] Burn oedema is maximal in the first 24 hours. Thereafter, fluid requirement is judged clinically by capillary refill, mental status, and urine output. Different regimes are used for intravascular resuscitation (Table 20.3). Glucose and electrolyte levels should be monitored and abnormalitie corrected. The burnt areas should be covered with a sterile non-adherent dressing and potent analgesics administered. This decreases heat loss, risk of infections and release of stress hormones.

Table 20.3	Various fluid resuscitation regimes in burn victims
Formula	**Recommended fluid**
Parkland	Ringer's lactate 4 ml/kg/% TBSA
Brooke	Ringer's lactate 1.5 ml/kg/% TBSA and colloid 0.5 ml/kg/% TBSA
Brooke (Modified)	Ringer's lactate 2 ml/kg/% TBSA
Evans	Normal saline 1.0 ml/kg/% TBSA and colloid 1.0 ml/kg/% TBSA
Demling	Dextran 40 in saline 2 ml/kg/h for 8 h Ringer's lactate maintain UO at 30 ml/h FFP 0.5 ml/kg/h for 18 h beginning 8 h post-burn
Warden	Lactated Ringer's + 50 mmol/l $NaHCO_3$ for 8 h to maintain UO at 30–50 ml/h Lactated Ringer's to maintain UO at 30–50 ml/h beginning 8 h post-burn

PERIOPERATIVE ANAESTHETIC CONSIDERATIONS

An anaesthesiologist plays important role in providing initial resuscitation, optimal analgesia, sedation, anaesthesia and intensive care management. Children have to be prepared physiologically and psychologically prior to any intervention. Burn patients require multiple dressings, burn wound excision, skin grafting and rehabilitation procedures. Adequate blood and blood products should be arranged and child premedicated with anxiolytics.

Preoperative fasting for more than 8 hours severely compromises the caloric intake of a child in catabolic phase. Therefore, enteral nutrition is discontinued about 4 hours before the surgical procedure in such patients.[59]

In the operating room, securing two large-bore intravenous cannula is essential before the procedure is started. Ultrasound guidance may be shought in difficult venous access. Intraosseous route or central venous catheter placement is considered when no peripheral veins are found.

Next important issue is airway management. Anticipate difficult airway and arrange difficult airway cart along with fibreoptic bronchoscope, small size tracheal tubes and be prepared for surgical airway. Once the airway is secured, the endotracheal tube should be firmly taped or sutured to prevent accidental extubation. Nowadays, availability of newer pediatric supraglottic airways has made airway management easier, as many cases do not actually require tracheal intubation.

Oesophageal stethoscope is most practical and useful tool of monitoring. Peripheral pulse oximetry, electrocardiography, capnography and temperature should be continuously monitored in all paediatric burns. Depending upon the haemodynamic status of child, invasive monitoring may be instituted. Ambient temperature should be maintained at 28–32°C and prevent hypothermia. Oxygen in sevoflurane is safe and preferred method of induction in small children. However, propofol and etomidate are also used for induction in titrated doses. Avoid succinylcholine 24 hours after burns and use rocuronium for RSI. Maintenance of anaesthesia is easily accomplished with N_2O, O_2, opioids, volatile agent and NDMR. It is advisable to use airway exchange catheter when extubating difficult airways. Arterial blood gas analysis is also essential, as these children exhibit high basal metabolic rate and thus increased CO_2 production. Monitoring of blood loss and its correction is another important aspect of large burn wound excisions. Blood and blood products should be administered as per the needs of the patient. Serum ionized calcium should be serially monitored and hypocalcaemia corrected, if any.

SPECIAL CONSIDERATIONS

Electrical Burns

Low voltage burns occur in domestic settings and passage of electrical current through cardiovascular system results in cardiac arrhythmias and cardiac arrest.[60] Children accidentally put electrical cords in mouth resulting in circumoral and lingual burns. High voltage current causes three types of injuries—entry and exit wounds, arc burns and surface burns. Electrical injuries cause deeper tissue and muscle damage. Myonecrosis and rhabdomyolysis are a common feature of electrical burns which may result in acute renal failure.

CONCLUSION

The management of major burns in children demands a protocol-based multidisciplinary approach with special skills and high quality care in burn centres. Aseptic handling, dynamic monitoring, goal-directed fluid therapy, targeted antibiotic therapy, nutritional support, effective analgesia and anxiolysis are the mainstays of burn management. Health care workers dealing with burn patients should have the knowledge of associated physiological and pharmacological alterations. Therefore, it is the need of the hour to have dedicated burn unit in hospitals to optimise management and improve outcome after burns.

REFERENCES

1. Romanelli T. Anaesthesia for burn injuries. In: Davis PJ (Ed). Smith's Anesthesia for Infants and Children, 8th edn. Mosby 2011;p 1003–1022.

2. Peddi M, Segu SS, Ramesha KT. The persistent paradigm of pediatric burnsin India: An epidemiological review. Indian Journal of Burns 2014;22(1):93–97.

3. Thombs BD, Singh VA, Milner SM. Children under 4 years are at greater risk of mortality following acute burn injury: evidence from a national sample of 12,902 pediatric admissions. Shock 2006;26(4):348–352.

4. Wachtel TL, Berry CC, Wachtel EE, Frank HA. The inter-rater reliability of estimating the size of burns from various burn area chart drawings. Burns 2000;26(2):156–170.

5. Lund CC, Browder NC Estimation of area of burns. Surgery, Gynecology and Obstetrics 1944;79;352–358.

6. Wallace AB. The exposure treatment of burns. Lancet 1951;257(6653):501–504.

7. Sheridan RL, Petras L, Basha G. Planimetry study of the percent of body surface area represented by the hand and palm. J Burn Care Rehabil 1995;16(6):605–606.

8. Rossiter ND, Chapman P, Haywood IA. How big is a hand? Burns 1996;22(3):230–231.

9. Neuwalder JM, Sampson C, Breuing KH, Orgill DP. A review of computer-aided body surface area determination: SAGE II and EPRI's 3D Burn Vision. J Burn Care Rehabil 2002;23(1):55–59.

10. Dirnberger J, Giretzlehner M, Ruhmer M, Haller H, Rodemund C. Modelling human burn injuries in a three-dimensional virtual environment. Stud Health Technol Inform 2003;94:52–58.

11. Palmieri TL, Greenhalgh DG. Topical treatment of pediatric patients with burns: a practical guide. Am J Clin Dermatol 2002;3(8):529–534.

12. Finnerty CC, Herndon DN, Przkora, et al. Cytokine expression profile over time in severely burned pediatric patients. Shock 2006;26:13–19.

13. Bernath MA, Stucki P, Berger MM. Burns and post-burn care: anesthetic considerations. In: Bissonnette B, Dalens B (Eds). Pediatric Anesthesia: Principles and Practice. McGraw-Hill 2001;p 2049–2069.

14. Gaissert HA, Lofgren RH, Grillo HC. Upper airway compromise after inhalation injury, complex strictures of the larynx and rachea and their management. Annals of Surgery 1993;218(5):672–678.

15. Fein A, Leff A, Hopewell PC. Pathophysiology and management of the complications resulting from fire and the inhaled products of combustion: Review of the literature. Critical Care Medicine 1980;8(2):55–112.

16. Kao LW, Nañagas KA. Carbon monoxide poisoning. Med Clin North Am 2005;89:1161–1194.

17. Suner S, Partridge R, Sucov A, Valente J, Chee K, Hughes A, Jay G. Non-invasive pulse co-oximetry screening in the emergency department identifies occult carbon monoxide toxicity. The Journal of Emergency Medicine 2008;34(4):441–450.

18. Hamel J. A Review of acute cyanide poisoning with a treatment update. Critical Care Nurse 2011;31(1):72–82.

19. MacLennan L, Moiemen N. Management of cyanide toxicity in patients with burns. Burns 2015;41(1):18–24.

20. Tokarik M, Sjöberg F, Vajtr D, Broz L, Balik M, Vranova J. Natriuretic peptide proANP (1–98), a biomarker of ALI/ARDS in burns. Burns 2013;39(2):243–248.

21. Maybauer MO, Rehberg S, Traber DL, Herndon DN, Maybauer DM. Pathophysiology of acute lung injury in severe burn and smoke inhalation injury. Anaesthesist 2009;58(8):805–812.

22. Demling RH. Smoke inhalation lung injury: an update. Eplasty 2008;8:e27.

23. Desai MH, Mlcak R, Richardson J, Nichols R, Herndon DN. Reduction in mortality in pediatric patients with inhalation injury with aerosolized heparin/N-acetyl-cystine therapy. J Burn Care Rehabil 1998;19(3):210–212.

24. Palmieri TL, Jackson WRR, Greenhalgh DG. Benefits of early tracheostomy in severely burned children. Critical Care Medicine 2002;30(4):922–924.

25. Huang YL, Yang Z. Roles of ischemia and hypoxia and the molecular pathogenesis of post-burn cardiac shock. Burns: Journal of the International Society for Burn Injuries 2003;29(8):828–833.

26. Zeng L, Chen Y, Wu M. Cardiac troponin I: a marker for detecting non-ischemic cardiac injury. Zhonghua Yi Xue Za Zhi 2001;81:393–395.

27. Xiao R, Huang YS. Cardiac function and organ blood flow at early stage following severe burn, Novel Strategies in ischemic heart disease. In Tech 2012;22:405–427.

28. Emara SS, Alzaylai AA. Renal failure in burn patients: a review. Ann Burns Fire Disasters 2013;26(1):12–15.

29. Mustonen KM, Vuola J. Acute renal failure in intensive care burn patients. J Burn Care Res 2008;29(1):227–237.

30. Oda J, Yamashita K, Inoue T, et al. Resuscitation fluid volume and abdominal compartment syndrome in patients with major burns. Burns 2006;32:151–154.

31. Burns GA, Caushaj PF. Abdominal compartment syndrome in patients with burns. J Burn Care Rehabil. 1999;20(5):351–353.

32. Ziegler TR, Smith RJ, O'Dwyer ST, Demling RH, Wilmore DW. Increased intestinal permeability associated with infection in burn patients. Arch Surg 1988;123(11):1313–1319.

33. Magnotti LJ, Deitch EA. Burns, bacterial translocation, gut barrier function and failure. J Burn Care Rehabil 2005; 26:383.

34. McDonald WS, Sharp CWJ, Deitch EA. Immediate enteral feeding in burn patients is safe and effective. Ann Surg 1991;213:177.

35. Atiyeh BS, Gunn SWA, Dibo SA. Nutritional and pharmacological modulation of the metabolic response of severely burned patients: Review of the literature (Part 1). Ann Burns Fire Disasters 2008;21(2):63–72.

36. Hart DW, Wolf SE, Mlcak R, et al. Persistence of muscle catabolism after severe burn. Surgery 2000;128:312.

37. Wolf SE, Debroy M, Herndon DN. The cornerstones and directions of pediatric burn care. Pediatr Surg Int 1997;12:312–320.

38. Jeschke MG. The hepatic response to thermal injury: is the liver important for postburn outcomes? Mol Med 2009;15(9–10):337–351.

39. Harries RHC, Phillips LG. Hematologic and acute phase response. In: Herndon D (Ed). Total Burn Care. London: Saunders 1996;p 293–301.

40. Housinger TA, Brinkerhoff C, Warden GD. The relationship between platelet count, sepsis and survival in pediatric burn patients. Arch Surg 1993;128:65–67.

41. Winkelman MD, Galloway PG. Central nervous system complications of thermal burns. A postmortem study of 139 patients. Medicine (Baltimore) 1992;71(5):271–283.

42. Fayazov AD, Shukurov SI, Shukurov BI, Sultanov BC, Namazov AN, Ruzimuratov DA. Disorders of the immune system in severely burned patients. Ann Burns Fire Disasters 2009 Sep 30;22(3):121–130.

43. Blanchet B, Julien V, Vinsonneau C, Tod M. Influence of burns on pharmacokinetics and pharmacodynamics of drugs used in the care of burn patients. Clin Pharmacokinet 2008;47(10):635–654.

44. Harbin KR, Norris TE. Anesthetic management of patients with major burn injury. AANA Journal 2012;80(6):430–439.

45. Green SM, Johnson NE. Ketamine sedation for paediatric procedures: Part 2, review and implications. Annals of Emergency Medicine 1990;19(9):1033–1046.

46. Canpolat DG, Esmaoglu A, Tosun Z, et.al. Ketamine-propofol vs ketamine-dexmedetomidine combinations in pediatric burn patients undergoing burn dressing changes. J Burn Care Res 2012:33:718–722.

47. Cancio LC, Cuenca PB, Walker SC, Shepherd JM. Total intravenous anesthesia for major burn surgery. Int J Burns Trauma 2013;3(2):108–114.

48. Bishop S, Maguire S. Anaesthesia and intensive care for major burns. Contin Educ Anaesth Crit Care Pain 2012. doi: 10.1093/bjaceaccp/mks001.

49. Martyn J, Goldhill DR, Goudsouzian NG. Clinical pharmacology of muscle relaxants in patients with burns. The Journal of Clinical Pharmacology 1986;26(8):680–685.

50. Osta WA, El-Osta MA, Pezhman EA, et al. Nicotinic acetylcholine receptor gene expression is altered in burn patients. Anesth Analg 2010;110(5):1355–1359.

51. Han T, Kim H, Bae J, Kim K, Martyn JA. Neuromuscular pharmacodynamics of rocuronium in patients with major burns. Anesth Analg 2004;99(2):386–392.

52. Gandhi M, Thomson C, Lord D, Enoch S. Management of Pain in Children with Burns. International Journal of Pediatrics 2010 Article ID 825657,doi:10.1155/2010/825657.

53. Merkel SI, Voepel-Lewis T, Shayevitz JR, et al. The FLACC: a behavioral scale for scoring post-operative pain in young children. Paediatr Nurs 1997;23(3):293–297.

54. Castro RJA, Leal PC, Sakata RK. Pain management in burn patients. Rev Bras Anestesiol 2013;63(1):154–158.

55. Asmussen S, Maybauer DM, Fraser JF, Jennings K, George S, Maybauer MO. A meta-analysis of analgesic and sedative effects of dexmedetomidine in burn patients. Burns 2013;39(4):625–31.

56. American College of Surgeons Committee on Trauma Initial Assessment and Management. Advance Trauma Life Support for Doctors, ATLS, Instructor Course Manual. Chicago: American College of Surgeons, 2011.

57. Dorsey DP, Bowman SM, Klein MB, Archer D, Sharar SR. Perioperative use of cuffed endotracheal tubes is advantageous in young pediatric burn patients. Burns 2010;36(6): 856–860.

58. Atiyeh BS, Dibo SA, Ibrahim AE, Zgheib ER. Acute burn resuscitation and fluid creep: it is time for colloid rehabilitation. Ann Burns Fire Disasters 2012;30;25(2): 59–65.

59. Pearson KS, From RP, Symreng T, Kealey GP. Continuous enteral feeding and short fasting periods enhance perioperative nutrition in patients with burns. J Burn Care Rehabil 1992;13(4):477–481.

60. Rabban JT, Blair JA, Rosen CL, Adler JN, Sheridan RL. Mechanisms of pediatric electrical injury. New implications for product safety and injury prevention. Arch Pediatr Adolesc Med 1997;151(7):696–700.

21

Neonatal Resuscitation

Rashmi Salhotra, Sujata Chaudhary

- ■ Anticipation of resuscitative need
- ■ Initial steps of resuscitation
  - • Temperature control
  - • Clearing the airway
  - • Assessment of need for oxygen and its administration
  - • Positive-pressure ventilation
  - • End-expiratory pressure
- ■ Assisted-ventilation device
- ■ Medications
- ■ Post-resuscitation care
- ■ Guidelines for withholding and discontinuing resuscitation

2010 AHA Guidelines for CPR and Emergency Cardiovascular Care

These guidelines apply to newly born infants but are also applicable to neonates requiring resuscitation during first few weeks to months following birth (newborn and neonates). About 10% of newborns/infants require assistance to begin breathing at birth, less than 1% require extensive resuscitative measures.[1] The requirement of resuscitation is generally identified by rapid assessment of three characteristics:

- ■ Term gestation
- ■ Crying or breathing
- ■ Good muscle tone

If the answer to all the three questions is "YES", then the baby does not require resuscitation and should not be separated from the mother. Such a baby should be observed for breathing, activity and colour and should be placed next to the mother after drying. If the answer to any of these is "NO", infant should receive one or more of the following four categories of actions in sequence:

a. Initial steps of stabilization

b. Ventilation

c. Chest compression

d. Administration of adrenaline and volume expansion

Approximately 60 sec (the "Golden minute") are required for completion of initial steps, re-evaluation and beginning ventilation. Decision to progress beyond initial steps is determined by simultaneous assessment of two vital characteristics:

1. Respiration: Apnoea, gasping, labored or unlabored breathing.

2. Heart rate (HR): >100/min or <100/min. HR is determined by intermittently auscultating the precordial pulse. Pulse oximetry is useful for continuous assessment of pulse with or without interruption of other resuscitative measures. The monitoring devices take 1–2 min to apply and may not function during poor cardiac output or perfusion.

Once positive pressure ventilation (PPV) or supplementary oxygen administration begins, assess three vital characteristics, i.e. HR, respiratory rate (RR) and oxygenation. An increase in HR is a sensitive indicator of a successful response to each step.

ANTICIPATION OF RESUSCITATIVE NEED

For successful resuscitation, it is vital to anticipate the need for resuscitation, make adequate preparations, do accurate evaluation and initiate support promptly. Majority of neonates requiring neonatal resuscitation can be identified before birth.

If the delivery is preterm (<37 weeks of gestation), the baby will have:

- Immature lungs which may be difficult to ventilate and are vulnerable to injury by PPV.
- Immature blood vessels in the brain which may rupture, thus prone to hemorrhage.
- Thin skin and large surface area leading to rapid heat loss.
- Increased susceptibility to infection.
- Increased risk of hypovolaemic shock, due to small blood volume.

INITIAL STEPS OF RESUSCITATION (Fig. 21.1)

1. Provide warmth by placing the baby under radiant heat source.
2. Position the head in sniffing position to open the airway.
3. Clear the airway, if necessary with a bulb syringe/suction catheter.
4. Dry the baby.
5. Stimulate breathing.

Temperature Control

Preterm babies (<1500 g) are more prone to develop hypothermia. Additional warming techniques are recommended, e.g. prewarming the room to 26°C, covering the baby in plastic wrapping, placing the baby on exothermic mattress, placing the baby under radiant heat, prewarming the linen, drying and placing the baby skin to skin with mother. Resuscitative measures, like endotracheal intubation and chest compression can be performed side by side with these manoeuvres.

Infants born to febrile mothers have higher incidence of perinatal respiratory depression, neonatal seizures, cerebral palsy and increased mortality.[2,3] Hyperthermia, during or after ischaemia is associated with progression of cerebral injury. Lowering temperature decreases the neuronal damage.[4] Iatrogenic hyperthermia needs to be avoided (Class IIb, LOE C) and normothermia should be aimed at.

Clearing the Airway

When Amniotic Fluid is Clear

Routine suctioning of trachea in intubated babies on mechanical ventilation can be associated with deterioration of pulmonary compliance and oxygenation and decreased cerebral blood flow.[5,6] Suctioning in the presence of secretions can decrease respiratory resistance.[7] Therefore, the recommendation is to perform suctioning only in babies who have obvious obstruction to spontaneous breathing or who require PPV (Class IIb, LOE C).

When Amniotic Fluid is Meconium-Stained

It is recommended that endotracheal suction should be performed in non-vigorous babies born to mothers with meconium-stained amniotic fluid (Class IIb, LOE C). If intubation attempts are prolonged and unsuccessful and there is persistent bradycardia, bag mask ventilation should be considered.

Assessment of Need for Oxygen and Its Administration

It is a known fact that blood oxygen levels in uncompromised babies generally do not reach extra-uterine value till approximately 10 min after birth. SpO_2 may remain 70–80% for several min after birth thus causing appearance of cyanosis. Skin colour is a very poor indicator of the state of oxygenation in an uncompromised baby following birth. Insufficient as well as excessive oxygenation can be harmful for newborn infant. Hypoxia and ischaemia are known to result in injury to multiple organs. Adverse outcomes have been reported even from brief exposure to excessive oxygenation during and following resuscitation.

Pulse Oximetry

Newer pulse oximetry probes are available which are designed specifically for neonates. They provide reliable readings within 1–2 min following birth.[8–10] They are reliable both in term as well as preterm neonates provided there is a pulse and perfusion.

Pulse-oximetry is recommended when:

1. Resuscitation is anticipated.[1]
2. PPV is administered for more than few breaths.
3. Cyanosis is persistent.

4. Supplementary oxygen is administered (Class I, LOE B).

The preferred location for probe placement is preductal or right upper limb, i.e. wrist or medial surface of the palm.[10]

Administration of Supplementary Oxygen

Meta-analysis of randomized controlled trials on the use of room air versus 100% oxygen for resuscitation showed increased survival when resuscitation was initiated with air.[11, 12] If air and blended oxygen is used, SpO_2 must be targeted in the range as described above (Class IIb, LOE C). If the HR remains <60/min after 90 sec of resuscitation with lower concentration of oxygen, it should be increased to 100% till HR returns to normal (Class IIb, LOE B).

Positive Pressure Ventilation (PPV)

Even after the initial steps of resuscitation, if the infants remain apnoeic or gasping or HR <100/min, PPV should be initiated.

Initial Breaths and Assisted Ventilation

Functional residual capacity (FRC) is created with either spontaneous or assisted inflations following birth. The optimal pressure, inflation time and flow rate required to establish an effective FRC with PPV during resuscitation is not defined. Assisted rate of 40–60/min are commonly used. The adequacy of initial ventilation is judged by an improvement in HR.[13] If the HR does not improve, chest wall movement should be assessed. Initial peak inflating pressures needed are variable and unpredictable and should be individualized to achieve an increase in HR or movement of chest with each breath. Inflation pressure should be monitored, initial inflation pressure of 20 cm H_2O (as high as >30–40 cm H_2O in term babies without spontaneous respiration) may be required (Class IIb, LOE C). CO_2 detectors may be used during mask ventilation.

End Expiratory Pressure

The use of continuous positive airway pressure (CPAP) has been studied in preterm infants and has been found to be beneficial. Experts recommend its use even in term infants who are breathing spontaneously but with difficulty. CPAP is beneficial as its use in infants has shown to decrease the rate of intubation and mechanical ventilation, surfactant use and duration of ventilation but increases the rate of pneumothorax.[14] It is recommended to use CPAP or intubation with mechanical ventilation in preterm infants who are spontaneously breathing but in respiratory distress (Class IIb, LOE B). Positive end expiratory pressure (PEEP) may also be beneficial and is also recommended in infants during mechanical ventilation. It can be given with T-piece and a flow-inflating bag.

ASSISTED VENTILATION DEVICE

Laryngeal Mask Airway (LMA)

It is recommended to use an LMA if face mask ventilation or endotracheal intubation is not possible, unsuccessful or feasible (Class IIa, LOE B). For newborns >2000 gm or delivered >34 weeks of gestation, LMA is safe and recommended for ventilation (Class IIb, LOE B), however, its use has not been studied much in small preterm babies <2000 gm or <34 weeks gestation.

Endotracheal Tube

Indications of endotracheal intubation during neonatal resuscitation are:

- Initial endotracheal suctioning of non-vigorous meconium-stained newborn
- If bag mask ventilation is ineffective or prolonged
- During performance of chest compressions
- Specific resuscitation circumstances, e.g. congenital diaphragmatic hernia, extremely low birth weight baby.

Timing of endotracheal intubation depends on skill and experience of available providers. As soon as intermittent positive pressure ventilation is initiated after intubation, there is a prompt increase in the HR. It is also one of the best indicators of effective ventilation and proper placement of the endotracheal tube.[13] End-tidal CO_2 ($EtCO_2$) detection in infants with an adequate cardiac output confirms the tracheal position and the absence denotes oesophageal intubation.[15–17] Other methods for confirmation of endotracheal placement of tube are condensation on the inside of endotracheal tube, chest movements and presence of bilateral breath sounds.

Chest Compressions

Chest compressions must be initiated in neonates with HR <60/min despite adequate ventilation with supplementary oxygen for 30 sec. Delivery of adequate ventilation is very important in the neonates. Therefore, assisted ventilations must be ensured prior to starting compressions in the newborns as ventilation is likely to be hampered during chest compressions.[18] The site of chest compressions is lower third of sternum and the depth is approximately one-third of A-P diameter of the chest (Class IIb, LOE C).[19, 20]

Two techniques of performing chest compressions have been described, 2 thumbs with fingers encircling the chest and 2 fingers with 2nd hand supporting the back technique. In the 2 thumbs with fingers encircling the chest technique, higher peak systolic and coronary perfusion pressure may be generated as compared to the other technique [21–25] and is, therefore, the preferred technique in newborns (Class IIb, LOE C). The ratio of compression to ventilation should be 3:1 with 90 compressions and 30 breaths/min. Compression and ventilation must be co-ordinated and chest recoil should be allowed in between the compressions. However, the compressing thumbs or the fingers must not be lifted from the chest (Class IIb, LOE C). Sustained compressions or a higher ratio of compression:ventilation of 15:2 or 30:2 is advocated if arrest is of primary cardiac etiology (Class IIb, LOE C). All the vital parameters including respiration, HR and oxygen are reassessed periodically and cycles of chest compressions and ventilation should be continued till spontaneous HR ≥60/min. Frequent interruptions of compressions and ventilations should be avoided.

MEDICATIONS

There are very few indications of medications in newborn babies during resuscitation. Most common cause of bradycardia in neonates is hypoxaemia or inadequate ventilation, which is corrected by establishing adequate ventilation and by provision of oxygen. If bradycardia does not resolve even after administration of 100% oxygen and chest compressions, adrenaline and volume expansion may be administered. Rarely, it may become necessary to administer buffers, narcotic antagonists or vasopressin.

Rate and Dose of Epinephrine

The recommended dose for epinephrine is 0.01–0.03 mg/kg IV. Higher doses (0.1 mg/kg) are not recommended because of risk of exaggerated hypertension, decreased myocardial function and worsening of neurological function. Previously, endotracheal route of administration of epinephrine was also advocated but there is lack of evidence to support its use via endotracheal route. But till the time IV access is obtained, 0.05–0.1 mg/kg epinephrine via endotracheal tube can be given (Class IIb, LOE C). Concentration of epinephrine for either IV or endotracheal route is 1:10,000 (0.1 mg/ml).

Volume Expansion

Administration of fluid for volume expansion is recommended only if there has been blood loss or it is suspected (pale skin, poor perfusion and weak pulses) or when there has been no response to other resuscitative measures (Class IIb, LOE C). Isotonic crystalloid solution or blood in a dose of 10 ml/kg may be given and the same amount may be repeated. Care must be taken to avoid rapid administration of volume expanders as it may lead to intraventricular haemorrhage (Class IIb, LOE C).

POST-RESUSCITATION CARE

Babies requiring resuscitation at birth are at high risk and may deteriorate any time after their vital signs have returned to normal. Maintenance of adequate ventilation and circulation and close monitoring are essential to detect deterioration early during the course so that prompt resuscitative measures can be re-initiated.

Naloxone

It is generally not required as a part of initial resuscitation in delivery room for newborn with respiratory depression. HR and oxygenation should be restored by supporting ventilation.

Glucose

Hypoglycaemia may lead to brain injury and such newborns may have hypoxic–ischaemic insult. Hyperglycaemia after ischaemia, on the other hand may have a protective effect. However, the blood glucose levels which may be associated with adverse outcomes are not known.[26, 27] It is recommended that IV glucose should be given as soon as possible after resuscitation to avoid hypoglycaemia (Class IIb, LOE C) and the consequences thereof.

Induced Therapeutic Hypothermia

In infants born at ≥36 weeks with evolving moderate to severe hypoxic–ischaemic encephalopathy, it has been found that therapeutic hypothermia (33.5–34.5°C) decreases mortality and degree of neuro-developmental disabilities.[28–30] Therefore, it is recommended that infants born at ≥36 weeks gestation should be offered induced hypothermia. Therapeutic hypothermia should be commenced within 6 hours following birth and should be continued for 72 hours, after which the infants should be rewarmed slowly over at least 4 hour.

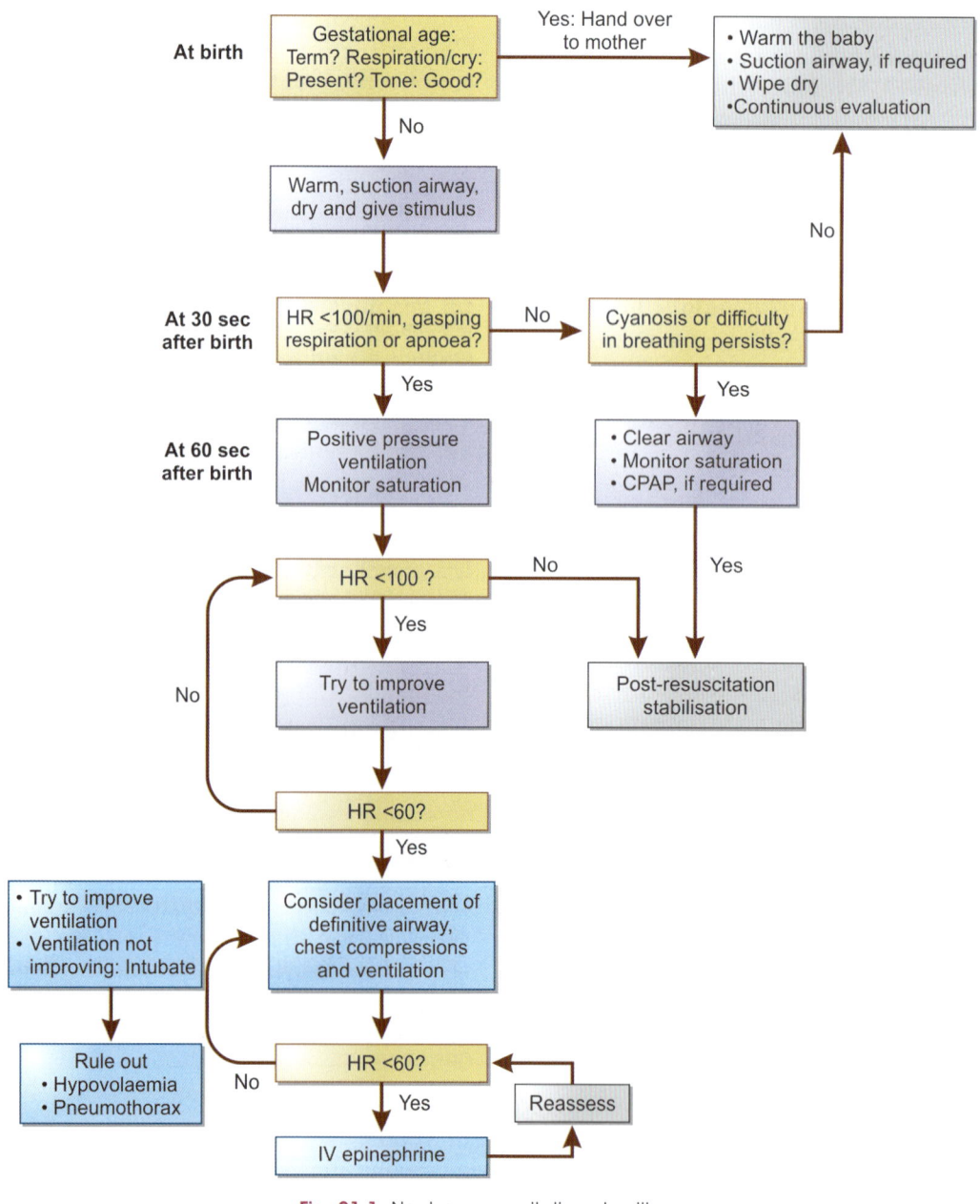

Fig. 21.1. Newborn resuscitation algorithm

GUIDELINES FOR WITHHOLDING AND DISCONTINUING RESUSCITATION

Withholding Resuscitation

When gestation age (<23 weeks), birth weight (<400 gm), or congenital anomalies (anencephaly, trisomy 13) are incompatible with life, or are associated with almost certain early death and when unacceptably high morbidity is likely among the rare survivors, resuscitation is not indicated (Class IIb, LOE C). Conditions associated with a high rate of survival and acceptable morbidity, resuscitation is indicated as in babies with gestational age >25 weeks and those with most congenital malformations (Class IIb, LOE C). Conditions that are associated with uncertain prognosis in which survival is borderline, the morbidity rate is relatively high and the anticipated burden to the child is high, parental desires concerning initiation of resuscitation should be supported (Class IIb, LOE C).[18]

Discontinuing Resuscitative Efforts

In a newly born baby with no detectable heart rate, resuscitation may be stopped, if the HR remains undetectable for 10 min (Class IIb, LOE C).[31-33]

REFERENCES

1. Perlman JM, Risser R. Cardiopulmonary resuscitation in the delivery room: associated clinical events. Arch Pediatr Adolesc Med 1995;149:20–25.
2. Petrova A, Demissie K, Rhoads GG, Smulian JC, Marcella S, Ananth CV. Association of maternal fever during labor with neonatal and infant morbidity and mortality. Obstet Gynecol 2001;98:20–27.
3. Lieberman E, Lang J, Richardson DK, Frigoletto FD, Heffner LJ, Cohen A. Intrapartum maternal fever and neonatal outcome. Pediatrics 2000;105(1 Pt 1):8–13.
4. Coimbra C, Boris-Moller F, Drake M, Wieloch T. Diminished neuronal damage in the rat brain by late treatment with the antipyretic drug dipyrone or cooling following cerebral ischemia. Acta Neuropathol 1996;92:447– 453.
5. Perlman JM, Volpe JJ. Suctioning in the preterm infant: effects on cerebral blood flow velocity, intracranial pressure, and arterial blood pressure. Pediatrics 1983;72:329–334.
6. Simbruner G, Coradello H, Fodor M, Havelec L, Lubec G, Pollak A. Effect of tracheal suction on oxygenation, circulation, and lung mechanics in newborn infants. Arch Dis Child 1981;56:326–330.
7. Prendiville A, Thomson A, Silverman M. Effect of tracheobronchial suction on respiratory resistance in intubated preterm babies. Arch Dis Child 1986;61:1178–1183.
8. Hay WW (Jr), Rodden DJ, Collins SM, Melara DL, Hale KA, Fashaw LM. Reliability of conventional and new pulse oximetry in neonatal patients. J Perinatol 2002;22:360–366.
9. O'Donnell CP, Kamlin CO, Davis PG, Morley CJ. Feasibility of and delay in obtaining pulse oximetry during neonatal resuscitation. J Pediatr 2005;147:698–699.
10. Dawson JA, Kamlin CO, Wong C, te Pas AB, O'Donnell CP, Donath SM, Davis PG, Morley CJ. Oxygen saturation and heart rate during delivery room resuscitation of infants_30 weeks' gestation with air or 100% oxygen. Arch Dis Child Fetal Neonatal Ed 2009;94:F87–F91.
11. Davis PG, Tan A, O'Donnell CP, Schulze A. Resuscitation of newborn infants with 100% oxygen or air: a systematic review and meta-analysis. Lancet 2004;364:1329–1333.
12. Rabi Y, Rabi D, Yee W. Room air resuscitation of the depressed newborn: a systematic review and meta-analysis. Resuscitation 2007;72:353–363.
13. Dawes GS. Foetal and Neonatal Physiology: A comparative study of the changes at birth. Chicago: Year Book Medical Publishers, Inc; 1968.
14. Morley CJ, Davis PG, Doyle LW, Brion LP, Hascoet JM, Carlin JB. Nasal CPAP or intubation at birth for very preterm infants. N Engl J Med 2008;358:700–708.
15. Hosono S, Inami I, Fujita H, Minato M, Takahashi S, Mugishima H. A role of end-tidal CO_2 monitoring for assessment of tracheal intubations in very low birth weight infants during neonatal resuscitation at birth. J Perinat Med 2009;37:79–84.
16. Roberts WA, Maniscalco WM, Cohen AR, Litman RS, Chhibber A. The use of capnography for recognition of esophageal intubation in the neonatal intensive care unit. Pediatr Pulmonol 1995;19:262–268.
17. Garey DM, Ward R, Rich W, Heldt G, Leone T, Finer NN. Tidal volume threshold for colorimetric carbon dioxide detectors available for use in neonates. Pediatrics 2008;121:e1524–1527.
18. Kattwinkel J, Perlman JM, Aziz K, Colby C, Fairchild K, Gallagher J, Hazinski MF, Halamek LP, Kumar P, Little G, McGowan JE, Nightengale B, Ramirez MM, Ringer S, Simon WM, Weiner GM, Wyckoff M, Zaichkin J. Part 15: neonatal resuscitation: 2010 American Heart Association Guidelines for Cardiopulmonary Resuscitation and Emergency Cardiovascular Care. Circulation 2010;122(Suppl 3):S909–S919.
19. Orlowski JP. Optimum position for external cardiac compression in infants and young children. Ann Emerg Med 1986;15:667–673.

20. Braga MS, Dominguez TE, Pollock AN, Niles D, Meyer A, Myklebust H, Nysaether J, Nadkarni V. Estimation of optimal CPR chest compression depth in children by using computer tomography. Pediatrics 2009;124:e69–e74.

21. Menegazzi JJ, Auble TE, Nicklas KA, Hosack GM, Rack L, Goode JS. Two-thumb versus two-finger chest compression during CRP in a swine infant model of cardiac arrest. Ann Emerg Med 1993;22:240–243.

22. Houri PK, Frank LR, Menegazzi JJ, Taylor R. A randomized, controlled trial of two-thumb vs two-finger chest compression in a swine infant model of cardiac arrest. Prehosp Emerg Care 1997;1:65–67.

23. Udassi JP, Udassi S, Theriaque DW, Shuster JJ, Zaritsky AL, Haque IU. Effect of alternative chest compression techniques in infant and child on rescuer performance. Pediatr Crit Care Med 2009;10:328–333.

24. David R. Closed chest cardiac massage in the newborn infant. Pediatrics 1988;81:552–554.

25. Thaler MM, Stobie GH. An improved technique of external cardiac compression in infants and young children. N Engl J Med 1963;269:606–610.

26. Salhab WA, Wyckoff MH, Laptook AR, Perlman JM. Initial hypoglycaemia and neonatal brain injury in term infants with severe fetal acidemia. Pediatrics 2004;114:361–366.

27. Ondoa-Onama C, Tumwine JK. Immediate outcome of babies with low Apgar score in Mulago Hospital, Uganda. East Afr Med J 2003;80:22–29.

28. Gluckman PD, Wyatt JS, Azzopardi D, Ballard R, Edwards AD, Ferriero DM, Polin RA, Robertson CM, Thoresen M, Whitelaw A, Gunn AJ. Selective head cooling with mild systemic hypothermia after neonatal encephalopathy: multicentre randomised trial. Lancet 2005;365:663–670.

29. Shankaran S, Laptook AR, Ehrenkranz RA, Tyson JE, McDonald SA, Donovan EF, Fanaroff AA, Poole WK, Wright LL, Higgins RD, Finer NN, Carlo WA, Duara S, Oh W, Cotten CM, Stevenson DK, Stoll BJ, Lemons JA, Guillet R, Jobe AH. Whole-body hypothermia for neonates with hypoxic-ischemic encephalopathy. N Engl J Med 2005;353:1574–1584.

30. Azzopardi DV, Strohm B, Edwards AD, Dyet L, Halliday HL, Juszczak E, Kapellou O, Levene M, Marlow N, Porter E, Thoresen M, Whitelaw A, Brocklehurst P. Moderate hypothermia to treat perinatal asphyxia encephalopathy. N Engl J Med 2009;361:1349–1358.

31. Jain L, Ferre C, Vidyasagar D, Nath S, Sheftel D. Cardiopulmonary resuscitation of apparently stillborn infants: survival and long-term outcome. J Pediatr 1991;118:778–782.

32. Casalaz DM, Marlow N, Speidel BD. Outcome of resuscitation following unexpected apparent stillbirth. Arch Dis Child Fetal Neonatal Ed 1998;78:F112–F115.

33. Laptook AR, Shankaran S, Ambalavanan N, Carlo WA, McDonald SA, Higgins RD, Das A. Outcome of term infants using apgar scores at 10 minutes following hypoxic-ischemic encephalopathy. Pediatrics 2009;124:1619–1626.

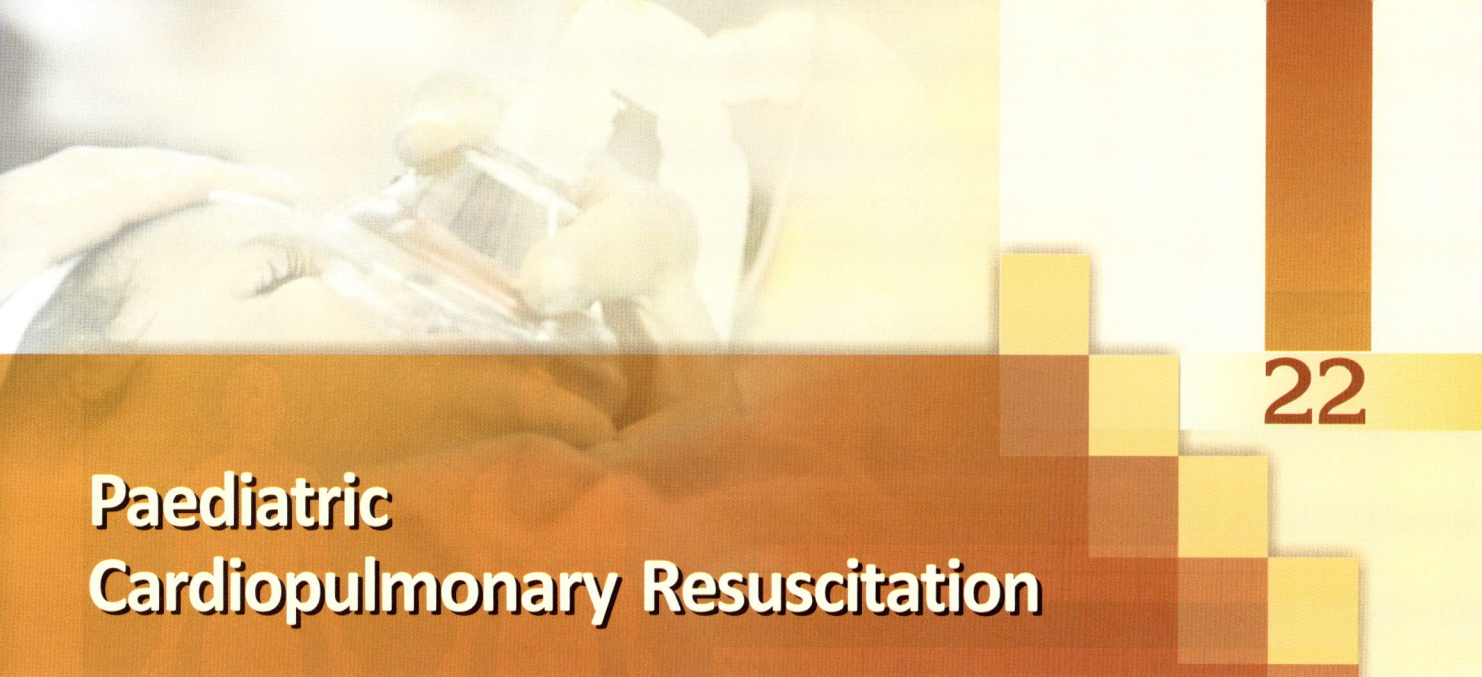

22

Paediatric Cardiopulmonary Resuscitation

Sujata Chaudhary, Rashmi Salhotra

- ▪ Paediatric basic life support
  - ● Chain of survival
  - ● Two-rescuer CPR for health care providers
  - ● Paediatric BLS algorithm
  - ● Breathing adjuncts
- ▪ Foreign body airway obstruction or choking
- ▪ Drowning
- ▪ Special situations
- ▪ Paediatric advanced life support
- ▪ Respiratory distress and failure
- ▪ Medications for paediatric resuscitation
- ▪ Cardiac arrest situations
- ▪ Special situations for resuscitation—shock
- ▪ Post-cardiac arrest care

PAEDIATRIC BASIC LIFE SUPPORT

Chain of Survival

According to 2010 American Heart Association guidelines for cardiopulmonary resuscitation and emergency cardiovascular care, paediatric basic life support (BLS) can be summarised as the pediatric chain of survival (Fig. 22.1) which consists of 5 links.

Prevention of Cardiopulmonary Arrest

Injury is the leading cause of death in children >1 year of age. Out of all the injuries, road traffic accident is the most common cause. Therefore, prevention is most vital as recovery from traumatic cardiac arrest is rare.

Due attention should be given to prevention with use of seat belts, close monitoring at home to prevent fall, electrocution, choking over a foreign body, etc.

Early Cardiopulmonary Resuscitation (CPR)

This is the second link in the paediatric chain of survival. The most common cause of cardiopulmonary arrest in paediatric age group is respiratory rather than cardiac. The 2010 AHA guidelines for CPR/ECC recommend a change from the previous ABC sequence to the CAB sequence. This is because the majority of victims who suffer cardiac arrest are adults, the commonest cause being ventricular fibrillation (VF). Therefore, chest compressions become most important. Secondly, obtaining an equipment, like a pocket mask or bag and mask resuscitator for initiating breaths or overcoming hesitation to initiate mouth-to-mouth breaths, takes time and hence causes delay in initiating chest compressions. However, in children, ventilations are vital to resuscitation as asphyxial arrests are more common. But initiating compressions before ventilation causes a delay of only 18 sec in case of one rescuer CPR and even lesser in case of 2 rescuer CPR. Thirdly, the CAB sequence ensures that more victims will receive bystander CPR. Fourthly, the change in the sequence from ABC to CAB in children also maintains uniformity for ease of remembering.

a. Scene safety: Before initiating BLS, the rescuer must ensure that the scene is safe for both the rescuer as well as the victim.

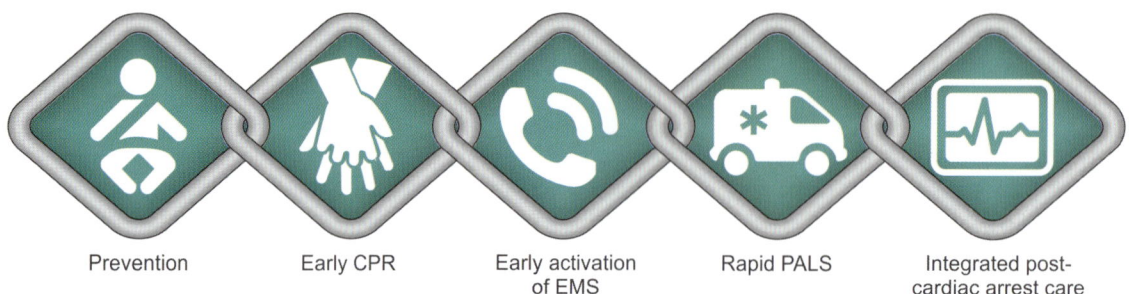

Prevention　　　Early CPR　　　Early activation　　　Rapid PALS　　　Integrated post-
of EMS　　　　　　　　　　cardiac arrest care

Fig. 22.1. Paediatric chain of survival

b. Check responsiveness: This should be done by giving two types of stimuli: auditory and tactile. Gently tap the victim on the shoulder without shaking vigorously and ask loudly, "Are you okay?" Look for movement or moaning or answering from the victim's side. A quick scan for any injuries should be performed at this time.

c. Check breathing: Scan the chest for respiratory movements. If there is regular breathing and no evidence of trauma, turn the child, should be put in the recovery position to maintain airway patency. At least 5 sec but not more than 10 sec should be taken for checking respiration. In case of no breathing or only gasping, CPR should be initiated.

d. Chest compressions: For a lone rescuer, give 30 compressions. For infants, use two fingers placed just below the intermammary line (Fig. 22.2) (Class IIb, LOE C). Compress for 4 cm (1.5 inch). For child, compress the lower half of the sternum with the heel of one or two hands (Fig. 22.3). Depth of compression should be at least one-third of the AP diameter of the chest or approximately 5 cm (2 inches). Allow complete chest recoil as incomplete recoil is associated with higher intra-thoracic pressures and significantly decreases venous return, coronary perfusion, blood flow and cerebral perfusion. Rescuer fatigue may be one of the reasons for incomplete chest recoil and, therefore, poor chest compressions. Thus it is advised that the compressors should rotate after 5 cycles of CPR or after 2 minutes.

e. Ventilations: Compression:ventilation (C:V) ratio for lone rescuer is 30:2. After 30 compressions, open the airway with head-tilt chin-lift and give two effective breaths. In case of trauma where cervical spine injury is suspected, only jaw thrust should

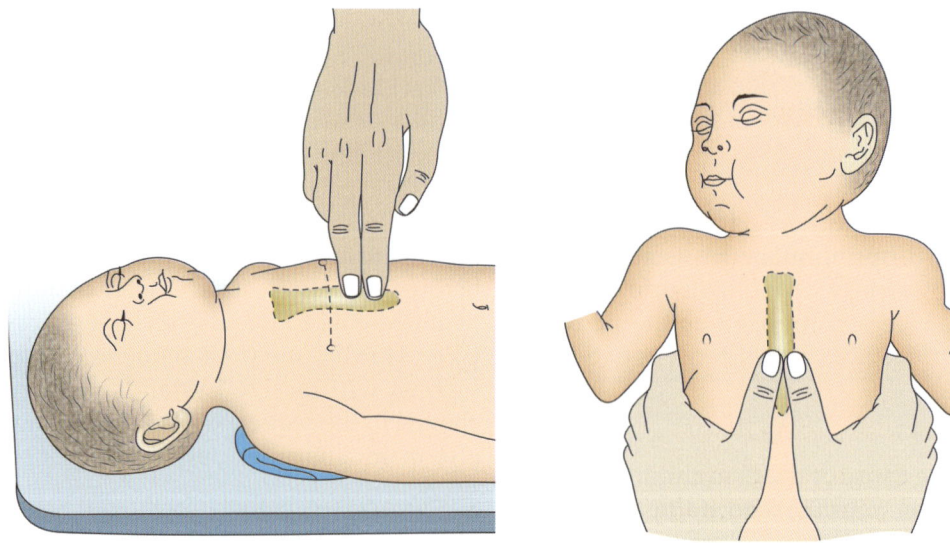

Fig. 22.2. Chest compression with two fingers on sternum of thumb with encircling hand technique

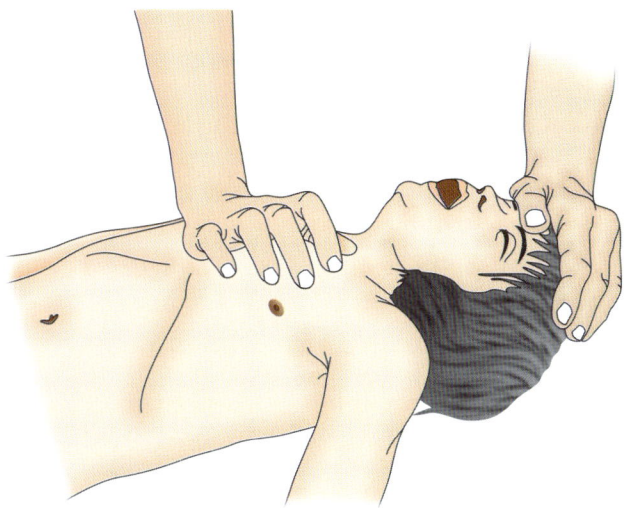

Fig. 22.3. Chest compression with heel of hands

be given. For infants, manoeuvres to provide ventilations may include: mouth-to-mouth, mouth-to-nose or mouth-to-mouth and nose technique. Each breath is to be delivered over a period of 1 sec allowing 1 sec for expiration. A tidal volume enough to produce a visible chest rise must be delivered. If chest does not rise after one breath, the airway must be repositioned so that the next breath is effective. After delivering two effective breaths, the rescuer should start chest compressions immediately. After 5 cycles of C:V, activate the emergency medical services (EMS) and ask for an automated external defibrillator (AED).

f. Activate EMS: If there are two rescuers, one of them should start CPR immediately and the other one should activate the EMS and call for AED. If there is only a single rescuer, then 2 min or 5 cycles of CPR should be delivered before activating the EMS because most of the infants and children have asphyxial arrests rather than VF arrests. C:V at the rate of 30:2 should be continued till the EMS personnel arrive or victim starts breathing spontaneously.

Quality of Chest Compressions

a. Push hard and push fast.
b. Give at least 100 compressions/min.
c. Depth of compression should be approximately 1½ inch (4 cm) in infants and 2 inches (5 cm) in children (Class I LOE C).

d. Allow complete chest recoil in between compressions.
e. Minimise interruptions between compressions to <10 sec.
f. Avoid excessive ventilations.

Two-Rescuer CPR for Health Care Providers (HCP)

In case of witnessed arrest, assume that it is due to VF. After ascertaining unresponsiveness and absent breathing, EMS should be activated before starting CPR. AED should be used as soon as it is available.

If the victim is unresponsive and not breathing, send someone to activate EMS. Take at least 5 sec and not more than 10 sec to feel for pulse (brachial in infants and carotid or femoral in a child). If no pulse felt within 10 sec or not sure about the presence of pulse, begin chest compressions (Class IIA, LOE C).

If there is inadequate breathing and pulse rate ≥ 60/min, give rescue breaths at the rate of 12–20 bpm (1 breath every 3–5 sec) till there is spontaneous respiration. Reassess the pulse every 2 min taking <10 sec. If pulse rate <60/min with inadequate breathing and signs of poor perfusion (pallor, mottling, cyanosis), begin chest compressions (Fig. 22.4).

If child is unresponsive, not breathing and pulse is absent, begin chest compressions. In case of lone HCP, two-finger chest compression technique is to be used (Fig. 22.2). In case of two-rescuer CPR, two-thumb encircling hand technique should be used (Fig. 22.2). This technique is preferred over two-finger technique as it produces higher coronary artery perfusion pressure, adequate depth and force of compression[1,2] and may generate higher systolic and diastolic pressures.[3,4]

After 15 compressions, give two ventilations. Use head-tilt chin-lift to open the airway, if no suspected trauma. In case of suspected cervical spine injury, use jaw thrust. If it is difficult to open the airway with jaw thrust, head-tilt chin-lift should be done.

If an advanced airway is in place, chest compressions should be given uninterruptedly at the rate of 100/min without pausing for ventilations. Ventilations should be given at the rate of 8–10 bpm (or 1 breath every 6–8 sec). Excessive ventilation should be avoided at all costs. Only as much tidal volume so as to produce a visible chest rise must be delivered. This is important because firstly, hyperventilation leads to rise in intrathoracic pressure and impedes

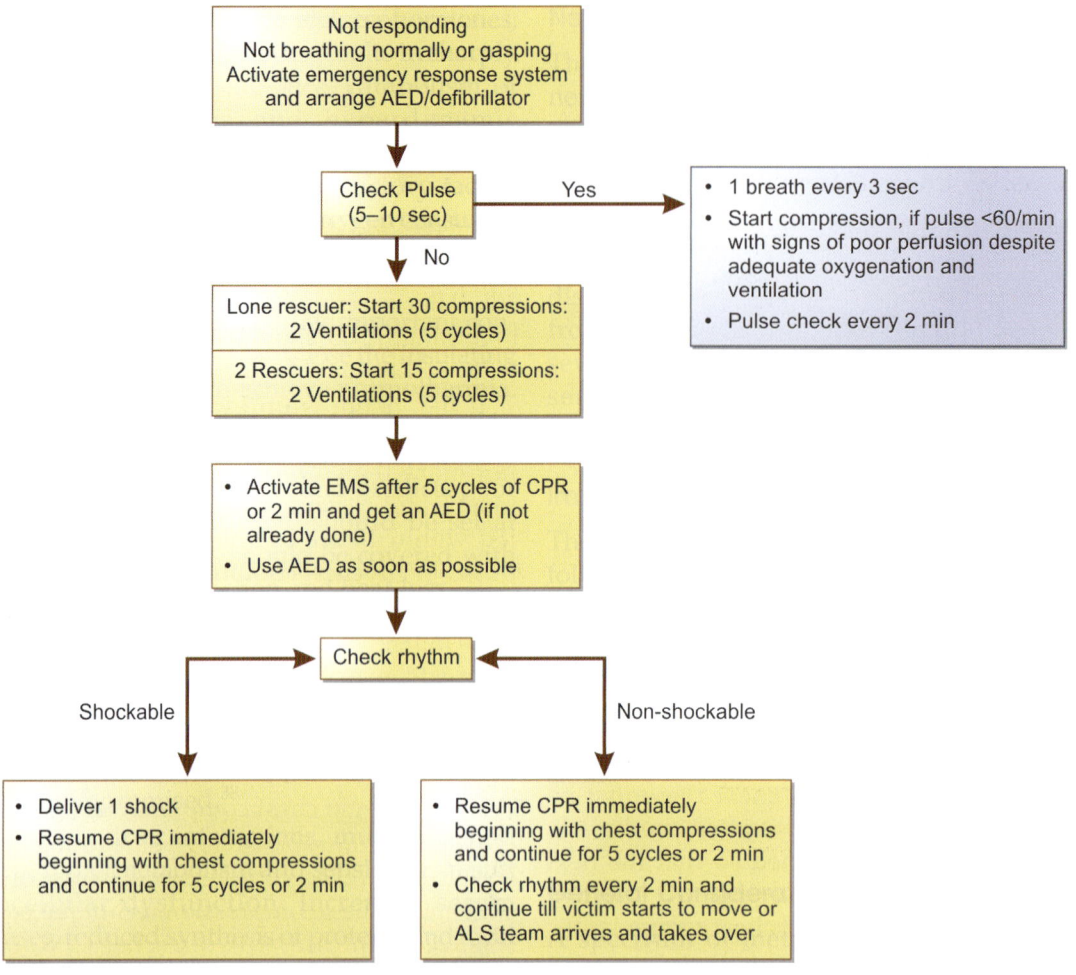

Fig. 22.4. Paediatric basic life support algorithm

venous return which leads to decreased cardiac output, cerebral blood flow and coronary perfusion pressure. Secondly, air trapping leads to barotraumas in victims with obstructive lung disease. Thirdly, some amount of air may pass into the stomach and may increase the risk of regurgitation and aspiration.

If the collapse is sudden, VF or pulseless ventricular tachycardia (VT) should be suspected. Both these are shockable rhythms. For infants, a manual defibrillator is preferred when a shockable rhythm is identified (Class IIb, LOE C). The energy dose for first shock is 2 J/kg and for 2nd shock is 4 J/kg.

If a manual defibrillator is not available, use AED with paediatric attenuator for infants and children up to <8 years of age. If neither is available, then use the defibrillator without attenuator (Class IIb, LOE C). The

AED reanalyses the rhythm automatically after every 2 min. It also advises whether shock needs to be delivered or not. If shock is advisable, it should be given and chest compressions should be resumed immediately after shock is delivered.

Hands Only (Compression only CPR)

Since asphyxia arrests are more common in paediatric age group, optimal CPR includes both compressions and ventilations. A large study in the paediatric population has revealed that bystander CPR with chest compression and ventilation is more effective than compression only CPR.[1] Guidelines recommend that optimal CPR in infants and children includes both compression and ventilation but compressions alone are preferable to no CPR at all (Class I LOE B).

Breathing Adjuncts

Barrier Devices

These are helpful to overcome the hesitation to give mouth-to-mouth rescue breathing without a barrier device. The risk of transmission of infection is very low even when these devices are not used. Some may even increase resistance to air flow.[5] The use of a barrier device, should not delay rescue breathing. If there is any delay in obtaining barrier device or ventilation equipment, mouth-to-mouth ventilation should be initiated (if willing and able) or chest compressions alone CPR should be continued.

Bag-Mask Ventilation

Proper size mask, airway and manual resuscitators need to be selected. For infants and children, a bag with volume of 450–500 ml and for older children, an adult bag with 1000 ml volume should be chosen. Supplementary oxygen should be attached along with an oxygen reservoir bag. O_2 flow rate should be adjusted to 10–15 L/min. Initially 100% O_2 should be given, but once the monitors are available, FiO_2 can be titrated such that oxyhaemoglobin saturation is ≥94%. Bag-mask ventilation is not recommended for lone rescuers or lay rescuer CPR. A lone rescuer should use a pocket mask or a barrier device for giving breaths. Hyperventilation should be avoided at all costs.

Two-person bag-mask ventilation: If skilled rescuers are available, a two-person technique is more effective than a single person bag-mask ventilation technique. It is especially beneficial when there is significant airway obstruction, poor lung compliance,[6] or poor mask seal. One of the rescuers opens the airway with both hands to maintain a tight mask-to-face seal while the other compresses the ventilation bag. There are higher chances of delivering larger volumes in the two person technique thus, resulting in excessive ventilation. Therefore, extra caution should be exercised to avoid hyperventilation because of reasons stated previously.

Gastric inflation and cricoid pressure: Gastric inflation may occur during ventilation and may interfere with effective ventilation[7] and cause regurgitation. It should be minimized by delivering each breath over a period of 1 sec.[8] Cricoid pressure may be considered in an unresponsive victim, if there is an additional health-care provider.[9] Excessive cricoid pressure should be avoided as it can obstruct the trachea.[10]

Oxygenation

100% oxygen should be used during resuscitation. After return of spontaneous circulation, oxygen saturation should be monitored. Oxyhaemoglobin saturation should be maintained ≥94% by adjusting the FiO_2. Humidified oxygen should be used whenever possible to prevent mucosal drying and thickening of pulmonary secretions.

Oxygen masks: Oxygen concentration of 30–50% can be provided with the help of simple face masks. For delivering higher concentration of oxygen, a tight-fitting non-rebreathing mask with a reservoir bag and an oxygen flow rate of approximately 15 L/min may be required.

Nasal cannulae: Appropriate sized nasal cannulas can be used for spontaneously breathing children. These are variable performance devices and FiO_2 delivered will not be constant at all the times.

Other CPR Techniques and Adjuncts

Mechanical devices for chest compression, active compression–decompression CPR, interposed abdominal compression CPR (IAC-CPR), the impedance threshold device or pressure sensor accelerometer (feedback) devices are other adjuncts which may be used but the evidence to recommended for or against the use of such devices is insufficient in infants and children.

FOREIGN BODY AIRWAY OBSTRUCTION (FBAO) OR CHOKING

In children (<5 years of age), foreign body aspiration is the cause of more than 90% of childhood mortality, out of which 65% of the victims are infants. The most common cause of choking in infants is liquids,[11] whereas in children, balloons, small objects and foods (e.g. hot dogs, round candies, nuts and grapes) are common causes.[12–15]

A *sudden* onset of respiratory distress with coughing, gagging, stridor, or wheezing is often the characteristic feature of FBAO.

Relief of FBAO

FBAO may be mild or severe. In mild airway obstruction, the child can cough and make some sounds. No interference should be done. The victim is allowed to clear the airway by coughing. A close watch is kept to see, if the obstruction becomes severe.

In severe type of obstruction, the victim will not be able to cough or make any sound. In a child, subdiaphragmatic abdominal thrusts (Heimlich manoeuvre, Fig. 22.5)[16,17] should be started immediately until the object is expelled or the victim becomes unresponsive.

For an infant, deliver repeated cycles of 5 back blows (back slaps) followed by 5 chest compressions[18] until the object is expelled or the victim becomes unresponsive (Fig. 22.6). Abdominal thrusts are not recommended for infants because they may damage the infant's liver. If the victim becomes unresponsive, lay the victim on a flat hard surface and start CPR with chest compressions (do not perform a pulse check). After 30 chest compressions, open the airway. If a foreign body is seen, remove it but blind finger sweeps are no more recommended as they may push the foreign body farther into the pharynx and injure the oropharynx.[19–21] This is followed by two breaths.

Chest compressions and ventilations should be continued until the object is expelled. After two min, activate the emergency response system, if not done earlier.

DROWNING

The duration of submersion, the water temperature and the promptness and efficacy of delivered CPR determines the outcome after drowning.[22–24] Neurologically, intact survival has been reported after prolonged submersion in icy waters.[25,26]

Resuscitation should be started immediately after the victim has been removed from water. If the rescuer has received special training, rescue breathing may be initiated while the victim is still in water.[27] Chest compressions should not be initiated in water. After removing the victim from the water and confirming for unresponsiveness and absent breathing, start CPR. In case of lone rescuer, continue with 5 cycles (about 2 min) of compressions and ventilations before activating the emergency response system and getting

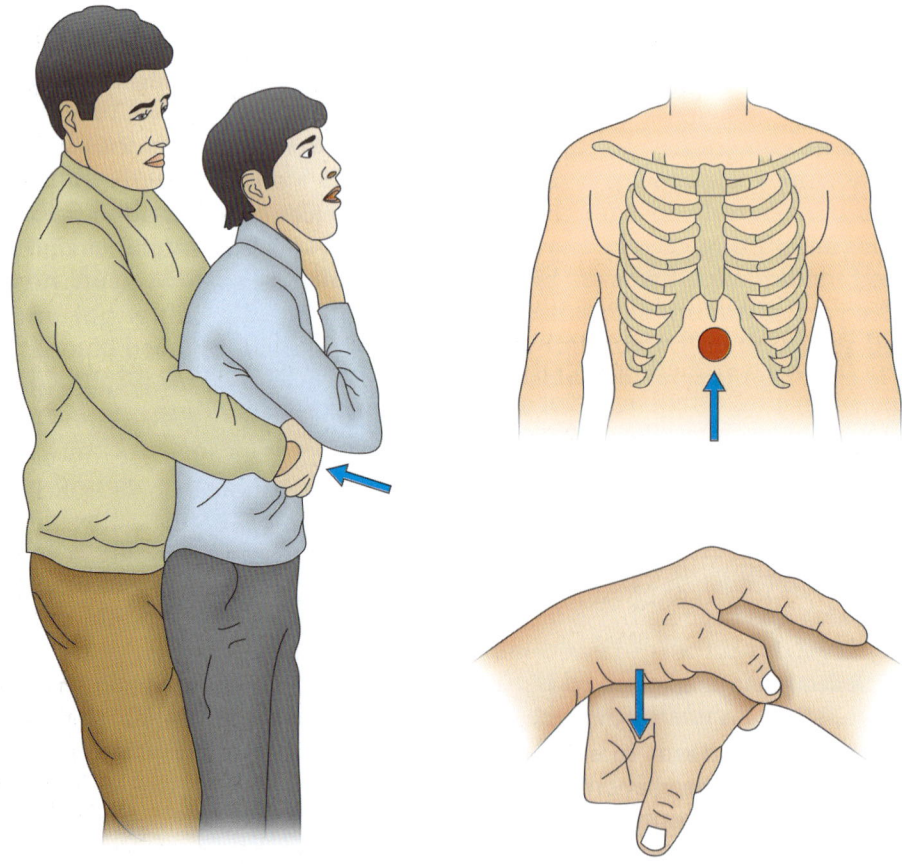

Fig. 22.5. Heimlich manoeuvre

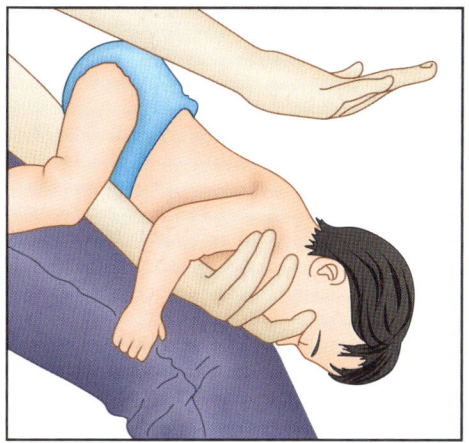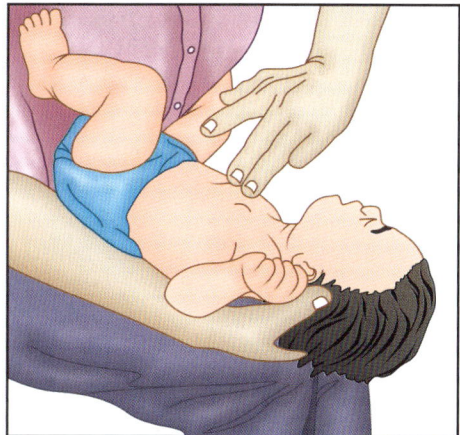

Fig. 22.6. Back slaps and chest thrusts

an AED. If there are two rescuers, the second rescuer can activate the emergency response system immediately and get the AED while the first rescuer continues CPR.

SPECIAL SITUATIONS

Do Not Attempt Resuscitation (DNAR)

"Do not attempt resuscitation" (DNAR) regulations are different in every part of the world. It is not legalized in India as of now. But where ever it is legal, the orders to such an effect must be written down in the case record form.

Ventilation with a Tracheostomy or Stoma

Whenever a child with a tracheostomy is discharged, the caregivers should be told as to how to assess the airway patency, suction and change of tracheostomy tube, recognition of complications with the tracheostomy and perform CPR with the tracheostomy. They must be taught that if there is insufficient chest rise after ventilation despite adequate suction or change of tube, mouth-to-stoma ventilation or bag-mask ventilation through the nose and mouth with the occluded tracheal stoma may be attempted.

Trauma

In a trauma victim, the type and site of injury must always be borne in mind and appropriate precautions must be taken during resuscitation. Specialized services of a trauma centre must be utilized in such cases. Cervical spine injury must be anticipated and

movements at the cervical spine must be avoided unless proven otherwise. Jaw thrust should be used to open the airway and head-tilt chin-lift is best avoided. Manual-in-line-stabilization of neck may be done, if there are two rescuers. During transport, the thighs, pelvis and the shoulders of the victim must be immobilized. The airway may be obstructed due to the blood, debris, foreign body or dental fragments. A suction device must always be kept handy in such cases. It is of foremost importance to expose the victim and look for active bleeding and apply pressure to stop the external bleeding.

PAEDIATRIC ADVANCED LIFE SUPPORT (PALS)

The most common cause of cardiac arrest in paediatric age group is respiratory rather than primary cardiac event as is the case in adult cardiac arrests.

Co-ordinated Team Work

PALS is normally delivered in the hospital settings where there is a team of trained personnel who work in a co-ordinated fashion. There are usually multiple rescuers or team members who have very defined tasks assigned to them by the team leader. He/she after ascertaining unresponsiveness and absence of pulse and respiration directs the other team members about their roles and responsibilities. They may have access to invasive monitoring which is helpful in providing real-time assessment and guide further action.

Chest compressions should be initiated immediately while a second rescuer prepares to start bag and mask ventilations. As already stated, hypoxic arrests are more common, consequently ventilation is extremely important in paediatrics. High-quality CPR, must be delivered as discussed above. Oxygen should be used, if available. In the meantime, other simultaneous actions, like procuring monitor/defibrillator, establishing vascular access and calculation of dosage of medicines, should be done by other team members.

RESPIRATORY DISTRESS AND FAILURE

Respiratory failure is characterized by inadequate ventilation, insufficient oxygenation, or both. Respiratory failure may be present, if there is an increased respiratory rate, particularly with signs of distress (e.g. increased respiratory effort including nasal flaring, retractions, seesaw breathing, or grunting), inadequate respiratory rate, effort, or chest excursion (e.g. diminished breath sounds or gasping), especially if mental status is depressed or cyanosis with abnormal breathing despite supplementary oxygen. This may be classified as:

a. Upper airway obstruction
b. Lower airway obstruction
c. Lung tissue (parenchymal) diseases
d. Disordered control of breathing

General Management

Support the airway, breathing and circulation.

Specific Management

Upper Airway Obstruction

Upper airway obstruction may be because of aspirated foreign body, tissue oedema, tongue fall, secretions, blood or debris in the nose, larynx and pharynx because of infection, inflammation or trauma.

1. Remove the foreign body.
2. Suction the mouth and nose.
3. Allow the child to assume a position of comfort.
4. Insert an airway adjunct or definitive airway device, if required.
5. Establishing a surgical airway may be required in some cases.
6. Reduce the airway oedema by epinephrine, nebulisation, administration of diphenhydramine or methyl prednisolone in cases of anaphylaxis.

Lower Airway Obstruction

The common causes of lower airway obstruction include bronchiolitis and acute asthma.

1. *Bronchiolitis:* Oral and nasal suctioning must be done as and when required. Viral studies, chest X-ray and ABG analysis must be done and appropriate therapy must be initiated.
2. *Asthma:* Humidified oxygen, bronchodilators, metered dose inhalers, nebulisations, steroid inhalations, mast cell inhibitors, mechanical ventilation must be provided in a stepwise fashion according to the severity of the disease and the level of consciousness.

Lung Tissue Disorders

1. *Pneumonia:* Complete blood count, ABG, viral studies, chest X-ray, sputum culture and sensitivity must be performed. Appropriate antibiotic therapy, nebulisation, steam inhalations, use of BiPAP, CPAP or mechanical ventilation must be instituted as required.
2. *Chemical pneumonitis:* Maintain ABC. Nebulisations with bronchodilators, CPAP or BiPAP, high frequency oscillations or extracorporeal membrane oxygenation (ECMO) may be required.
3. *Aspiration pneumonitis:* Maintain ABC. Use CPAP, BiPAP and appropriate antibiotics.
4. *Cardiogenic pulmonary oedema:* Ventilatory support, medical therapy to support cardiovascular functions, reduction of metabolic demand by reducing the temperature and work of breathing are some of the measures. Expert consultation must be sought.
5. *Non-cardiogenic pulmonary oedema (ARDS):* Maintain ABC. Small tidal volumes with high respiratory rates should be used. Peak and plateau pressures must not exceed the safe upper limits.

Disordered Control of Breathing

1. *Respiratory distress/failure with increased ICP:* Manual stabilisation of cervical spine in cases of trauma, provision of jaw thrust while avoiding head-tilt chin-lift, administration of hypertonic saline for increased ICP, avoidance of hyperthermia and treatment of agitation.
2. *Respiratory distress or failure in poisoning or drug overdose:* Maintain ABC. Administer specific

antidote, suctioning of the airway to remove the vomitus and support the vitals.

3. *Neuromuscular disease:* For children with advanced neuromuscular disease induced restrictive lung disease, non-invasive positive pressure ventilation may be required.

Airway

Maintain the patency of the airway by displacing the tongue or soft palate from the pharyngeal air passages. Useful in situations where the victim is unresponsive and gag reflex is absent. Proper size should be selected otherwise it may itself be a cause of obstruction. If the gag reflex is present, a nasopharyngeal airways can be used instead of an oropharyngeal airway.

Laryngeal mask airway (LMA): It is a useful rescue device when bag-mask ventilation is unsuccessful or when intubation is not possible (Class IIa, LOE C).[28,29]

Oxygen Therapy

Till sufficient data is obtained, it is reasonable to ventilate with 100% oxygen during CPR (Class IIa, LOE C). After the ROSC and availability of monitoring facility, the oxygen may be titrated to maintain the oxyhaemoglobin saturation at least 94%.

Pulse oximetry should always be monitored, if the equipment is available and the victim has a perfusing rhythm. But the limitations of pulse oximetry are patients with poor peripheral perfusion, carbon monoxide poisoning, or methaemoglobinaemia.

Bag-Mask Ventilation

For short periods of out-of hospital resuscitation scenarios, bag and mask ventilations are as effective and may be even safer than endotracheal tube ventilation.[30,31] Properly sized mask and a good seal are important factors during bag-mask ventilations. Hyperventilations must be avoided. Each breath must be delivered over a period of 1 sec allowing another 1 sec for exhalation. If the endotracheal tube or other definitive airway devices have been placed, ventilations must be delivered at a rate of about 1 breath every 6 to 8 sec (8 to 10/min) without interrupting chest compressions (Class I, LOE C). In the victim with pure respiratory arrest but absent or inadequate respiratory effort, give 1 breath every 3 to 5 sec (12 to 20 breaths/min).

Rapid Sequence Intubation (RSI)

RSI is recommended only if the rescuer is trained and is experienced in the use of the requisite medications, like opioids, inducing agents and neuromuscular blocking drugs.

Cricoid Pressure

It is not routinely recommended due to lack of sufficient evidence. However, if it is being applied, it must be released, if it is interfering with the ease or speed of intubation (Class III, LOE C).[32,33]

Cuffed versus Uncuffed Endotracheal Tubes

Both cuffed and uncuffed endotracheal tubes may be used for securing the airway, however, the use of cuffed tubes are associated with better protection against aspiration.[34] The intracuff pressure should be measured and should not exceed 20 to 25 cm H_2O.

Endotracheal Tube Size

Length-based resuscitation tapes are available and are helpful and more accurate than age-based formula in estimating the size of the endotracheal tube for children up to approximately 35 kg,[35,36] and even for children with short stature.[37]

After age 2, uncuffed endotracheal tube size can be estimated by the following formula:

Uncuffed endotracheal tube ID (mm) = 4 + (age/4)

A 3.0 mm ID cuffed tube is a good choice for emergency intubation of an infant less than 1 year of age. For children between 1 and 2 years of age, a cuffed endotracheal tube of 3.5 mm ID is sufficient (Class IIa, LOE B).[38, 39]

After age 2, the size can be determined using the formula (Class IIa, LOE B):[38–40]

Cuffed endotracheal tube ID (mm) = 3.5 + (age/4)

Verification of Endotracheal Tube Placement

The ETT can be misplaced during the patient transport[41] or during CPR. It may get displaced or obstructed.[42,43] Clinical assessment and other confirmatory devices should be used to confirm the proper placement. Frequent assessment of the tube position including immediately after intubation, after securing the endotracheal tube, during transport and after each movement of the patient is recommended (Class I, LOE B).

The confirmation of the proper position must be done by looking for bilateral chest movement and listening for equal breath sounds over both lung fields. Epigastrium must be auscultated to rule out oesophageal intubation. Exhaled or end-tidal CO_2 must be monitored. If there is a perfusing rhythm (ROSC or in pure respiratory arrest cases), oxyhaemoglobin saturation must be checked with a pulse oximeter. A direct laryngoscopy and visualization of the endotracheal tube is the most confirmatory test for the correct position of the ETT. A chest X-ray is also helpful. After intubation, the ETT should be secured with tapes with the patient's head in the neutral position. A DOPE protocol must always be followed whenever there is difficulty in ventilating an intubated patient.

- Displacement of the tube
- Obstruction of the tube
- Pneumothorax
- Equipment failure

Exhaled or End-Tidal CO_2 Monitoring

Exhaled CO_2 detection (capnography or colorimetry) is recommended for the confirmation of tracheal tube position for neonates, infants, and children with a perfusing cardiac rhythm in all settings (e.g. pre-hospital, emergency department [ED], ICU, ward, operating room) (Class I, LOE C)[44,45] and during intra-hospital or interhospital transport (Class IIb, LOE C).[46,47] The shortcoming of capnography or colorimetry is that it cannot differentiate between tracheal or right mainstem bronchial intubation. During cardiac arrest, the absence of CO_2 may reflect very low pulmonary blood flow rather than tube misplacement. Therefore, a direct laryngoscopic examination must be undertaken to confirm the correct tube position. Fallacies of colorimetric end-tidal CO_2 detection method include:

1. Contamination with gastric contents or acidic drugs (e.g. endotracheally administered epinephrine), which may lead to a consistent colour rather than a breath-to-breath colour change.
2. An intravenous (IV) bolus of epinephrine[48] may transiently reduce pulmonary blood flow and exhaled CO_2 below the limits of detection.[49]
3. Severe airway obstruction (e.g. status asthmaticus) and pulmonary oedema may impair CO_2 elimination below the limits of detection.[49–52]

4. A large glottic air leak may reduce exhaled tidal volume through the tube and dilute CO_2 concentration.

Oesophageal Detector Device (EDD)

An EDD is a good alternative to confirm endotracheal tube placement in children weighing >20 kg with a perfusing rhythm (Class IIb, LOE B)[53,54] where capnography is not available.

Transtracheal Catheter Oxygenation and Ventilation

When there is a severe airway obstruction above the level of the cricoid cartilage and the standard methods to manage the airway are unsuccessful transtracheal catheter oxygenation and ventilation may be considered for securing the airway. It is a crisis management technique since the tidal volumes delivered are usually too small to effectively remove carbon dioxide. The method only maintains oxygenation and hence an alternative technique for definitive airway management needs to be in place.

Suction Devices

A properly sized and functioning suction device with an adjustable suction regulator should be used. The length of the suction catheter to be inserted must be marked and care should be taken to avoid inserting it beyond the end of the endotracheal tube, lest mucosal injury may occur.

Monitoring

Electrocardiography

As soon as the monitors are available, they must be used. Cardiac rhythm should be monitored continuously to identify the rhythm and make management decisions accordingly.

Echocardiography

It can identify the possible causes of arrest and appropriate management of potentially treatable causes of arrest, like pericardial tamponade and inadequate ventricular filling (Class IIb, LOE C).[55,56]

End-Tidal CO_2 ($EtCO_2$).

It is a good guide to the efficacy of CPR and also a guide to the quality of chest compressions. (Class IIa,

LOE C). If the $EtCO_2$ is consistently <10 to 15 mm Hg, it implies that the chest compressions are poor. An abrupt and sustained rise in $EtCO_2$ in adults[57,58] is observed just prior to clinical identification of ROSC.

Vascular Access: Intravascular (IV)/Intraosseous (IO) Access

An IV line should be obtained early in the course of resuscitation to administer medications and draw blood samples. If securing IV line is difficult, especially in infants and children, an intraosseous (IO) access can be quickly established. IO access is a rapid, safe, effective, and acceptable route for vascular access in children,[59] and it is useful as the initial vascular access in cases of cardiac arrest (Class I, LOE C). All intravenous medications can be administered intraosseously, including epinephrine, adenosine, fluids, blood products,[60,61] and catecholamines.[62] Onset of action and drug levels for most drugs are comparable to venous administration.[63] Central venous access is not recommended as the initial route of vascular access during an emergency as it can be time consuming, difficult and may require higher levels of skill. If both central and peripheral accesses are available, then medications, like adenosine, are more effective when administered closer to the heart, and others (e.g. calcium, amiodarone, procainamide, sympathomimetics) may be irritant when infused into a peripheral vein. All the drugs administered during CPR must be flushed with 10 ml bolus of saline to push the drug into the circulation and the limb should be raised above the level of the heart.

Endotracheal Drug Administration

If it is not possible, to secure the IV/IO access rapidly, then lipid-soluble drugs, such as lidocaine, epinephrine, atropine, and naloxone (mnemonic "LEAN")[64, 65] can be administered via an endotracheal tube.[66] However, the effects may not be uniform with tracheal as compared with intravenous administration. During CPR, the chest compressions should be briefly withheld, drugs should be administered and should be followed with a flush of at least 5 ml of normal saline and 5 consecutive positive-pressure ventilations.[67] There is uncertainty as to how much dose should be administered through the endotracheal route, experts recommend doubling or tripling the dose of lidocaine, atropine or naloxone given via the ETT. For epinephrine, a dose ten times the intravenous

Table 22.1	Medications for paediatric resuscitation[68]
Name of the medication	**Dose and special considerations**
Adenosine	0.1 mg/kg (max. 6 mg) Second dose: 0.2 mg/kg (max. 12 mg) ECG monitoring Rapid IV/IO bolus with fast push
Amiodarone	5 mg/kg IV/IO; may repeat twice up to 15 mg/kg Maximum single dose 300 mg Under ECG and BP monitoring
Atropine	0.02 mg/kg IV/IO 0.04–0.06 mg/kg ET Repeat once, if needed Minimum dose: 0.1 mg Maximum single dose: 0.5 mg
Calcium chloride (10%)	20 mg/kg IV/IO (0.2 ml/kg) slow injection over 10 min Maximum single dose 2 g
Epinephrine (adrenaline)	0.01 mg/kg (0.1 ml/kg 1:10,000) IV/IO Maximum dose 1 mg IV/IO Repeat every 3–5 min
Glucose	0.5–1 g/kg IV/IO Newborn: 5–10 ml/kg D10 W Infants and children: 2–4 ml/kg D25 W Adolescents: 1–2 ml/kg D50 W
Lidocaine	Bolus: 1 mg/kg IV/IO Infusion: 20–50 µg/kg/min
Magnesium sulphate	25–50 mg/kg IV/IO over 10–20 min Maximum dose 2 g
Naloxone IV/IO	Full reversal: >5 year or <20 kg: 0.1 mg/kg >5 year or >20 kg: 2 mg IV/IO
Procainamide	15 mg/kg IV/IO Slow injection over 30–60 min Monitor ECG and BP Expert consultation
Sodium bicarbonate	1 mEq/kg per dose IV/IO slowly

IV: intravenous; IO: intraosseous; ET: endotracheal tube

dose (0.1 mg/kg or 0.1 ml/kg of 1:1000 concentration) is recommended. Non-lipid-soluble drugs (e.g. sodium bicarbonate and calcium) should not be administered via the endotracheal route as they may injure the airway (Table 22.1).

CARDIAC ARREST SITUATIONS

Shockable Rhythm: VF/Pulseless VT

If a shockable rhythm is identified, one shock of 2 J/kg is delivered after clearing everybody from the victim. After shock delivery, chest compressions should be resumed immediately with minimal interruption between the last compression and shock delivery. CPR should be continued for 2 min or 5 cycles. Simultaneous IV/IO access can be obtained, if multiple rescuers are present (Fig. 22.7).

After 2 min, the rhythm is reanalysed and a second shock (4 J/kg), if advisable, is given. This sequence of re-analysing the rhythm and delivering of shock (4 J/kg from the second shock onwards to a maximum of 10 J/kg or the adult dose, whichever is lower) should be continued every 2 min till the child becomes responsive or the rhythm becomes non-shockable. Epinephrine 0.01 mg/kg (0.1 ml/kg of 1:10000 epinephrine) should be repeated every 3–5 min to a maximum of 1 mg (Class I LOE B).

Amiodarone can be given during CPR (Class IIb LOE C) in place of the first or second dose of epinephrine. If at any time, the rhythm becomes non-shockable, follow the right limb of the algorithm (Fig. 22.7).

Once an advanced airway is in place, the compressing rescuer should deliver continuous chest compressions at the rate of 100/min without pausing for ventilations. Ventilation should be provided at the rate of about 1 breath every 6–8 sec or 8–10 breaths/min.

Rhythm Check

This should be done only when there is a change in the rhythm, an organised rhythm or there is evidence of return of spontaneous circulation (ROSC), such as

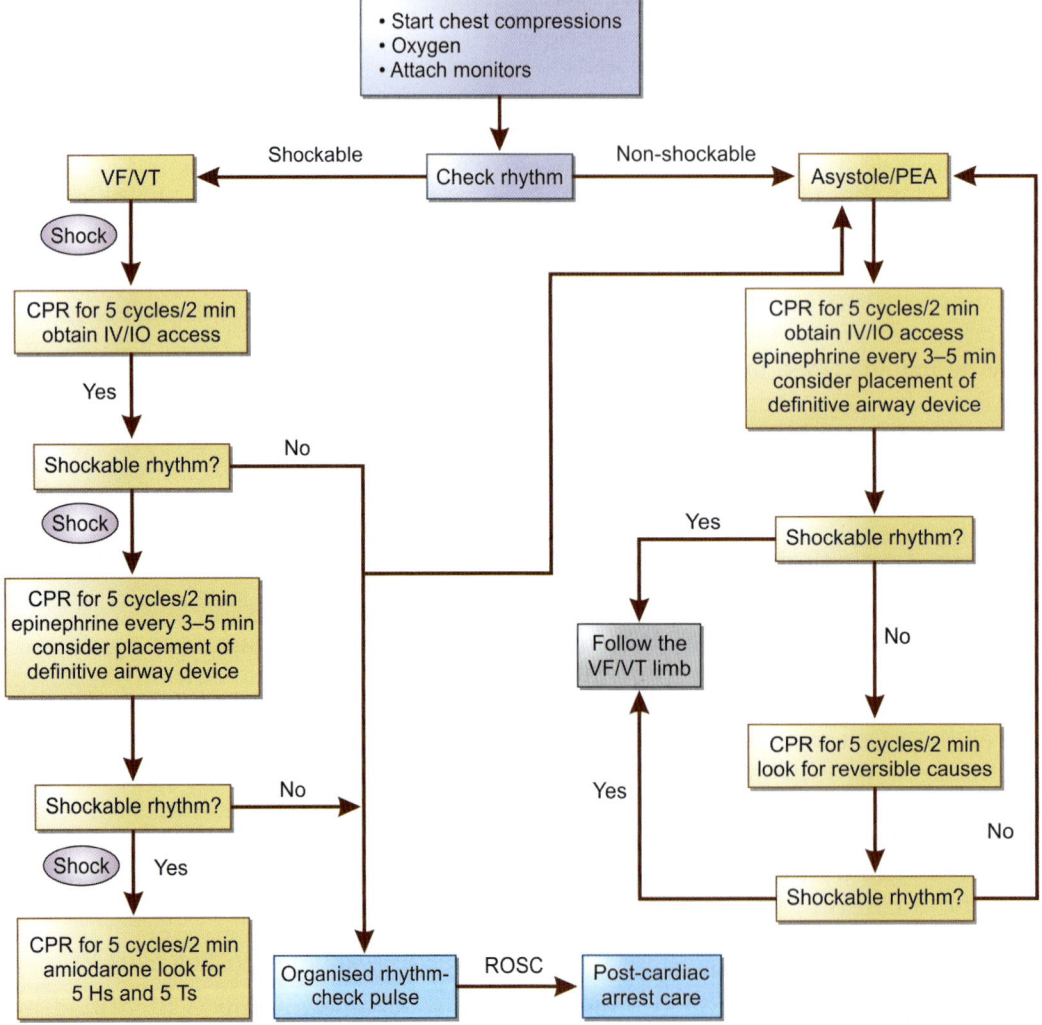

Fig. 22.7. Paediatric cardiac arrest

an abrupt increase in $EtCO_2$ or arterial waveform pulsations. This should be followed by post-resuscitation care.

If VF recurs, resume CPR and give a bolus of amiodarone before attempting defibrillation. Look for the reversible causes and treat them.

Torsades de pointes or polymorphic VT rapidly deteriorates to VF or pulseless VT. It may be congenital or due to drug toxicity. Rapid initiation of CPR and delivering of defibrillation should be done. Treatment is with rapid IV infusion of magnesium sulphate 25–50 mg/kg to a maximum dose of 2 g.

Non-shockable Rhythm: Asystole/Pulseless Electrical Activity (PEA)

Continue CPR with minimal interruptions in chest compression. Epinephrine 0.01 mg/kg (0.1 ml/kg of 1:10000) to a maximum of 1 mg/kg should be administered every 3–5 min (Class I, LOE B). The high doses of epinephrine previously administered have been found to be of no additional benefit and it may actually be harmful in cases of asphyxia (Class III, LOE B). It may, however, be considered in case of β blocker overdose (Class IIb, LOE C).

Pulse should be checked only when there is a change in rhythm or there is presence of organised electrical activity. In case of PEA, pulse should be checked every 2 min. If the rhythm remains nonshockable, continue with CPR. If at any time the rhythm becomes shockable, follow the left limb of the algorithm. One must always be on a look out for reversible causes of arrest and treat them—call for help/activate the emergency response system.

Reversible causes of cardiac arrest

6Hs	5Ts
1. Hypoxia	1. Tension pneumothorax
2. Hypoglycaemia	2. Toxins
3. Hypotension	3. Tamponade
4. Hypo-/hyperkalaemia	4. Thrombosis cardiac
5. H^+ ion (acidosis)	5. Thrombosis pulmonary
6. Hypothermia	

Defibrillators

Defibrillators can be either manual or automated (AED) with monophasic or biphasic waveforms.

Manual Defibrillators

Manual defibrillators have two sizes of hand-held paddles: adult (8–10 cm) and infant. Adult size is used for adults and children >10 kg (>approximately 1 year). Infant paddles are used for infants <10 kg. The infant paddles may slide over or be located under the adult paddles. Manual defibrillators can also be used with self-adhesive pads. Largest paddles or self-adhering electrodes[69–71] that fit on the child's chest without touching each other (when possible, leave about 3 cm between the paddles or electrodes) must be selected. Self-adhering pads should be pressed firmly on the chest so that the gel on the pad completely touches the child's chest. Appropriate paddle size for electrode gel must be applied liberally on manually applied paddles for proper conduction of the delivered energy. Saline-soaked pads, ultrasound gel, bare paddles or alcohol pads should not be used.

For proper placement of self-adhesive AED or monitor/defibrillator pads, follow the written instructions on the pads. Manual paddles are marked as sternum and apex. These are to be placed over the right side of the upper chest and the apex of the heart (to the left of the nipple over the left lower ribs) so that the heart is between two paddles. A firm pressure so as to produce a mild deformity in the chest wall should be applied. An anterior-posterior position of the paddles has not been shown to have any advantage over the conventional position.[72]

In children with VF, an initial monophonic dose of 2 J/kg effectively terminates ventricular fibrillation 18 to 50% times only,[73,74] while similar doses of biphasic shocks are effective 48% of the time.[72] Energy doses >4 J/kg (up to 9 J/kg) have been shown to be effective in children[75–77] and pediatric animals.[78] Some adult studies[79,80] and paediatric animal models[81–83] have shown that biphasic shock is as effective and less harmful than monophasic shocks. An initial dose of 2 J/kg may be considered (Class IIb, LOE C) for the first shock and for subsequent shocks and refractory VF, the dose may be increased to 4 J/kg (Class IIa, LOE C). Subsequent energy levels should be at least 4 J/kg. Higher energy up to a maximum of 10 J/kg or the adult maximum dose (Class IIb, LOE C) may be considered.

AEDs

Many AEDs can accurately detect VF in children of all ages.[84–87] They have a high degree of sensitivity and specificity to differentiate "shockable" from "nonshockable" rhythms.[85,86] For infants and children up to approximately 25 kg (approximately 8 years of age), a paediatric dose attenuator must be used.[77,88] If an AED with a dose attenuator is not available, the one with standard electrodes must be used. An AED without a dose attenuator may be used, if neither a manual defibrillator nor one with a dose attenuator is available (Class IIb, LOE C).

Bradycardia

The bradycardia algorithm (Fig. 22.8) applies to the care of an infant or child with bradycardia and cardiorespiratory compromise, but with a palpable pulse. If at any time during the course of action, the victim becomes pulseless, immediately the management should switch over to the pulseless arrest algorithm (Fig. 22.7). Treatment of bradycardia is indicated whenever the rhythm results in haemodynamic compromise.

The airway, breathing and circulation should be supported. Support the airway by positioning the child or allowing the child to assume a comfortable position or by opening the airway with manoeuvres. Supplemental oxygen should be provided and ventilation should be assisted, if required. A pulse oximeter should be attached to assess oxygenation. ECG and defibrillator should be attached. IV/IO access should be secured.

Management will depend upon whether bradycardia is persisting and causing cardiorespiratory symptoms despite adequate oxygenation and ventilation (Fig. 22.8).

If pulses, perfusion, and respirations are adequate, no emergency treatment is necessary. Close monitoring and further evaluation must be done. If heart rate is <60 beats/min with poor perfusion despite effective ventilation and oxygenation, start CPR. After 2 min or 5 cycles of CPR, re-evaluate to determine, if bradycardia and signs of haemodynamic compromise persist.

Continue to support airway, ventilation and oxygenation. Continue chest compressions (Class I, LOE B). If bradycardia still persists or responds only transiently, administer epinephrine IV (or IO) 0.01 mg/kg (0.1 ml/kg of 1:10,000 solution) or if IV/IO access not available, give endotracheally 0.1 mg/kg (0.1 ml/kg of 1:1,000 solution) (Class I, LOE B).

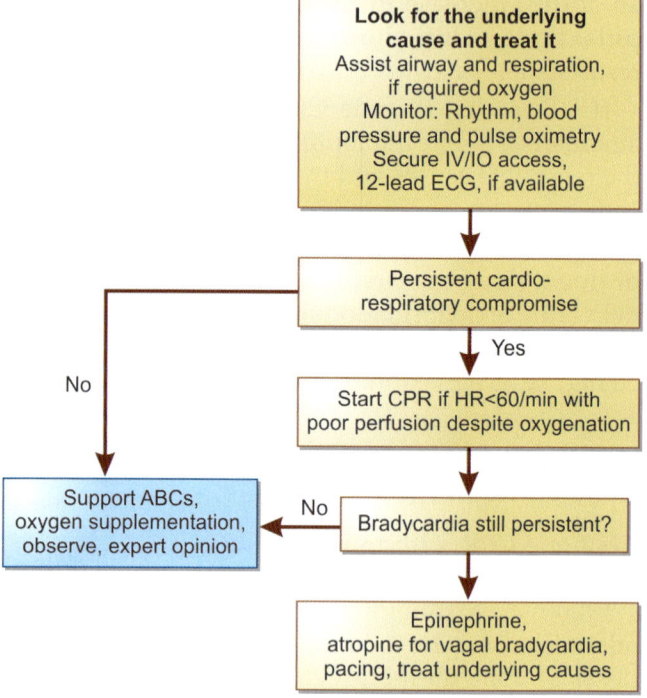

Fig. 22.8. PALS bradycardia algorithm

- If bradycardia is due to increased vagal tone or primary AV conduction block (i.e. not secondary to hypoxia), give IV/IO atropine 0.02 mg/kg or an endotracheal dose of 0.04 to 0.06 mg/kg (Class I, LOE C).

- Emergency transcutaneous pacing may be life-saving, if bradycardia is due to complete heart block or sinus node dysfunction unresponsive to ventilation, oxygenation, chest compressions and medications, especially if it is associated with congenital or acquired heart disease (Class IIb, LOE C).[89] Pacing is not useful for asystole[89,90] or bradycardia due to post-arrest hypoxic/ischaemic myocardial insult or respiratory failure.

Tachycardia

This algorithm (Fig. 22.9) applies whenever there is tachycardia with pulse in paediatric population. If there are signs of poor perfusion and pulses are not palpable, immediately switch over to the Pulseless Arrest Algorithm (Fig. 22.7).

If pulses are palpable and the patient has adequate perfusion, support ABC and provide supplemental oxygen. Attach monitor/defibrillator and pulse

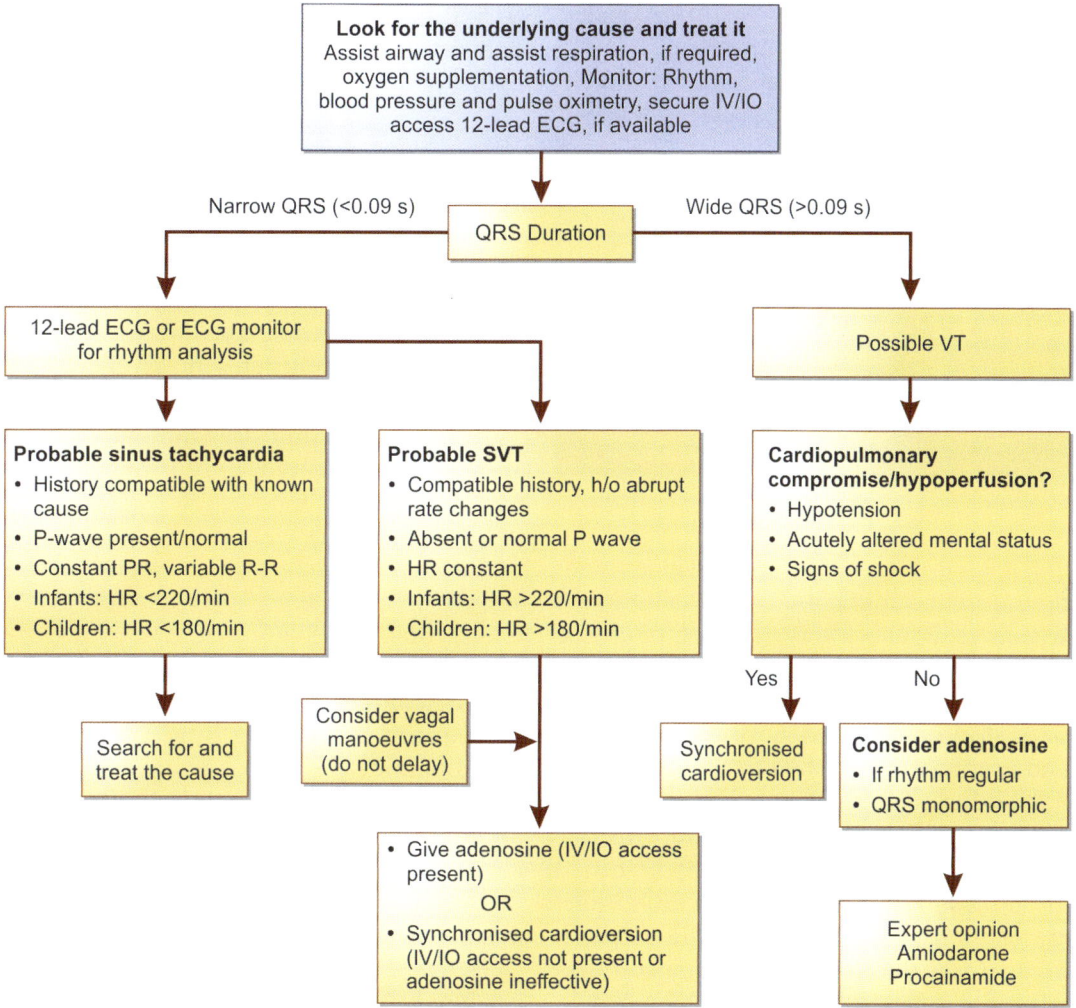

Fig. 22.9. PALS tachycardia algorithm

oximeter. Obtain vascular access. Evaluate 12-lead ECG and assess QRS duration (Fig. 22.9).

Narrow-Complex (<0.09 Second) Tachycardia

A 12-lead ECG (Fig. 22.9) and the patient's clinical presentation and history usually helps in differentiating sinus tachycardia from supraventricular tachycardia (SVT). If the rhythm is sinus tachycardia, search for and treat reversible causes.

Supraventricular Tachycardia

Close monitoring of the rhythm during therapy should be done to evaluate the effect of interventions. The patient's degree of haemodynamic compromise determines the type of further interventions.

If the patient is haemodynamically stable, attempt vagal manoeuvres (Class IIa, LOE C). If the first attempt is unsuccessful and the patient remains stable, a repeat attempt at vagal manoeuvres may be done. If the second attempt also fails, alternative method or pharmacologic techniques must be used to revert the rhythm. If the patient is unstable, vagal manoeuvres must be used only while preparing for electrical cardioversion or pharmacological medications. In infants and young children, ice may be applied to the face without occluding the airway.[91,92] In older children, carotid sinus massage or Valsalva manoeuvres may be performed.[93–95]

If IV/IO access is available and two attempts to revert the rhythm with vagal manoeuvres have failed, pharmacologic cardioversion with adenosine should

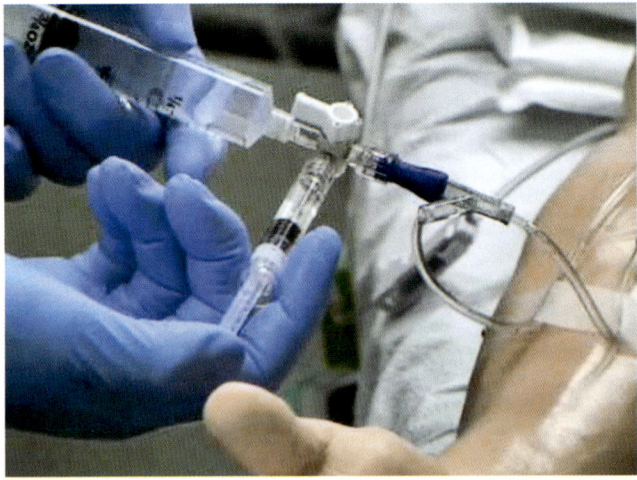

Fig. 22.10 Administration of adenosine using two syringe method

be attempted. It is a proven and effective remedy with minimal and transient side effects.[96–100] If IV/IO access is readily available, adenosine is the drug of choice (Class I, LOE C). IV/IO adenosine 0.1 mg/kg should be administered using 2 syringes connected to a T-connector or stopcock; give adenosine rapidly with 1 syringe and immediately flush with 5 ml of normal saline with the other (Fig. 22.10).

Verapamil, 0.1 to 0.3 mg/kg IV/IO is also effective in terminating SVT in older children,[101,102] but it should not be used in infants without expert consultation (Class III, LOE C) as it has the potential to cause myocardial depression, hypotension and cardiac arrest.[102,103]

If the patient is haemodynamically unstable or if adenosine is ineffective, electrical synchronized cardioversion should be attempted. The patient should be sedated, if possible. Initially a dose of 0.5 to 1 J/kg should be used. If unsuccessful, the dose may be increased to 2 J/kg (Class IIb, LOE C). If a second shock is unsuccessful or the tachycardia recurs quickly, amiodarone or procainamide should be considered before delivering a third shock.

Amiodarone 5 mg/kg IO/IV[104,105] or procainamide 15 mg/kg IO/IV[106] may be considered for a patient with SVT unresponsive to vagal manoeuvres and adenosine and/or electric cardioversion. These drugs should not be used for haemodynamically stable patients where there is time to wait for expert consultation prior to administration (Class IIb, LOE C) (Fig. 22.9). Both amiodarone and procainamide must be infused slowly (amiodarone over 20 to 60 minutes and procainamide over 30 to 60 minutes), depending on the urgency, while the ECG and blood pressure are monitored.

Wide-Complex (>0.09 Second) Tachycardia

Wide-complex tachycardia is usually ventricular in origin (ventricular tachycardia) but occasionally may be supraventricular.[107] Because all anti-arrhythmic therapies have a potential for serious adverse effects, consultation with an expert is strongly recommended before treating children who are haemodynamically stable.

In haemodynamically stable patients, adenosine should be considered, only if the rhythm is regular and the QRS is monomorphic. It is contraindicated in patients with Wolff-Parkinson-White syndrome and wide-complex tachycardia. Electrical cardioversion should be considered after sedation using a starting energy dose of 0.5 to 1 J/kg. If that fails, the dose may be increased to 2 J/kg (Class IIb, LOE C) (Fig. 22.9). Pharmacologic conversion with either intravenous amiodarone (5 mg/kg over 20 to 60 minutes) or procainamide (15 mg/kg given over 30 to 60 minutes) while monitoring ECG and blood pressure may be attempted. This must be stopped or infusion must be slowed down, if there is a decline in blood pressure or the QRS widens (Fig. 22.9). Expert consultation is strongly recommended prior to administration.

In haemodynamically unstable patients, electrical cardioversion is recommended using a starting energy dose of 0.5 to 1 J/kg. Dose may be increased to 2 J/kg for subsequent shocks (Class I, LOE C).

SPECIAL SITUATIONS FOR RESUSCITATION—SHOCK

Septic Shock

Survival after a septic shock does not bear any correlation with treatment of the condition with colloids or crystalloids.[108–111] Although colloid may be beneficial,[112] isotonic crystalloid solution may be used as the initial fluid for septic shock (Class IIa, LOE C). Central venous oxygen saturation ($ScvO_2$) should be monitored to titrate therapy. "Goal-directed" therapy, with a target $ScvO_2 \geq 70\%$ improves patient survival in severe sepsis (Class IIb, LOE B).[113–115] Ventilation should be assisted and it should be taken as an early measure during management (Class IIb, LOE C).[112,116]

Hypovolaemic Shock

Whenever there is grossly inadequate blood flow and oxygen delivery to meet tissue metabolic demands, a shock, like state may occur. Hypovolaemic shock is the most commonly encountered type in children. It may fall anywhere on the spectrum between compensated to a decompensated state. In the initial stages, compensatory mechanisms, like tachycardia and increased systemic vascular resistance (vasoconstriction), help to maintain the cardiac output and perfusion pressure, respectively. But eventually if supportive management fails or no measures are taken to improve the situation, decompensation and hypotensive shock state occurs, resulting in inadequate tissue perfusion.

Signs of compensated shock:
- Tachycardia
- Cool and pale distal extremities
- Prolonged (>2 seconds) capillary refill (despite warm ambient temperature)
- Weak peripheral pulses
- Normal systolic blood pressure

Signs of inadequate end-organ perfusion:
- Depressed mental status
- Decreased urine output
- Metabolic acidosis
- Tachypnoea
- Weak central pulses
- Deterioration in colour (e.g. mottling)

An isotonic crystalloid solution as a bolus of 20 ml/kg (e.g. Ringer's lactate or normal saline)[117,118] should be used as the initial fluid for the treatment of shock (Class I, LOE A). Colloid administration has no additional benefit during the early phase of resuscitation.[119,120] Additional boluses (20 ml/kg) may be given, if systemic perfusion does not improve.

Trauma

If a cervical spine injury is suspected, the neck movements must be restricted and traction over the head and neck must be strictly avoided. Head-ilt must be avoided and only jaw thrust should be used to open the airway. If the airway cannot be opened with a jaw thrust only then a head-tilt chin-lift manoeuvre must be performed. Hyperventilation must be avoided at all costs even in case of head injury (Class III, LOE C).[121,122] Tension pneumothorax, hemothorax, or pulmonary contusion can impair oxygenation and ventilation and must be suspected and ruled out in all thoraco-abdominal trauma cases. Nasogastric tube should be avoided in a case of maxillofacial trauma or suspected basilar skull fracture. An orogastric tube may be inserted in these patients (Class IIa, LOE C).[123]

POST-RESUSCITATION STABILIZATION (POST-CARDIAC ARREST CARE)

Post-resuscitation care has been introduced as the fifth link of the chain of survival in 2010 guidelines of resuscitation. It is aimed at preserving the neurologic function, prevent secondary organ injury, diagnose and treat the cause of illness and enable the patient to arrive at a paediatric tertiary-care facility in an optimal physiologic state.

Respiratory System

FiO_2 must be reduced to reduce the PaO_2 while ensuring adequate arterial oxygen content as hyperoxaemia enhances the oxidative injury observed following reperfusion. FiO_2 must be adjusted to maintain the arterial oxyhaemoglobin saturation ≥94%. Assisted ventilation should be given, if there is significant respiratory compromise. If the patient is already intubated, DOPE protocol must be followed to check for displacement, obstruction, pneumothorax, equipment failure. In the hospital setting, arterial blood gases must be obtained 10 to 15 min after establishing the initial mechanical ventilator settings and further ventilatory adjustment must be made accordingly.

Appropriate analgesia and adequate sedation or respiratory paralysis to facilitate mechanical ventilation must be provided, if required. Neuromuscular blockers, however, can mask seizures and impede neurologic examinations. Exhaled CO_2 ($EtCO_2$) must be monitored especially during transport and diagnostic procedures (Class IIa, LOE B).[124–126]

Cardiovascular System

Continuous monitoring of heart rate and blood pressure must be established. Clinical evaluations at frequent intervals must be done until the patient is stable. A urinary catheter must be inserted for monitoring urine output. A 12-lead ECG may help to establish the cause of cardiac arrest. Arterial blood gas analysis, serum electrolytes, glucose and calcium

Table 22.2 Medications to maintain cardiac output and for post-resuscitation stabilization[68]	
Medication	**Dose range**
Clear runny nose	Child < 1 year
Inamrinone (inodilator)	0.75–1 mg/kg IV/IO over 5 minutes; may repeat at 2 minutes then: 5–10 µg/kg per minute
Dobutamine (inotrope; vasodilator)	2–20 µg/kg per minute IV/IO
Dopamine (inotrope, chronotrope; pressor in high doses)	2–20 µg/kg per minute IV/IO
Epinephrine (inotrope, chronotrope; pressor in high doses)	0.1–1 µg/kg per minute IV/IO
Milrinone (inodilator)	Loading dose: 50 µg/kg IV/IO over 10–60 min then 0.25–0.75 µg/kg per minute
Norepinephrine (vasopressor)	0.1–2 µg/kg per min
Sodium nitroprusside (vasodilator)	Initial: 0.5–1 µg/kg per minute; titrate to effect up to 8 µg/kg per minute

IV, intravenous; IO, intraosseous.

concentrations must be monitored at regular intervals. A chest X-ray should be performed to evaluate endotracheal tube position, heart size, and pulmonary status. Arterial lactate and central venous oxygen saturation should be monitored to assess adequacy of tissue oxygen delivery.

Myocardial dysfunction and vascular instability must be treated with vasoactive drugs. The doses of these drugs may be titrated to improve myocardial function and organ perfusion. Epinephrine, norepinephrine, dopamine, dobutamine, sodium nitroprusside, inodilators, such as inamrinone, milrinone, may be required in appropriate doses (Table 22.2).

Neurologic System

One of the primary goals of resuscitation is to preserve neurological status. This may be done by avoiding excessive ventilation or hyperventilation. Hyperventilation may impair neurologic outcome by adversely affecting cerebral perfusion.[127]

Therapeutic hypothermia (32°C to 34°C) has been induced for comatose children (Class IIb, LOE C).[128,129] The ideal method and duration of cooling and rewarming are yet not known. Shivering should be prevented by providing sedation and neuromuscular blockade. Temperature must be monitored continuously and fever (>38°C) must be treated aggressively with antipyretics and cooling devices because it adversely influences recovery from ischaemic brain injury (Class IIa, LOE C).[130–135]

Post-ischaemic seizures must be treated aggressively and correctable causes must be managed. Rate of rewarming from 32 to 34°C must not be done faster than 0.5°C per 2 hours unless indicated for clinical reasons.

Renal System

Urine output must be maintained at >1 ml/kg per hour in infants and children or >30 ml/hour in adolescents. Dehydration, inadequate systemic perfusion precipitate renal ischaemic damage and must be aggressively managed with fluid therapy. Nephrotoxic medications must be avoided and doses must be modified accordingly.

Termination of Resuscitative Efforts

There are no set guidelines or reliable predictors to guide the termination of resuscitative efforts in children. Clinical variables associated with survival include length of CPR, number of doses of epinephrine, age, witnessed versus unwitnessed cardiac arrest, and the first and subsequent rhythm.[136–148] None of these associations, however, predict outcome. Witnessed collapse, bystander CPR, and a short interval from collapse to arrival of professionals improve the chances of a successful resuscitation.

REFERENCES

1. Dorfsman ML, Menegazzi JJ, Wadas RJ, Auble TE. Two-thumb vs two-finger chest compression in an infant model of prolonged cardiopulmonary resuscitation. Acad Emerg Med 2000;7:1077–1082.

2. Whitelaw CC, Slywka B, Goldsmith LJ. Comparison of a two-finger versus two-thumb method for chest compres-

sions by healthcare providers in an infant mechanical model. Resuscitation 2000;43:213–216.

3. David R. Closed chest cardiac massage in the newborn infant. Pediatrics 1988;81:552–554.

4. Ishimine P, Menegazzi J, Weinstein D. Evaluation of two-thumb chest compression with thoracic squeeze in a swine model of infant cardiac arrest. Acad Emerg Med 1998;5:397.

5. Terndrup TE, Warner DA. Infant ventilation and oxygenation by basic life support providers: comparison of methods. Prehospital Disaster Med 1992;7:35– 40.

6. Hirschman AM, Kravath RE. Venting vs ventilating. A danger of manual resuscitation bags. Chest 1982;82: 369–370.

7. Berg MD, Idris AH, Berg RA. Severe ventilatory compromise due to gastric distention during pediatric cardiopulmonary resuscitation. Resuscitation 1998;36:71–73.

8. Gausche M, Lewis RJ, Stratton SJ, Haynes BE, Gunter CS, Goodrich SM, Poore PD, McCollough MD, Henderson DP, Pratt FD, Seidel JS. Effect of out-of-hospital pediatric endotracheal intubation on survival and neurological outcome: a controlled clinical trial. JAMA 2000;283: 783–790.

9. Moynihan RJ, Brock-Utne JG, Archer JH, Feld LH, Kreitzman TR. The effect of cricoid pressure on preventing gastric insufflation in infants and children. Anesthesiology 1993;78:652–656.

10. Hartsilver EL, Vanner RG. Airway obstruction with cricoid pressure. Anaesthesia 2000;55:208–211.

11. Vilke GM, Smith AM, Ray LU, Steen PJ, Murrin PA, Chan TC. Airway obstruction in children aged less than 5 years: the prehospital experience. Prehosp Emerg Care 2004;8: 196–199.

12. Morley RE, Ludemann JP, Moxham JP, Kozak FK, Riding KH. Foreign body aspiration in infants and toddlers: recent trends in British Columbia. J Otolaryngol 2004;33:37– 41.

13. Harris CS, Baker SP, Smith GA, Harris RM. Childhood asphyxiation by food. A national analysis and overview. JAMA 1984;251:2231–2235.

14. Rimell FL, Thome AJ, Stool S, Reilly JS, Rider G, Stool D, et al. Characteristics of objects that cause choking in children. JAMA 1995; 274:1763–1766.

15. Committee on Injury, Violence and Poison Prevention, et al. Prevention of choking among children. Pediatrics 2010;125:601–607.

16. Heimlich HJ. A life-saving maneuver to prevent food-choking. JAMA 1975;234:398–401.

17. Sternbach G, Kiskaddon RT. Henry Heimlich: a life-saving maneuver for food choking. J Emerg Med 1985;3:143–148.

18. Langhelle A, Sunde K, Wik L, Steen PA. Airway pressure with chest compressions versus Heimlich manoeuvre in recently dead adults with complete airway obstruction. Resuscitation 2000;44:105–108.

19. Kabbani M, Goodwin SR. Traumatic epiglottis following blind finger sweep to remove a pharyngeal foreign body. Clin Pediatr (Phila) 1995;34:495–497.

20. Hartrey R, Bingham RM. Pharyngeal trauma as a result of blind finger sweeps in the choking child. J Accid Emerg Med 1995;12:52–54.

21. Gjoni D, Mbamalu D, Banerjee A, James K. An unusual complication of an attempt to open the airway in a choking child. Br J Hosp ed (Lond) 2009;70:595.

22. Kyriacou DN, Arcinue EL, Peek C, Kraus JF. Effect of immediate resuscitation on children with submersion injury. Pediatrics 1994;94:137–142.

23. Suominen P, Baillie C, Korpela R, Rautanen S, Ranta S, Olkkola KT. Impact of age, submersion time and water temperature on outcome in near-drowning. Resuscitation 2002;52:247–254.

24. Graf WD, Cummings P, Quan L, Brutocao D. Predicting outcome in pediatric submersion victims. Ann Emerg Med 1995;26:312–319.

25. Modell JH, Idris AH, Pineda JA, Silverstein JH. Survival after prolonged submersion in freshwater in Florida. Chest 2004;125:1948–1951.

26. Mehta SR, Srinivasan KV, Bindra MS, Kumar MR, Lahiri AK. Near drowning in cold water. J Assoc Physicians India 2000;48:674–676.

27. Szpilman D, Soares M. In-water resuscitation–is it worthwhile? Resuscitation 2004;63:25–31.

28. Russell P, Chambers N, du Plessis J, Vijayasekeran S. Emergency use of a size 1 laryngeal mask airway in a ventilated neonate with an undiagnosed type IV laryngotracheo-oesophageal cleft. Paediatr Anaesth 2008;18:658–662.

29. Scheller B, Schalk R, Byhahn C, Peter N, L'Allemand N, Kessler P, Meininger D. Laryngeal tube suction II for difficult airway management in neonates and small infants. Resuscitation 2009;80:805–810.

30. Gerritse BM, Draaisma JM, Schalkwijk A, van Grunsven PM, Scheffer GJ. Should EMS-paramedics perform paediatric tracheal intubation in the field? Resuscitation 2008;79:225–229.

31. A prospective multicenter evaluation of prehospital airway management performance in a large metropolitan region. Denver Metro Airway Study Group, et al. Prehosp Emerg Care 2009;13:304–310.

32. Ellis DY, Harris T, Zideman D. Cricoid pressure in emergency department rapid sequence tracheal intubations: a risk-benefit analysis. Ann Emerg Med 2007;50: 653–665.

33. Walker RW, Ravi R, Haylett K. Effect of cricoid force on airway calibre in children: a bronchoscopic assessment. Br J Anaesth 2010;104:71–74.

34. Browning DH, Graves SA. Incidence of aspiration with endotracheal tubes in children. J Pediatr 1983;102: 582–584.

35. Luten RC, Wears RL, Broselow J, Zaritsky A, Barnett TM, Lee T, Bailey A, Vally R, Brown R, Rosenthal B. Length-based endotracheal tube and emergency equipment in pediatrics. Ann Emerg Med 1992;21:900–904.

36. Davis D, Barbee L, Ririe D. Pediatric endotracheal tube selection: a comparison of age-based and height-based criteria. AANA J 1998;66:299–303.

37. Daugherty RJ, Nadkarni V, Brenn BR. Endotracheal tube size estimation for children with pathological short stature. Pediatr Emerg Care 2006;22:710–717.

38. Dullenkopf A, Kretschmar O, Knirsch W, Tomaske M, Hug M, Stutz K, Berger F, Weiss M. Comparison of tracheal tube cuff diameters with internal transverse diameters of the trachea in children. Acta Anaesthesiol Scand 2006;50:201–205.

39. Salgo B, Schmitz A, Henze G, Stutz K, Dullenkopf A, Neff S, Gerber AC, Weiss M. Evaluation of a new recommendation for improved cuffed tracheal tube size selection in infants and small children. Acta Anaesthesiol Scand 2006;50:557–561.

40. Duracher C, Schmautz E, Martinon C, Faivre J, Carli P, Orliaguet G. Evaluation of cuffed tracheal tube size predicted using the Khine formula in children. Paediatr Anaesth 2008;18:113–118.

41. Beyer AJd, Land G, Zaritsky A. Nonphysician transport of intubated pediatric patients: a system evaluation. Crit Care Med 1992;20:961–966.

42. Gausche M, Lewis RJ, Stratton SJ, Haynes BE, Gunter CS, Goodrich SM, Poore PD, McCollough MD, Henderson DP, Pratt FD, Seidel JS. Effect of out-of-hospital pediatric endotracheal intubation on survival and neurological outcome: a controlled clinical trial. JAMA 2000;283: 783–790.

43. Katz SH, Falk JL. Misplaced endotracheal tubes by paramedics in an urban emergency medical services system. Ann Emerg Med 2001;37:32–37.

44. Hosono S, Inami I, Fujita H, Minato M, Takahashi S, Mugishima H. A role of end-tidal CO_2 monitoring for assessment of tracheal intubations in very low birth weight infants during neonatal resuscitation at birth. J Perinat Med 2009;37:79–84.

45. Salthe J, Kristiansen SM, Sollid S, Oglaend B, Soreide E. Capnography rapidly confirmed correct endotracheal tube placement during resuscitation of extremely low birthweight babies (<1000 g). Acta Anaesthesiol Scand 2006;50:1033–1036.

46. Campbell RC, Boyd CR, Shields RO, Odom JW, Corse KM. Evaluation of an end-tidal carbon dioxide detector in the aeromedical setting. J Air Med Transp 1990;9: 13–15.

47. Bhende MS, Allen WD, Jr. Evaluation of a Capno-Flo resuscitator during transport of critically ill children. Pediatr Emerg Care 2002;18:414–416.

48. Cantineau JP, Merckx P, Lambert Y, Sorkine M, Bertrand C, Duvaldestin P. Effect of epinephrine on end-tidal carbon dioxide pressure during prehospital cardiopulmonary resuscitation. Am J Emerg Med 1994;12:267–270.

49. Ornato JP, Shipley JB, Racht EM, Slovis CM, Wrenn KD, Pepe PE, Almeida SL, Ginger VF, Fotre TV. Multicenter study of a portable, hand-size, colorimetric end-tidal carbon dioxide detection device. Ann Emerg Med 1992;21:518–523.

50. Ward KR, Yealy DM. End-tidal carbon dioxide monitoring in emergency medicine. Part 2: Clinical applications. Acad Emerg Med 1998;5:637–646.

51. Hand IL, Shepard EK, Krauss AN, Auld PA. Discrepancies between transcutaneous and end-tidal carbon dioxide monitoring in the critically ill neonate with respiratory distress syndrome. Crit Care Med 1989;17:556–559.

52. Tobias JD, Meyer DJ. Noninvasive monitoring of carbon dioxide during respiratory failure in toddlers and infants: end-tidal versus transcutaneous carbon dioxide. Anesth Analg 1997;85:55–58.

53. Sharieff GQ, Rodarte A, Wilton N, Bleyle D. The self-inflating bulb as an airway adjunct: is it reliable in children weighing less than 20 kilograms? Acad Emerg Med 2003;10:303–308.

54. Sharieff GQ, Rodarte A, Wilton N, Silva PD, Bleyle D. The self inflating bulb as an esophageal detector device in children weighing more than twenty kilograms: A comparison of two techniques. Ann Emerg Med 2003;41:623–629.

55. Tayal VS, Kline JA. Emergency echocardiography to detect pericardial effusion in patients in PEA and near-PEA states. Resuscitation 2003;59:315–318.

56. Varriale P, Maldonado JM. Echocardiographic observations during inhospital cardiopulmonary resuscitation. Crit Care Med 1997;25:1717–1720.

57. Grmec S, Krizmaric M, Mally S, Kozelj A, Spindler M, Lesnik B. Utstein style analysis of out-of-hospital cardiac arrest–bystander CPR and end expired carbon dioxide. Resuscitation 2007;72:404–414.

58. Pokorna M, Necas E, Kratochvil J, Skripsky R, Andrlik M, Franek O. A sudden increase in partial pressure end-tidal carbon dioxide (P(ET)CO_2) at the moment of return of spontaneous circulation. J Emerg Med 2009.

59. Horton MA, Beamer C. Powered intraosseous insertion provides safe and effective vascular access for pediatric emergency patients. Pediatr Emerg Care 2008;24:347–350.

60. Fiser DH. Intraosseous infusion. N Engl J Med 1990;322:1579–1581.

61. Guy J, Haley K, Zuspan SJ. Use of intraosseous infusion in the pediatric trauma patient. J Pediatr Surg 1993;28: 158–161.

62. Berg RA. Emergency infusion of catecholamines into bone marrow. Am J Dis Child 1984;138:810–811.

63. Andropoulos DB, Soifer SJ, Schreiber MD. Plasma epinephrine concentrations after intraosseous and central venous injection during cardiopulmonary resuscitation in the lamb. J Pediatr 1990;116:312–315.

64. Ward JTJ. Endotracheal drug therapy. Am J Emerg Med 1983;1:71– 82.

65. Johnston C. Endotracheal drug delivery. Pediatr Emerg Care. 1992;8:94–97.

66. Efrati O, Ben-Abraham R, Barak A, Modan-Moses D, Augarten A, Manisterski Y, Barzilay Z, Paret G. Endo-bronchial adrenaline: should be reconsidered? Dose response and haemodynamic effect in dogs. Resuscitation 2003;59:117–122.

67. Jasani MS, Nadkarni VM, Finkelstein MS, Mandell GA, Salzman SK, Norman ME. Effects of different techniques of endotracheal epinephrine administration in pediatric porcine hypoxic-hypercarbic cardiopulmonary arrest. Crit Care Med 1994;22:1174–1180.

68. Kleinman ME, Chameides L, Schexnayder SM, Samson RA, Hazinski MF, Atkins DL, Berg MD, de Caen AR, Fink EL, Freid EB, Hickey RW, Marino BS, Nadkarni VM, Proctor LT, Qureshi FA, Sartorelli K, Topjian A, van der Jagt EW, Zaritsky AL. Part 14: Pediatric advanced life support: 2010 American Heart Association Guidelines for Cardiopulmonary Resuscitation and Emergency Cardiovascular Care. Circulation 2010;122(Suppl 3): S876–S908.

69. Atkins DL, Sirna S, Kieso R, Charbonnier F, Kerber RE. Pediatric defibrillation: importance of paddle size in determining transthoracic impedance. Pediatrics 1988;82:914–918.

70. Atkins DL, Kerber RE. Pediatric defibrillation: current flow is improved by using "adult" electrode paddles. Pediatrics 1994;94:90–93.

71. Samson RA, Atkins DL, Kerber RE. Optimal size of self-adhesive preapplied electrode pads in pediatric defibrillation. Am J Cardiol 1995;75:544 –545.

72. Tibballs J, Carter B, Kiraly NJ, Ragg P, Clifford M. External and internal biphasic direct current shock doses for pediatric ventricular fibrillation and pulseless ventricular tachycardia. Pediatr Crit Care Med 2010. In press.

73. Berg MD, Samson RA, Meyer RJ, Clark LL, Valenzuela TD, Berg RA. Pediatric defibrillation doses often fail to terminate prolonged out-of hospital ventricular fibrillation in children. Resuscitation 2005;67:63–67.

74. Rodriguez-Nunez A, Lopez-Herce J, Garcia C, Dominguez P, Carrillo A, Bellon JM. Pediatric

defibrillation after cardiac arrest: initial response and outcome. Crit Care 2006;10:R113.

75. Rossano JW, Quan L, Kenney MA, Rea TD, Atkins DL. Energy doses for treatment of out-of-hospital pediatric ventricular fibrillation. Resuscitation 2006;70:80–89.

76. Gurnett CA, Atkins DL. Successful use of a biphasic waveform automated external defibrillator in a high-risk child. Am J Cardiol 2000;86:1051–1053.

77. Atkins DL, Jorgenson DB. Attenuated pediatric electrode pads for automated external defibrillator use in children. Resuscitation 2005;66:31–37.

78. Berg RA, Chapman FW, Berg MD, Hilwig RW, Banville I, Walker RG, et al. Attenuated adult biphasic shocks compared with weight-based monophasic shocks in a swine model of prolonged pediatric ventricular fibril-lation. Resuscitation 2004;61:189–197.

79. Schneider T, Martens PR, Paschen H, Kuisma M, Wolcke B, Gliner BE, et al. Multicenter, randomized, controlled trial of 150-J biphasic shocks compared with 200-J to 360-J monophasic shocks in the resuscitation of out-of-hospital cardiac arrest victims. Optimized Response to Cardiac Arrest (ORCA) Investigators. Circulation 2000;102:1780–1787.

80. van Alem AP, Chapman FW, Lank P, Hart AA, Koster RW. A prospective, randomised and blinded comparison of first shock success of monophasic and biphasic waveforms in out-of-hospital cardiac arrest. Resuscitation 2003;58:17–24.

81. Berg RA, Samson RA, Berg MD, Chapman FW, Hilwig RW, Banville I, et al. Better outcome after pediatric defibrillation dosage than adult dosage in a swine model of pediatric ventricular fibrillation. J Am Coll Cardiol 2005;45:786–789.

82. Clark CB, Zhang Y, Davies LR, Karlsson G, Kerber RE. Pediatric transthoracic defibrillation: biphasic versus monophasic waveforms in an experimental model. Resuscitation 2001;51:159–163.

83. Tang W, Weil MH, Jorgenson D, Klouche K, Morgan C, Yu T, et al. Fixed-energy biphasic waveform defibrillation in a pediatric model of cardiac arrest and resuscitation. Crit Care Med 2002;30:2736–2741.

84. Atkins DL, Hartley LL, York DK. Accurate recognition and effective treatment of ventricular fibrillation by automated external defibrillators in adolescents. Pediatrics 1998;101:393–397.

85. Atkinson E, Mikysa B, Conway JA, Parker M, Christian K, Deshpande J, et al. Specificity and sensitivity of automated external defibrillator rhythm analysis in infants and children. Ann Emerg Med 2003;42:185–196.

86. Cecchin F, Jorgenson DB, Berul CI, Perry JC, Zimmerman AA, Duncan BW, et al. Is arrhythmia detection by automatic external defibrillator accurate for children? Sensitivity and specificity of an automatic external

defibrillator algorithm in 696 pediatric arrhythmias. Circulation 2001;103:2483–2488.

87. Atkins DL, Scott WA, Blaufox AD, Law IH, Dick M, II, Geheb F, et al. Sensitivity and specificity of an automated external defibrillator algorithm designed for pediatric patients. Resuscitation 2008;76:168 –174.

88. Samson RA, Berg RA, Bingham R, Biarent D, Coovadia A, Hazinski MF, et al. Use of automated external defibrillators for children: an update: an advisory statement from the pediatric advanced life support task force, International Liaison Committee on Resuscitation. Circulation 2003;107:3250–3255.

89. Beland MJ, Hesslein PS, Finlay CD, Faerron-Angel JE, Williams WG, Rowe RD. Noninvasive transcutaneous cardiac pacing in children. Pacing Clin Electrophysiol 1987;10:1262–1270.

90. Quan L, Graves JR, Kinder DR, Horan S, Cummins RO. Transcutaneous cardiac pacing in the treatment of out-of-hospital pediatric cardiac arrests. Ann Emerg Med 1992;21:905–909.

91. Sreeram N, Wren C. Supraventricular tachycardia in infants: response to initial treatment. Arch Dis Child 1990;65:127–129.

92. Aydin M, Baysal K, Kucukoduk S, Cetinkaya F, Yaman S. Application of ice water to the face in initial treatment of supraventricular tachycardia. Turk J Pediatr 1995;37: 15–17.

93. Ornato JP, Hallagan LF, Reese WA, Clark RF, Tayal VS, Garnett AR, et al. Treatment of paroxysmal supraventricular tachycardia in the emergency department by clinical decision analysis [published correction appears in Am J Emerg Med 1990;8:85]. Am J Emerg Med 1988;6:555–560.

94. Lim SH, Anantharaman V, Teo WS, Goh PP, Tan AT. Comparison of treatment of supraventricular tachycardia by Valsalva maneuver and carotid sinus massage. Ann Emerg Med 1998;31:30–35.

95. Waxman MB, Wald RW, Sharma AD, Huerta F, Cameron DA. Vagal techniques for termination of paroxysmal supraventricular tachycardia. Am J Cardiol 1980;46:655–664.

96. Balaguer Gargallo M, Jordan Garcia I, Caritg Bosch J, Cambra Lasaosa FJ, Prada Hermogenes F, Palomaque Rico A. Supraventricular tachycardia in infants and children. An Pediatr (Barc) 2007;67:133–138.

97. Dixon J, Foster K, Wyllie J, Wren C. Guidelines and adenosine dosing in supraventricular tachycardia. Arch Dis Child 2005;90:1190–1191.

98. Moghaddam M, Mohammad Dalili S, Emkanjoo Z. Efficacy of adenosine for acute treatment of supraventricular tachycardia in infants and children. J Teh Univ Heart Ctr 2008;3:157–162.

99. Riccardi A, Arboscello E, Ghinatti M, Minuto P, Lerza R. Adenosine in the treatment of supraventricular tachy-

cardia: 5 years of experience (2002–2006). Am J Emerg Med 2008;26:879–882.

100. Lim SH, Anantharaman V, Teo WS, Chan YH. Slow infusion of calcium channel blockers compared with intravenous adenosine in the emergency treatment of supraventricular tachycardia. Resuscitation 2009;80: 523–528.

101. Holdgate A, Foo A. Adenosine versus intravenous calcium channel antagonists for the treatment of supraventricular tachycardia in adults. Cochrane Database Syst Rev 2006;CD005154.

102. Ng GY, Hampson Evans DC, Murdoch LJ. Cardiovascular collapse after amiodarone administration in neonatal supraventicular tachycardia. Eur J Emerg Med 2003;10: 323–325.

103. Saul JP, Scott WA, Brown S, Marantz P, Acevedo V, Etheridge SP, et al. Intravenous amiodarone for incessant tachyarrhythmias in children: a randomized, double-blind, antiarrhythmic drug trial. Circulation 2005;112: 3470–3477.

104. Haas NA, Camphausen CK. Acute hemodynamic effects of intravenous amiodarone treatment in pediatric patients with cardiac surgery. Clin Res Cardiol 2008;97:801–810.

105. Chang PM, Silka MJ, Moromisato DY, Bar-Cohen Y. Amiodarone versus procainamide for the acute treatment of recurrent supraventricular tachycardia in pediatric patients. Circ Arrhythm Electrophysiol 2010;3:134–140.

106. Benson D (Jr), Smith W, Dunnigan A, Sterba R, Gallagher J. Mechanisms of regular wide QRS tachycardia in infants and children. Am J Cardiol 1982;49:1778–1788.

107. Dung NM, Day NPJ, Tam DTH, Loan HT, Chau HTT, Minh LN, et al. Fluid replacement in dengue shock syndrome: A randomized, double-blind comparison of four intravenous-fluid regimens. Clin Infect Dis 1999; 29:787–794.

108. Ngo NT, Cao XT, Kneen R, Wills B, Nguyen VM, Nguyen TQ, et al. Acute management of dengue shock syndrome: a randomized double-blind comparison of 4 intravenous fluid regimens in the first hour. Clin Infect Dis 2001;32: 204–213.

109. Wills BA, Nguyen MD, Ha TL, Dong TH, Tran TN, Le TT, et al. Comparison of three fluid solutions for resuscitation in dengue shock syndrome. N Engl J Med 2005;353:877–89.

110. Upadhyay M, Singhi S, Murlidharan J, Kaur N, Majumdar S. Randomized evaluation of fluid resuscitation with crystalloid (saline) and colloid (polymer from degraded gelatin in saline) in pediatric septic shock. Indian Pediatr 2005;42:223–231.

111. Booy R, Habibi P, Nadel S, de Munter C, Britto J, Morrison A, et al. Reduction in case fatality rate from meningococcal disease associated with improved healthcare delivery. Arch Dis Child 2001;85:386–390.

112. de Oliveira CF, de Oliveira DS, Gottschald AF, Moura JD, Costa GA, Ventura AC, et al. ACCM/PALS haemodynamic support guidelines for paediatric septic shock: an outcomes comparison with and without monitoring central venous oxygen saturation. Intensive Care Med 2008;34:1065–1075.

113. Rivers E, Nguyen B, Havstad S, Ressler J, Muzzin A, Knoblich B, et al. Early goal-directed therapy in the treatment of severe sepsis and septic shock. N Engl J Med 2001;345:1368–1377.

114. Nguyen HB, Corbett SW, Steele R, Banta J, Clark RT, Hayes SR, et al. Implementation of a bundle of quality indicators for the early management of severe sepsis and septic shock is associated with decreased mortality. Crit Care Med 2007;35:1105–1112.

115. Ledingham IM, McArdle CS. Prospective study of the treatment of septic shock. Lancet 1978;1:1194–1197.

116. Schierhout G, Roberts I. Fluid resuscitation with colloid or crystalloid solutions in critically ill patients: a systematic review of randomised trials. Br Med J 1998;316:961–964.

117. Human albumin administration in critically ill patients: systematic review of randomised controlled trials. Cochrane Injuries Group Albumin Reviewers, et al. Br Med J 1998;317:235–240.

118. Alderson P, Schierhout G, Roberts I, Bunn F. Colloids versus crystalloids for fluid resuscitation in critically ill patients. In: The Cochrane Library. Oxford: Update Software. 2003(Issue 3).

119. Finfer S, Bellomo R, Boyce N, French J, Myburgh J, Norton R. A comparison of albumin and saline for fluid resuscitation in the intensive care unit. N Engl J Med 2004;350:2247–2256.

120. Muizelaar JP, Marmarou A, Ward JD, Kontos HA, Choi SC, Becker DP, et al. Adverse effects of prolonged hyperventilation in patients with severe head injury: a randomized clinical trial. J Neurosurg 1991;75:731–739.

121. Skippen P, Seear M, Poskitt K, Kestle J, Cochrane D, Annich G, et al. Effect of hyperventilation on regional cerebral blood flow in headinjured children. Crit Care Med 1997;25:1402–1409.

122. Baskaya MK. Inadvertent intracranial placement of a nasogastric tube in patients with head injuries. Surg Neurol 1999;52:426–427.

123. Bhende MS, Allen WD, Jr. Evaluation of a Capno-Flo resuscitator during transport of critically ill children. Pediatr Emerg Care 2002;18:414–416.

124. Tobias JD, Lynch A, Garrett J. Alterations of end-tidal carbon dioxide during the intrahospital transport of children. Pediatr Emerg Care 1996;12:249–251.

125. Singh S, Allen WD (Jr), Venkataraman ST, Bhende MS. Utility of a novel quantitative handheld microstream capnometer during transport of critically ill children. Am J Emerg Med 2006;24:302–307.

126. Buunk G, van der Hoeven JG, Meinders AE. Cerebrovascular reactivity in comatose patients resuscitated from a cardiac arrest. Stroke 1997;28:1569–1573.

127. Doherty DR, Parshuram CS, Gaboury I, Hoskote A, Lacroix J, Tucci M, et al. Hypothermia therapy after pediatric cardiac arrest. Circulation 2009;119:1492–1500.

128. Fink EL, Clark RS, Kochanek PM, Bell MJ, Watson RS. A tertiary care center's experience with therapeutic hypothermia after pediatric cardiac arrest. Pediatr Crit Care Med 2010;11:66–74.

129. Zeiner A, Holzer M, Sterz F, Schorkhuber W, Eisenburger P, Havel C, et al. Hyperthermia after cardiac arrest is associated with an unfavorable neurologic outcome. Arch Intern Med 2001;161: 2007–2012.

130. Takasu A, Saitoh D, Kaneko N, Sakamoto T, Okada Y. Hyperthermia: is it an ominous sign after cardiac arrest? Resuscitation 2001;49:273–277.

131. Ginsberg MD, Busto R. Combating hyperthermia in acute stroke: a significant clinical concern. Stroke 1998;29: 529–534.

132. Hickey RW, Kochanek PM, Ferimer H, Alexander HL, Garman RH, Graham SH. Induced hyperthermia exacerbates neurologic neuronal histologic damage after asphyxial cardiac arrest in rats. Crit Care Med 2003;31:531–535.

133. Laptook A, Tyson J, Shankaran S, McDonald S, Ehrenkranz R, Fanaroff A, et al. Elevated temperature after hypoxic-ischemic encephalopathy: risk factor for adverse outcomes. Pediatrics 2008;122:491–499.

134. Kim Y, Busto R, Dietrich WD, Kraydieh S, Ginsberg MD. Delayed postischemic hyperthermia in awake rats worsens the histopathological outcome of transient focal cerebral ischemia. Stroke 27:2274–2280, 1996; discussion 2281.

135. Baena RC, Busto R, Dietrich WD, Globus MY, Ginsberg MD. Hyperthermia delayed by 24 hours aggravates neuronal damage in rat hippocampus following global ischemia. Neurology 1997;48:768–773.

136. Samson RA, Nadkarni VM, Meaney PA, Carey SM, Berg MD, Berg RA. Outcomes of in-hospital ventricular fibrillation in children. N Engl J Med 2006;354:2328–2339.

137. Atkins DL, Everson-Stewart S, Sears GK, Daya M, Osmond MH, Warden CR, et al. Epidemiology and outcomes from out-of-hospital cardiac arrest in children: the Resuscitation Outcomes Consortium Epistry-Cardiac Arrest. Circulation 2009;119:1484–1491.

138. Zaritsky A, Nadkarni V, Getson P, Kuehl K. CPR in children. Ann Emerg Med 1987;16:1107–1111.

139. Gillis J, Dickson D, Rieder M, Steward D, Edmonds J. Results of inpatient pediatric resuscitation. Crit Care Med 1986;14:469–471.

140. Reis AG, Nadkarni V, Perondi MB, Grisi S, Berg RA. A prospective investigation into the epidemiology of in-hospital pediatric cardiopulmonary resuscitation using the international Utstein reporting style. Pediatrics 2002;109:200–209.

141. Nadkarni VM, Larkin GL, Peberdy MA, Carey SM, Kaye W, Mancini ME, et al. First documented rhythm and clinical outcome from in-hospital cardiac arrest among children and adults. JAMA 2006;295:50–57.

142. Meaney PA, Nadkarni VM, Cook EF, Testa M, Helfaer M, Kaye W, et al. Higher survival rates among younger patients after pediatric intensive care unit cardiac arrests. Pediatrics 2006;118:2424–2433.

143. Parra DA, Totapally BR, Zahn E, Jacobs J, Aldousany A, Burke RP, et al. Outcome of cardiopulmonary resuscitation in a pediatric cardiac intensive care unit. Crit Care Med 2000;28:3296–3300.

144. Innes PA, Summers CA, Boyd IM, Molyneux EM. Audit of paediatric cardiopulmonary resuscitation. Arch Dis Child 1993;68:487–491.

145. Slonim AD, Patel KM, Ruttimann UE, Pollack MM. Cardiopulmonary resuscitation in pediatric intensive care units. Crit Care Med 1997;25:1951–1955.

146. Young KD, Gausche-Hill M, McClung CD, Lewis RJ. A prospective, population-based study of the epidemiology and outcome of out-ofhospital pediatric cardiopulmonary arrest. Pediatrics 2004;114: 157–164.

147. Suominen P, Baillie C, Korpela R, Rautanen S, Ranta S, Olkkola KT. Impact of age, submersion time and water temperature on outcome in near-drowning. Resuscitation 2002;52:247–254.

148. Rodriguez-Nunez A, Lopez-Herce J, Garcia C, Carrillo A, Dominguez P, Calvo C, et al. Effectiveness and long-term outcome of cardiopulmonary resuscitation in paediatric intensive care units in Spain. Resuscitation 2006;71:301–309.

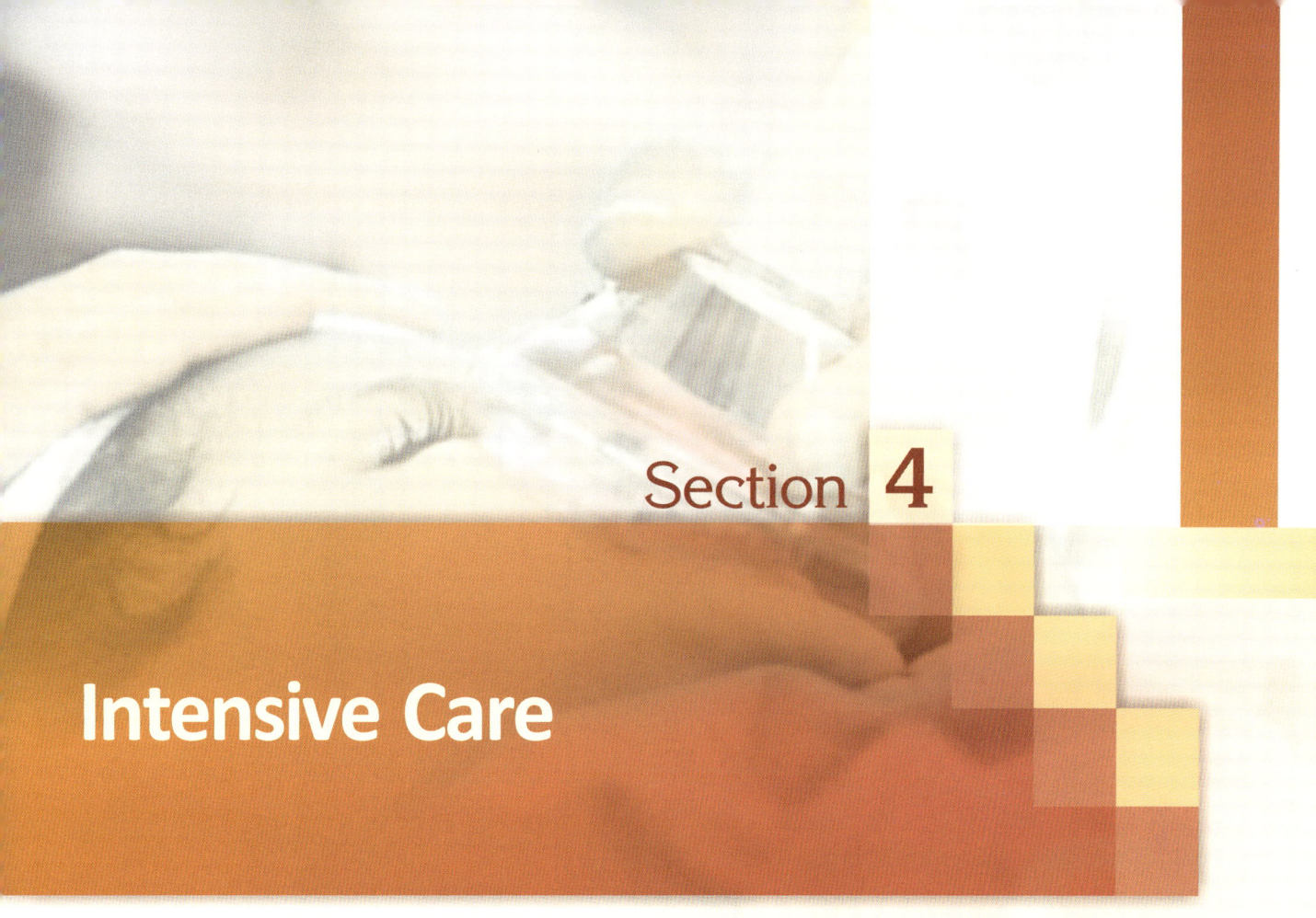

Section 4

Intensive Care

23

Organisation of a Paediatric Intensive Care Unit

Asha Tyagi, Abhijit Bhattacharya

- Need for intensive care in resourace-limited developing countries
- Guideline recommendations for designing a PICU
- Challenges in setting up of PICU in resource-limited situations

The mortality rate in children aged "Under-5 years" is an accurate predictor of child survival. There is a wide disparity in the "Under-5" mortality rates for developed countries versus developing ones, such as India. While Under-5 mortality rate is only 3/1000 in Japan, it is one of the highest at 59/1000 live births in India.[1] This contrast is a grim pointer to the third world's need for concentrated efforts in the area of health care.[1]

IS THERE A NEED FOR PAEDIATRIC ICUs IN INDIA?

India remains one of the countries with the lowest percentage of its GDP, only a meager 1%, being spent on public healthcare services.[2] Non-availability of quality health services is one of the reasons for high mortality amongst children.

In developing countries, it is the treatable and preventable infectious diseases that remain the leading cause of death for infants. Even for neonatal deaths, sepsis remains an important cause of in developing countries. While on one hand the presence of sepsis and infectious diseases demands larger availability of interventional health care, there is a paucity of available resources on the other. The preliminary question

regarding organisation of intensive care units (ICUs) in developing countries is whether it is justified to invest into such high-cost facilities in an already resource-limited setting. Critical care in a resource poor or constrained setting has been defined as the provision of care for life-threatening illness without regard to the location, including the pre-hospital, emergency, hospital wards, and intensive care setting.[3]

It has been argued in favour of setting up paediatric ICUs (PICUs) that if we are adequately geared to salvage an 80-year-old with acute myocardial infarction in intensive care services, why should a 4-year-old suffering with sepsis deserve any lesser.[4] Also, not only is the percentage of critically ill children higher in developing countries, the plight of these patients is likely to be worse.[5] Thus ICUs catering to critically ill children may well be a need of the hour. Critical care is a labour-intense way of caring for the extremely sick patients that goes much beyond the use of fancy expensive gadgets and equipment. Setting up ICUs may help to train health staff for early recognition, stabilisation and management of sick children, bringing about a ripple effect towards improvement of basic health services, bringing down the need for more invasive interventions, and improving overall outcomes in hospitalized children.[5–7] There is also evidence to show that the sickest subgroup of critically ill children is less likely to die, if treated in PICU in a tertiary care hospital.[8] Lastly, advancements in medicine and surgery have led to complex surgeries and interventions in sick children that demand intensive care of these patients.

RECOMMENDATIONS FOR SETTING UP OF A PAEDIATRIC ICU

A paediatric ICU usually needs to take care of critically ill children. Herein there may be slight variation in the inclusive ages of children, including references of up to 16 years age,[9] 0 to 18 years,[10] or all those except adults and newborns.[4] "Critically ill" implies patients whose homeostasis is compromised such that they require intensive monitoring and organ support by way of equipment and medications to restore and/or maintain body functions; or those who require or potentially require high dependency or intensive care whether medically, surgically or trauma-related.[10]

Various levels of ICU care have been defined and include level 1 care: High dependency care; level 2 care: Simple intensive care; level 3 care: Complex intensive care; and level 4 care: Highly specialised intensive care.[9,10] In developed countries, standards of care in paediatric intensive care suggest all levels of care to be provided within the PICU.[10] This may not be feasible in developing countries. Setting up of ICU should be according to needs of the patients being catered to. In case specialized care is not being offered, arrangements for the transfer of children to higher levels of ICU whenever required should be provided. Guidelines/recommendations and texts regarding organisation of PICUs are widely available. The guidelines given by paediatric section of Indian Society for Critical Care Medicine (ISCCM) is one such document in the Indian context.[9] International standards are also readily accessible.[10,11] Detailing of layout, designing, and availability of manpower, equipment and drugs can be readily referenced from these documents.[9–11]

Most documentations regarding setting up of ICUs deal with establishing the "structure" within which, patients who are critically ill will be looked after. While the goals of this development are spelt out in varying details in available guidelines/recommendations, the processes and anticipated challenges or difficulties in achieving them in resource-limited situations are not dwelt upon. In India, there remains a very wide disparity between standards of health care in various parts of the country, and even within a city or geographical part.

The profit-generating corporate hospitals caring for economically well-off patients usually have high revenue-generating, well-equipped ICUs. This is in contrast to the larger number of resource-crunched, overcrowded ICUs in government hospitals rendering free health services to the poor patients.

Thus, in certain situations in developing countries like ours, it may not be possible to completely adhere to existing guideline/recommendations. The need of setting up paediatric ICUs may often encourage accepting a certain amount of flexibility in the recommendations, more so since the guidelines for Indian scenario are not accepted as standards of care as yet.[9]

The following section gives a brief insight into salient features for setting up a PICU from pre-existing recommendations/guidelines.[9–11]

Preliminary Step

Before designing any PICU, an assessment of the perceived health needs of the patient population must include the expected estimate of the case-mix, i.e. type of cases, the level of interventions required, and nature of admissions (planned following surgical or non-surgical reasons, or unplanned emergency care). This data is likely to be peculiar for each PICU, irrespective of the common indications for ICU admission remaining as cardiovascular, respiratory or neurologic support. An assessment of the need of ICU has then to be weighed along with available resources.

Usual Location of ICU

Location of ICU should not be dictated merely by the availability of a vacant section of hospital premises. It must be in proximity to possible ingress and egress pathways, i.e. operation theatres, emergency department, wards, and high dependency units; as well as lift, radiology and laboratory. It should be isolated from frequent human traffic as well.

Staff

There is a common recommendation in all the relevant documents to promote availability of adequate dedicated staff for PICUs. By dedicated, it is implied that they should not be looking after other clinical areas and rather be available for the PICU at all times. Since it is doctors and nurses who run the machines and ultimately care for patients in ICU, in certain developed countries as much as 80% of the budget is diverted to personnel development.

The medical director/intensivist in-charge should be a paediatrician trained and experienced in critical care of children.

Consultants should be with regular daytime commitment at all times, for ensuring that quality assurance, training, protocols and audits are in place. One consultant must be available at all times for every 8 or 10 PICU beds.

Medical trainee: Patient ratio should not exceed 1:5, and a senior resident must be available outside routine working hours, for every 8 beds at all times.

Nurse: Patient ratio can vary from 0.5:1 to 1:1 (ventilated patient) to even 2:1 (ventilated patient also on ECMO support), depending on the level of care required. *Customary rotation of ICU nursing staff to wards and other hospital outlets should be desisted from and completely discouraged.*

Ancillary staff posted exclusively for the ICU should include physiotherapist, dietician, technician, radiographer, cleaning staff, secretarial/clerical staff and preferably a biomedical engineer.

Design and Bed Strength

For a paediatric ward of 25 beds, a PICU with 6–8 beds is recommended. Bed strength of 6 to 10 is desirable for a single unit since less than 4 and more than 16 beds risk inefficiency. The calculated bed-strength should aim to achieve an annual average occupancy of around 80%. Contingency plan to accommodate flexible staffing during increased occupancy times must be in place.

Surface area of 150 to 200 square feet is recommended for an open design PICU, while larger space of 200 to 250 square feet is desirable, if cubicles are planned. It should be ensured that there is ample vacant area to allow easy access to patient head, and perform routine ICU procedures and radiologic imaging.

At least one, preferably two isolation rooms with a separate area of 250 square feet along with an anteroom of at least 20 square feet for hand washing and wearing mask and gown, and separate ventilation should be planned for.

Space for all concerned staff, storage of supplies and medications, and dirty and clean linen segregation should be arranged within the complex.

The PICU should be designed to accommodate at least one washbasin for every two beds. For each bed, there should be two wall outlets for oxygen, one for air, two for suction, and at least ten electrical outlets. Windows should be incorporated to prevent a sense of isolation. An uninterrupted power supply in accordance with electrical load of various equipments must be ensured, and there should preferably be centrally controlled air conditioning, and central heating/overhead warmers for temperature control.

Equipment

The equipment required for setting up of a PICU extends along a continuum starting from most basic ones, such as oxygen delivery masks, intravenous catheters, intravenous sets, to multipara monitors, and specialized ones, such as ultrasound and echo machines depending on the level of care being planned. Details of such equipment can be perused elsewhere.[9–11]

A mini-laboratory with arterial blood gas, electrolyte, blood sugar, urea, creatinine, prothrombin time, partial thromboplastin time, complete blood count, and urine examination with Gram stain should be considered adjacent to the PICU. Twenty-four-hour availability of on site or in hospital arterial blood gas is essential. As an alternative to stat laboratory adjacent to PICU, a central main laboratory facility with a turn around time (reporting time) of less than one hour for stat laboratory test results is acceptable.

A refrigerator is essential for some pharmaceuticals.

Drugs

A mobile crash cart with emergency drugs and portable monitor/defibrillator must be present. A detailed list of required drugs may be accessed elsewhere.[9] The emergency and essential drugs remain a must in any ICU while the requirement of others can depend on the expected patient type and has to be tailored for each ICU.

CHALLENGES TURNED TO OPPORTUNITIES: LESSONS LEARNT

Having thus made a case for advocating setting up of PICUs even in resource-limited countries, it is worthwhile to envisage the challenges that can be expected in the process. That challenges may well turn into opportunities for achieving the seemingly uphill task of setting up an ICU in a resource-limited situation is exemplified by the setting up of a PICU in resource-limited Nepal by a dedicated team.[5] The entire exercise is a lesson in will, motivation and managerial expertise besides the clinical skills.

During development and implementation phases, the challenges faced resulted in scaling down on the goals and expectations according to the available resources, and training of the existing manpower by experienced staff through an International collaboration. While assessing the needs, resources that were available were taken into due consideration, local staff and administration were collaborated with and most importantly an attempt to understand local medical culture and common practices was made. Enforcing international or even national guidelines to places seeped in their own culture may not only be inappropriate, but impossible as well. Guidelines have to be customized and improvised to suite the needs and available resources. It is interesting to note that no compromise was made on designated space (650 square feet for 6 bedded facility), a decision especially pertinent in the face of communicable diseases and overcrowding expected in the area. Cognizance was also taken of the long hours of lack of electrical supply and investment made into two independent power lines and generators. Even ventilators with long battery-lives up to 2–3 hours were preferentially sought. Availability of clean water was accepted as a challenge and its supply ensured by a dedicated dug-well, hospital's chlorination plant and a monthly surveillance for coliform bacteria.

Shortage of funds was circumvented by successfully seeking grants from international collaborators. The effort and motivation required for garnering such support is commendable and well elaborated in concerned text.[5] Equipment were purchased in USA and then sent to the hospital as donations, some was even shipped, taking several months. International experts who worked entirely on a voluntary service even paying their own travel expenses trained the doctors and nursing staff already employed in the hospital in critical care. The commitment that led to setting up of the ICU is a worthy lesson even though it is not part of any guideline or recommendation.

During maintenance phase, the team perceived loss of trained staff to other lucrative jobs, and forced rationing of ICU admission as the greatest challenges. The latter is also a common challenge in most Indian hospitals that are funded by the government for free health care to the poor.

Our national guidelines should be able to incorporate a framework of criteria for granting and denying admission based on available resources and expected patient functionality. To adhere to such guidelines will of course prove to be an ongoing challenge given the grey areas of practice of medicine, and an increasingly aware patient population.[5]

CONCLUSION

Organisation of a PICU should look much beyond setting up of an equipped building as per existing guidelines/recommendations. The entire pathway of looking after sick children will have to be strengthened. This should start from the child's arrival in hospital at emergency or non-emergency areas and include retrieval services within or outside the hospital. In developing countries, like ours, it also needs to be thought over whether building of large number of basic level intensive care units would be more productive than fewer fancier, costlier, highly equipped PICUs at tertiary centers. There is evidence to show that some of the most effective critical care interventions, including rapid fluid resuscitation, early antibiotics, and patient monitoring are relatively inexpensive[12] and can produce tremendous benefits as evidenced in the "surviving sepsis campaign guidelines".[13]

REFERENCES

1. Park K. Preventive Medicine in Obstetrics, Paediatrics and Geriatrics. In: Park's textbook of Preventive and Social Medicine, 22nd edn; Banarsidas Bhanot Publishers, Jabalpur; pp 480–562.

2. http://in.reuters.com/article/2014/12/23/india-health-budget-idINKBN0K10Y020141223. Accessed on 26.4.15.

3. Geiling J, Burkle FM Jr, Amundson D. Task Force for Mass Critical Care. Resource-poorsettings: infrastructure and capacity building: care of the critically ill and injured during pandemics and disasters: CHEST consensus statement. Chest 2014;146(4 Suppl):e156S–67S.

4. Ramesh S. Paediatric intensive care—update. Indian J Anaesth 2003;47(5):338–344.

5. Basnet S, Adhikari N, Koirala J. Challenges in setting up pediatric and neonatal intensive care units in a resource-limited country. Pediatrics 2011;128(4):e986–992.

6. Kissoon N, Argent A, Devictor D, et al. World Federation of Pediatric Intensive and Critical Care Societies: its global agenda. Pediatr Crit Care Med 2009;10(5):597–600.

7. Advanced Life Support Group. Advanced Paediatric Life Support, 3rd edn. London: British Medical Journal Publishing Group;2001.

8. Pollack MM, Alexandwr SR, Clark N, et al. Improved outcomes from tertiary centre paediatric intensive care: a statewide comparison of tertiary and non-tertiary facilities. Critical Care Med 1991;19:150–159.

9. Khilnani P. Indian Society of Critical Care Medicine (Pediatric Section); Indian Academy of Pediatrics (Intensive care Chapter). Consensus guidelines for pediatric intensive care units in India. Indian Pediatr 2002;39(1):43–50.

10. PICS. Standards for the Care of Critically Ill Children, 4th edn. London: Paediatric Intensive Care Society, 2010.

11. Rosenberg DI, Moss MM. American College of Critical Care Medicine of the Society of Critical Care Medicine. Guidelines and levels of care for pediatric intensive care units. Crit Care Med 2004;32(10):2117–2127.

12. Riviello ED, Letchford S, Achieng L, Newton MW. Critical care in resource-poor settings: lessons learned and future directions. Crit Care Med 2011;39(4):860–867.

13. Dellinger RP, Levy MM, Rhodes A, et al. Surviving Sepsis Campaign Guidelines Committee including. The Pediatric Subgroup. Surviving Sepsis Campaign: international guidelines for management of severe sepsis and septic shock, 2012. Intensive Care Med 2013;39(2):165–228.

24

The Critically Ill Septic Child— Role of Anaesthesiologist

Balakrishnan Ashokka, Abhijit Bhattacharya

- ▪ Introduction to sepsis, definitions
- ▪ Prevalence, patterns in paediatric sepsis
- ▪ Sepsis in children peculiarity
- ▪ Grades and clinical spectrum of sepsis
- ▪ Anaesthetist's role in septic children
- ▪ Preoperative preparation
- ▪ Intraoperative anaesthetic conduct
- ▪ Postoperative management
- ▪ Evidence based practice in pediatric sepsis management
- ▪ Multidisciplinary team roles and resource management

INTRODUCTION TO SEPSIS, DEFINITIONS

Sepsis is the systemic manifestation of infection. In its severe forms, septic shock is the presence of hemodynamic compromise despite fluid resuscitation. The international paediatric consensus conference (2007) defined **sepsis** as *'systemic inflammatory response syndrome (SIRS) in the presence of or as a result of suspected or proven infection'*. **Severe sepsis** was defined to be *'sepsis with one of the following: cardiovascular organ dysfunction; acute respiratory syndrome; 2 or more organ dysfunction'* while **septic shock** was defined as *'sepsis with cardiovascular failure'*. Current understanding of sepsis suggests the presence of homeostatic imbalance between inflammation, coagulation and fibrinolysis.[1]

The early goal directed therapy and the surviving sepsis guidelines have revolutionized the early aggressive management of septic shock. In this chapter, we provide an overview of the early diagnosis of sepsis, deductive approach to early management in the first hour and an overview of the scope and prospect of the existing management protocols in the approach to management of anaesthetic care of septic children.

PREVALENCE, PATTERNS IN PAEDIATRIC SEPSIS

The prevalence of sepsis has been on a steady rise in the past two decades. A recent study from USA showed that the prevalence in paediatrics rose from 0.56 to 0.89 cases per 1000, with a corresponding increase in paediatric severe sepsis. This trend has been attributed chiefly to increase in neonatal sepsis. Source of infection could be identified only in less than 30% of all cases and *Staphylococcus aureus* was identified as the most common pathogen.[2] The overall mortality rate of sepsis is 4.2% and is one of the commonest causes of death in children. Sepsis accounts for 10% of ICU admissions.

SEPSIS IN CHILDREN PECULIARITY

Sepsis contrasts the adults in its initial presentation and rapid progression downhill to refractory shock. A systematic approach to cardinal symptoms of sepsis is essential. The chief presenting features in children and neonates are shown in Table 24.1.

GRADES AND CLINICAL SPECTRUM OF SEPSIS

Understanding Type of Shock and Planning Management

Diagnosing and managing the degree of sepsis is more to do with understanding the type of shock, such as

Table 24.1	Chief presenting features in children and neonates
Children	**Neonates**
Triad of fever, tachycardia and vasodilatation and	▪ Tachycardia
1. Mental status alteration	▪ Respiratory distress
2. Suspected infection with hypo- or hyperthermia	▪ Poor feeding
3. Clinically inadequate perfusion with:	▪ Poor tone
▪ Altered/decreased mental status	▪ Poor colour
▪ Prolonged capillary refill >2 min	▪ Diarrhoea
▪ Mottled cool extremities	▪ Reduced perfusion with a h/o maternal chorioamnionitis or PROM
▪ Flash capp refill when in shock	
▪ Bounding pulse wide pulse pressure	
▪ Decreased UOP <1 ml/ kg/hour	

hypovolaemic, cardiogenic and distributive shock features. Three distinct patterns of clinical presentation of sepsis are known.[3]

1. Low cardiac output state with low volume, minimum SVR change
2. Low cardiac output state with low volume, low SVR.
3. Low cardiac output state with high SVR

More often the picture is complex with a combination of the patterns of shock and simultaneous management of all etiopathologies might be required. The earliest signs of clinical sepsis would include the drop in mentation, poor feeding and reduced physical activity of the child with a corresponding fall in blood pressure. The presence of temperature change and warm peripheries though indicate the presence of sepsis, are not specific in identifying the pattern of septic shock.

ANAESTHETIST'S ROLE IN SEPTIC CHILDREN

Most of the anaesthetist's involvement in management of septic children will depend on the existing infrastructure of the hospital. Some centers require the early expert assessment of the septic child by the anaesthetists in the emergency units for airway management, venous access, early ambulation to paediatric critical care units managed with active collaboration with paediatric intensivists. The role of presence of well-trained practicing paediatric anaesthetists in all acute care management areas is heavily debated.[4] Fully structured hospitals are well equipped with specialty services that chiefly require the perioperative role of anaesthetists for the surgical care of the patient, while the system is well-trained to support and manage sick and septic children.

Chief reasons for intraoperative surgical care of paediatric patients will be for *source control,* such as drainage of septic loculi or abdominal sepsis with bowel resection. As these are emergent surgeries with compromised critically ill children, the anaesthetists have to reach out to expedite early goal directed management of the septic child adhering to current international guidelines (Table 24.2). Adherence to international guidelines such as surviving sepsis (2012), American College of Critical Care Medicine (ACCM)-AHA-PALS guidelines, (2010) with a system-based practice on aggressive management in the first hour of presentation has been known to improve outcomes and reduce length of hospital stay.[5]

PREOPERATIVE PREPARATION

Effective perioperative care of septic patients starts with adequate preoperative preparation. Early goal-directed therapy and simultaneous assessment and co-management of sepsis is recommended. In addition, care should be given for administration of prokinetics and antacids or acid suppressors to reduce the risks of aspiration pneumonitis.

Early Recognition of Shock

The first hour of the patient's presentation is known to be most precious phase for improving outcomes. Every hour wasted without prompt institution of aggressive management has known to be increase in mortality by 40%. A time-sensitive goal-directed stepwise management of shock in children and infants was outlined by Zawistowski.[6] The author suggested 4 time zones and management protocols, such as 0–5 mins (recognition of shock, high flow

Table 24.2   Goals for early aggressive therapy

- **Early goal-directed therapy**
  - MAP >65 or age adjusted perfusion pressure
  - CVP >8
  - Lactate <2
  - $ScvO_2$ 70%
- **Early fluid resuscitation**
  - Bolus: 20 ml/ kg of crystalloids
  - Start inotropes when 40 ml/ kg given
  - Intubation and ventilation, if >60 ml/ kg
  - Crystalloids based
  - No colloids (to avoid starch-based solutions)
  - Albumin equivocal
- **Early inotropy (CATS study)**
  - No need to wait for CVP—peripheral dopamine or IO routes
  - Noradrenaline in warm shock
  - Dobutamine plus noradrenaline, if cardiogenic
  - Choice of inotropy
    - Vasopressin role, if refractory to noradrenaline
    - Dopamine role in inotropy without central line
    - Milrinone and vasodilators, like SNP for pulmonary hypertension and RV failure
- **Early intubation and ventilation**
  - Low threshold for intubation, if fluids >40–60 ml/kg
  - If refractory to catecholamine needs ventilation
  - Ventilation
    - 6–7 ml/kg
    - Peep 8–10
    - Plateau <30
- **Perfusion indices and end points for oxygenation**
  - Lactate
  - $ScvO_2$
  - Capillary refill return
  - Hypotension resolving with inotropy reduction
  - Return of mentation
- **Early source control and antibiotics**
  - Early investigations and surgical roles
  - First hour empirical antibiotics: follow local antibiogram and follow up sensitivity

oxygen and IV/IO access); 5–15 min (initial resuscitation); 15–60 min (fluid refractory shock, inotropes titration); >60 min (catecholamine-resistant shock, paediatric intensive care management, cold and warm shock approaches) and advanced monitoring and management (persistent catecholamine-resistant shock, ECMO).

Management of paediatric sepsis and emergencies should be with adherence to international guidelines, such as the ACCM-PALS with appropriate evaluation of local practices and possibilities. Practice of implementation of protocols based recognition of sepsis and adherence to guidelines have proven to show substantial reductions in *'time to receipt of time-sensitive interventions and a decrement in variations of treatment'.*[7] Main barriers in adherence to recommendations have been shown to be the absence of locally written protocols embracing the principles of the surviving sepsis guidelines and unavailability of devices that could measure continuously or serially the central venous oxygen saturation ($ScvO_2$) and hence the use of stepwise approach in the management of sepsis in children.[8]

The chief aims of management should resonate the core concepts, such as:

1. Prompt meticulous rapid assessment
2. Early goal-directed aggressive therapy (Fig. 24.1)
3. Early source control
4. Continued advanced support and
5. Definitive goals for management for the next 48 hours.

Prompt Rapid Assessment

This includes promptly identifying early signs of circulatory failure, triage of children who need immediate ventilatory support and quick identification of type of shock (cold, warm, cold and failed heart). Warm shock refers to distributive shock seen in early phases where there is peripheral vasodilation and low blood pressure chiefly from endotoxaemia. Cold shock is more common in later stages of sepsis with cardiodepression or some variations in paediatric sepsis presentation and in the immunocompromised children and in neonates.

Almost all of the variants of sepsis are qualified by a fall in blood pressure. Understanding the relationship between preload, contractility and after-load will help in effective early management of sepsis. It is known that in children **oxygen delivery**, rather than the presence of excessive oxygen extraction is the major determinant of oxygen consumption.[3] Improved outcomes are probable, if a goal of oxygen consumption more than 200 ml/ min/sq.m could be achieved. So attention is directed towards assessment and management of cardiac output (CO) and cardiac index (CI). Use of ultrasonography (transthroacic, transoesophageal) has revolutionized the scientific

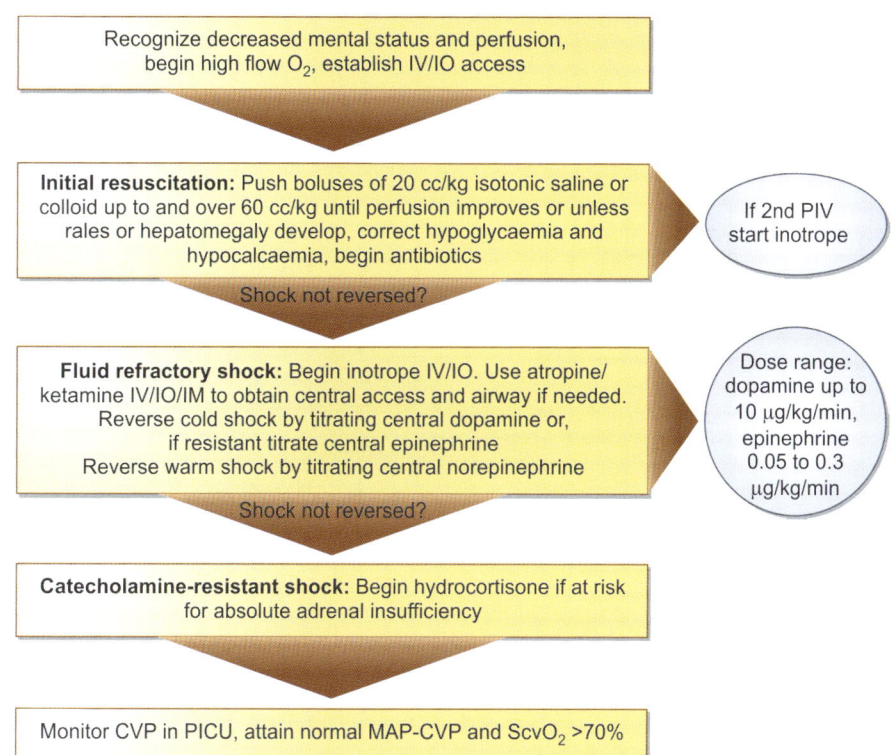

Recognize decreased mental status and perfusion, begin high flow O$_2$, establish IV/IO access

Initial resuscitation: Push boluses of 20 cc/kg isotonic saline or colloid up to and over 60 cc/kg until perfusion improves or unless rales or hepatomegaly develop, correct hypoglycaemia and hypocalcaemia, begin antibiotics

If 2nd PIV start inotrope

Shock not reversed?

Fluid refractory shock: Begin inotrope IV/IO. Use atropine/ketamine IV/IO/IM to obtain central access and airway if needed. Reverse cold shock by titrating central dopamine or, if resistant titrate central epinephrine Reverse warm shock by titrating central norepinephrine

Dose range: dopamine up to 10 μg/kg/min, epinephrine 0.05 to 0.3 μg/kg/min

Shock not reversed?

Catecholamine-resistant shock: Begin hydrocortisone if at risk for absolute adrenal insufficiency

Monitor CVP in PICU, attain normal MAP-CVP and ScvO$_2$ >70%

Fig. 24.1. Early goal directed management[9](ACCM-PALS guidelines suggesting the therapies to achieve normal blood pressure and capillary filling time <= 2 seconds)

approach to management of critically ill patients. Transthoracic echo can identify the presence of underfilled ventricles, compromised cardiac contractility and poor venous filling through IVC windows. While the diagnostic value of these techniques is commendable, the *scope of continuous monitoring and meticulously trending of progress* is not practically possible. Use of pulmonary artery catheter in the critical care setup is nearly obsolete. Semi-invasive cardiac output measurements can add valuable information in the management of septic children. Split connectors assembled on to peripheral arterial cannulae (Flo trac 4.0, Edward Lifesciences) can be one of the simplest tools to obtain holistic performance indices of the cardiac function. Our simplified approach to the management of septic shock with the use of systolic volume variation (SVV) is described in Fig. 24.2.

The presence of systolic volume variation more than 12 suggests the presence of poor volume status and the need for improvement of the volume. Upon optimizing the volume with SVV correction, then we deduce information from cardiac output (CO) measurement and systemic vascular resistance to diagnose the presence of cardiogenic shock for use inotropy or distributive shock for commencing vaso-pressors. This less invasive approach to management of haemodynamics is not reliable in the presence of arrhythmias.

INTRAOPERATIVE ANAESTHETIC CONDUCT

Intraoperative care of septic patient starts with *careful planning* of various stages of the actual conduct of anaesthesia: safe transfer of critically ill patient to operation theatre, adequate prior preparation of operating theatre for paediatric anaesthetic manage-ment, such as airway equipment, pre-calculated resuscitation drugs, appropriate fluids pre-warmed and surgical and scrub teams prepared and ready to minimize time under anaesthetics.

While sedation might be required for procedures, such as endoscopy, CT scan or MRI, the septic child is at a potential risk for pulmonary aspiration. Hence early definitive access of the airway with endotracheal

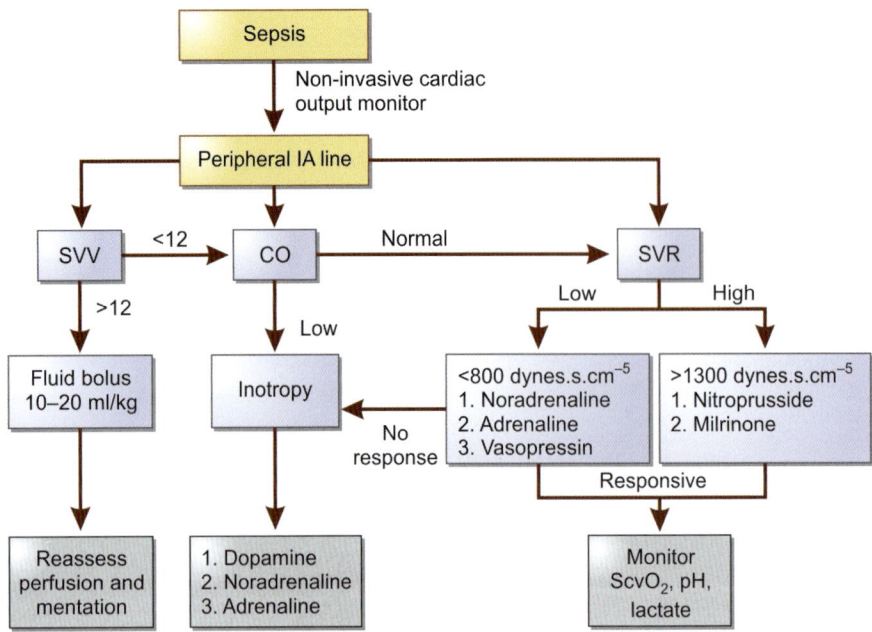

Fig. 24.2. A deductive approach to management of patient with sepsis with use of systolic volume variation (SVV), cardiac output (CO) and systemic vascular resistance (SVR)

intubation under rapid sequence intubation might be the safest option.

Peripheral venous access might have been established in the preoperative resuscitation period. But for the actual conduct of anaesthetic in septic children, large bore free flowing venous access will be required. With peripheral shut down in septic shock, intraosseous route might come in handy for the early phase of resuscitation. The use of external jugular vein (EJV) will come in handy and fairly spared by the parent teams for anaesthetists to use. When required the EJV peripheral lines can be used to rail road with a 2–3 lumen large venous central lines for post-op inotropy, fluid, blood sampling and parenteral nutrition. This technique does spare the central vein for vascular sheaths for dialysis in the long run or for portacath or Hickman lines. Central venous cannulation when done in trained hands under absolute sterile conditions is an important tool for executing goal-directed fluid management, frequent measurement of central venous oxygen saturation (ScvO$_2$) as indices of global perfusion and for administration of inotropes in refractory shock.

Of the options for drugs used in actual conduct of anaesthetic (Table 24.3), cardiostable induction agents are more commonly used. Combination of ketamine,

midazolam and opioids is safer alternative to thiopentone, propofol (hypotension) and etomidate (adrenal axis suppression). Muscle relaxant use is variable; rocuronium is increasingly popular for RSI, with concerns of hyperkalaemia with suxamethonium, given the background of acidosis of severe sepsis. Analgesia is usually multimodal. Central neuraxial blockade is limited by white cell counts >15000 and coagulopathy of sepsis. Short-acting cardiostable opioids, such as fentanyl, are a safer option. NSAID use is influenced by presence of pre-existing coagulopathy and chance of platelet dysfunction. Role of peripheral neural blocks in paediatric anaesthesia for sepsis is fairly limited.

Particular care for preoperative decompression of stomach with gastric tubes whenever possible is done preinduction. Large bore Yankauer suction should be checked and ready for induction. Cricoid pressure provided by trained dedicated assistant from the patient's left side aids intubation with no limitation of making an arc-like movement of laryngoscope from right side of the mouth to left. Pre-styleted ETTs are a better option to minimize intubation attempts. Use of paediatric airway adjuncts, such as intubating bougies, might be required.

Rapid desaturation is more common in septic children owing to a multitude of factors. Younger

Table 24.3	Summary of anaesthetic management, drugs and rationale	
Steps	**Drugs**	**Feature**
Induction	Thiopentone	Precipitous fall in BP
		Fastest induction agent
	Propofol	Fall in BP, organ metab
		Not approved in <2 years
	Ketamine	Cardiostable
		Caution in high SVR sepsis groups
		Maintains SVR, reducing reversal of shunt
	Midazolam + fentanyl	Onset not predictable
		Post-op ICU ventilation might be needed
	Inhalational	Very limited role; IV induction safer
Maintenance	Inhalationals	Avoid halothane— cardiodepressant
	Ketamine	Infusions or repeat bolus could be the safest in unstable patients
	Opioids	Fentanyl more predictable
		Morphine needs titration to haemodynamics, liver kidney function issues
	Muscle relaxants	Rocuronium for RSI better
		Suxamethonium, if difficult airway
		Atracurium—might require frequent bolus
	Fluids	Crystalloids safest
		Colloids: albumin > gelo > starch
	Monitoring	▪ Invasive arterial BP
		▪ UOP for perfusion
		▪ $ScvO_2$—global perfusion
		▪ Temperature; high or low
		▪ Blood gases: lactate, P/F
		▪ Non-invasive CO, SVV,
Postoperative	Pain management	▪ Spinal/epidural relative C/I
		▪ NSAIDs
		▪ Platelet dysfunction
		▪ Opioids: hampers mental status assessment for sepsis progress
		▪ Difficult to assess, evaluate in critically ill children
Common targets	MAP	Age adjusted equivalent of 65 mm Hg
	CVP	8–10 cm H_2O (at least >5 cm H_2O)
	Lactate	<2
	Base deficit	<5
	Non-invasive CO	SVV <12; SVR >800 <1300 dynes.s.cm^{-5}
	$ScvO_2$	70%

children have poor chest mechanics and discordance of breathing. The FRC is further reduced by distended abdomen with splinting of the diaphragm. Immune-mediated SIRS can result in early acute lung injury resulting in perfusion defects and shunt fraction worsening. The oxygen consumption is nearly double that of adults (adults 3–4 ml/kg/min vs neonates— 6–7 ml/kg/min) resulting in rapid desaturation during apnoea of general anaesthetic induction.

POSTOPERATIVE MANAGEMENT

Post-anaesthetic care of septic patients can be very stormy in the first 24–48 hours. These could be due to septic flare up by systemic seeding of the pathogens and inflammatory mediators after the septic foci are explored. Early mucosal ischaemia from hypo-perfusion of bowels results in systemic translocation of gut commensals. Early enteral feeding is known to minimize this peril. Stress of anaesthesia and surgery can result in worsening of the clinical picture. Most paediatric septic patients would require to be nursed in the high dependency equipped with trained staff familiar with 'early goal-directed therapy'.

Intubated patients may require to be electively ventilated in postoperative period for allowing the body to acclimatize to large fluid translocations and

SIRS response in the immediate postoperative period. Monitoring of intra-abdominal pressure (IAP) would detect early and prevent perioperative kidney failure. Staged abdominal closure may be needed to prevent excessive increase in intra-abdominal pressures, especially in the presence of ileus, sepsis, perioperative stress and catecholamine infusion use. Special efforts are needed to seek for fluid and electrolyte management, correction of coagulopathy. Point of care testing, such as thromboelastography (TEG), has revolutionized the practice of component therapy of blood and blood products usage. Multi-organ dysfunction syndrome (MODS) would be a common occurrence in the first 24–72 hours after abdominal surgeries for source control for sepsis. This requires setting of specific targets for optimization of target organ function meticulous early resolution of issues. All the targets of sepsis management in the goal-directed therapy with antibiotic coverage for the surgical intervention continued for first 24–48 hours or until clinical resolution of symptoms are noticed. It is well-known that adherence to established guidelines, such as the PALS, is known to improve patient outcomes especially shorter length of stay in hospital.[5]

Pain assessment and management might be a very challenging issue in paediatric septic patients. Where possible, postoperative pain management with neuraxial blockade, such as caudal, lumbar and thoracic epidural infusion, has very favourable postoperative outcome mainly by reduction of ilues, reduced intra-abdominal tension, obtunded systemic stress response and opioid-sparing effects. More often use of central neuraxial blockade usage is limited by presence of systemic sepsis with the presence of high white cell counts, coagulopathy and background hypotension. While use of NSAIDs might be limited by coagulopathy and renal compromise, opioid infusion might be the mainstay of postoperative pain relief.

Neonatal Sepsis Management

Special emphasis is given for the care of neonates with sepsis. Neonatal sepsis has been shown to be the reason for increase in prevalence of paediatric sepsis. The clinical picture is very delicate and challenging to deduce what type of sepsis is ongoing in a neonate-cold, warm or mixed shock. The prime evil is the clinical inability to differentiate between shock of septic origin and cardiac failure. The clinical picture is more complicated as the presentation of the both situations can have peripheral shut down, hypothermia, poor feeding and dusky skin. The newborns (first 7 days of life) are at risk of reversal of shunt to fetal circulation from failing systemic blood pressure and increasing pulmonary blood pressures due to acidosis, anoxia, and hypercarbia. This situation results in fairly high mortality. This catastrophic condition should be prevented or at least recognized early and systemic blood pressures supported with inotropes and judicious fluid management with ventilatory support. Neonatal lines and perioperative management are advanced specialty services that are best handled by trained team of specialists to improve outcomes.

EVIDENCE-BASED PRACTICE IN PAEDIATRIC SEPSIS MANAGEMENT

Adjuvant Therapy and Evidence

Debate exists on what would be the ideal fluid of choice, the role of steroids, suppressors of endotoxaemia, early renal replacement therapy and use of newer advanced modalities for deduction and management of sepsis. A few of the areas of interest in the past decade have been listed in Table 24.4.

MULTIDISCIPLINARY TEAM ROLES AND RESOURCE MANAGEMENT

Team-based management is paramount in the early recognition and prompt initiation of therapy of sepsis. Precious time and muscle is lost on paperwork referring to specialties and the supporting experts to initiate management. The key to efficient outcomes is *"simultaneous assessment and co-management"* irrespective of the diagnosis and source of infection. The principles of early management should be the same and protocol based, adjusted every hour akin to the clinical status of the patient situation with a chronological log of interventions and management reinstated. The team that would be involved in care of septic child would include:

- Emergency medicine or casualty services: Early recognition and prompt initiation
- Paediatric medicine: Specialty expert management
- Nursing and allied support: Completion of orders, prompt coordination with teams, specialists, investigations, report of critical alerts in clinical and investigations.

Table 24.4	Evidence based practice in paediatric sepsis management
■ **Steroids (corticus trial)**	• Low dose steroids in refractory shock
	• High dose steroids increase secondary infection and mortality
■ **Immunotherapy**	• Immunosuppression vs immunostimulation: not significant
	• TNF and IL-1 antagonists
	• TLR (toll like receptor) antagonists
■ **Nutritional support**	• Early enteral nutrition has proven to have better outcomes
■ **Glucose management**	• Tight vs non-tight glucose control
	• NICE sugar trial and non-tight strategy for glucose control (target <200 mg%) has proven to be better in reducing mortality.
■ **Activated protein C**	• **Drotrecogin alfa** (activated)—DrotAA (PROWESS trial)—increased bleeding risks
	• **PROWESS-SHOCK** trial in progress
■ **Sepsis and ALI/ ARDS:** ARDSNet protocol for lung protective strategy. Prevention of barotraumas, volutrauma, atelectotrauma and biotrauma	

Box 24.1: Surviving sepsis campaign: International guidelines for severe sepsis management 2012[10]

■ Early quantitative resuscitation of the septic patient during the first 6 hours after recognition (1C);
blood cultures before antibiotic therapy (1C);

■ Imaging studies performed promptly to confirm a potential source of infection (UG); administration of broad-spectrum antimicrobials therapy within 1 hour of recognition of septic shock (1B) and severe sepsis without septic shock (1C) as the goal of therapy;

■ Reassessment of antimicrobial therapy daily for de-escalation, when appropriate (1B); infection source control with attention to the balance of risks and benefits of the chosen method within 12 hours of diagnosis (1C);

■ Initial fluid resuscitation with crystalloid (1B) and consideration of the addition of albumin in patients who continue to require substantial amounts of crystalloid to maintain adequate mean arterial pressure (2C) and the avoidance of hetastarch formulations (1B);

■ Initial fluid challenge in patients with sepsis-induced tissue hypoperfusion and suspicion of hypovolaemia to achieve a minimum of 30 ml/kg of crystalloids (more rapid administration and greater amounts of fluid may be needed in some patients (1C);

■ Fluid challenge technique continued as long as haemodynamic improvement is based on either dynamic or static variables (UG);

■ Norepinephrine as the first-choice vasopressor to maintain mean arterial pressure >65 mm Hg (1B); epinephrine when an additional agent is needed to maintain adequate blood pressure (2B); vasopressin (0.03 U/min) can be added to norepinephrine to either raise mean arterial pressure to target or to decrease norepinephrine dose but should not be used as the initial vasopressor (UG); dopamine is not recommended except in highly selected circumstances (2C); dobutamine infusion administered or added to vasopressor in the presence of:
  • Myocardial dysfunction as suggested by elevated cardiac filling pressures and low cardiac output, or
  • Ongoing signs of hypoperfusion despite achieving adequate intravascular volume and adequate mean arterial pressure (1C); avoiding use of intravenous hydrocortisone in adult septic shock patients, if adequate fluid resuscitation and vasopressor therapy are able to restore haemodynamic stability (2C);

■ Haemoglobin target of 7–9 g/dl in the absence of tissue hypoperfusion, ischaemic coronary artery disease, or acute haemorrhage (1B).

Recommendations specific to paediatric severe sepsis include:

■ Therapy with face mask oxygen, high flow nasal cannula oxygen, or nasopharyngeal continuous PEEP in the presence of respiratory distress and hypoxemia (2C);

■ Use of physical examination therapeutic end points, such as capillary refill (2C); for septic shock associated with hypovolaemia, the use of crystalloids or albumin to deliver a bolus of 20 ml/kg of crystalloids (or albumin equivalent) over 5–10 min (2C);

■ More common use of inotropes and vasodilators for low cardiac output septic shock associated with elevated systemic vascular resistance (2C);

■ And use of hydrocortisone only in children with suspected or proven "absolute" adrenal insufficiency

■ Intensive care team: As part of reach out and early assessment before admission to prevent delays in acute care services, not staying cocooned inside the walls of the ICU.

- Anaesthesia services: Coordinating actively with medical and surgical specialties when there is a need for source control and surgical drainage of infection; prompt decision making on postoperative disposition, need for invasive monitoring, prolonged and intensive support in refractory cases requiring advanced monitoring interpretation and access.

- Administrative support in coordination of care, processes and protocol: Nurse manager and directors of the clinical specialties performing quality assurance.

REFERENCES

1. Skrupky LP, Kerby PW, Hotchkiss RS. Advances in the management of sepsis and in the understanding of key immunologic defects of the disorder. Anesthesiology 2011; 115(6):1349–1362. DOI: 10.1097/ALN.0b013e31823422e8.

2. Hartman ME, Linde-Zwirble W, Angus DC, et al. Trends in the epidemiology of pediatric severe sepsis. Pediatr Crit Care Med 2013;14:686–693. DOI: 10.1097/PCC.0b013e 3182917fad.

3. Playfor S. Management of critically ill child with sepsis. Contin Educ Anaesth Crit Care Pain 2005;4(1):12–15. DOI: 10.1093/bjaceaccp/mkh004.

4. Tomlinson A. Anaesthetists and care of critically ill child. Anaesthesia 2003;58:309–311.

5. Paul R, Neuman MI, Monuteaux MC, Melendez. Adherence to PALS sepsis guidelines and hospital length of stay. Pediatrics 2012;130:273–280. DOI:10.1542/peds.2012-0094.

6. Zawistowski CA. The management of sepsis. Curr Probl Pediatr Adolesc Health Care 2013;43:285–291. DOI: 10.1016/j.cppeds.2013.10.005.

7. Cruz AT, Perry AM, Williams EA, et al. Implementation of goal-directed therapy for children with suspected sepsis in the emergency department. Pediatrics 2011;127:758–766. DOI:10.1542/peds.2010-2895.

8. Santschi M, Leclerc F. Management of children with sepsis and septic shock: a survey among pediatric intensivists of the Reseau Mere-Enfant de la Francophonie. Ann Intensive Care 2013;3:7. Open access, downloaded 22 July 2014.

9. Kissoon N, Orr RA, Carcillo JA. Updated American college of critical care medicine—Pediatric advanced life support guidelines for managment of pediatric and neonatal septic shock. *Relevance to the emergency care clinician.* Pediatr Emerg Care 2010;26(11):867–869.

10. Dellinger RP, Levy MM, Rhodes A, et al. Surviving sepsis campaign: international guidelines for management of severe sepsis and septic shock, 2012. Intensive Care Med 2013;39:165–228. DOI 10.1007/s00134-012-2769-8.

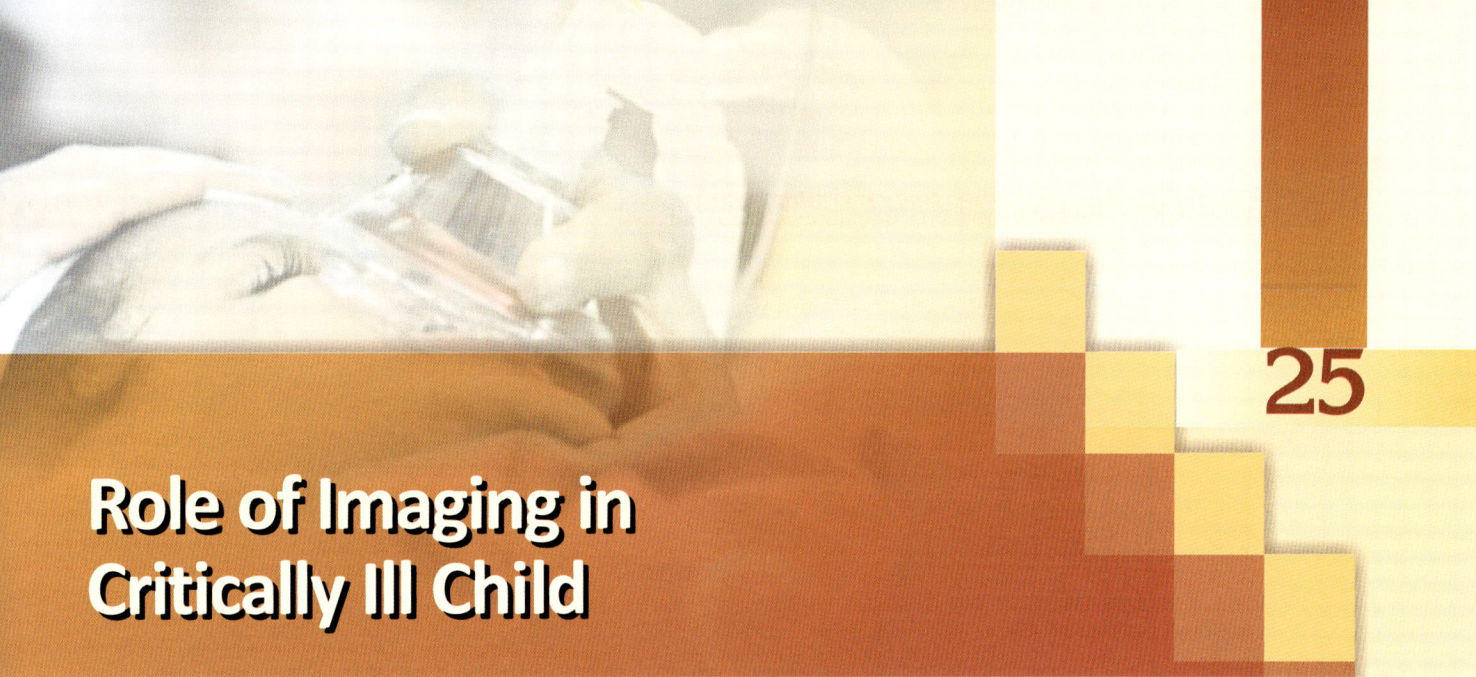

25

Role of Imaging in Critically Ill Child

Karuna Taneja

- Radiation concerns for patients and caregivers
- Imaging techniques available
- Computed tomography
- Imaging in the ICU
- General imaging
- Chest X-ray
- Specific pulmonary condition requiring imaging
- Imaging-guided intervention

We have not dealt with disease conditions and situations of neonates in this chapter.

The intensive care unit is a very special environment requiring expertise from the technicians and radiologists who have to work in a challenging situation. Patients are typically very sick, frequently unconscious, and almost always connected to life-support and monitoring equipment. As a result of this, the majority of imaging examinations are performed on patients with limited ability to cooperate and often at the bedside.

No specialised training is required to become an ICU radiologist. Expertise can be achieved, inclose cooperation with the ICU and emergency physicians.

RADIATION CONCERNS FOR PATIENTS AND CAREGIVERS (STAFF ON DUTY)

Diagnostic medical radiation (X-rays, fluoroscopy, CT, radionuclide imaging) has traditionally been responsible for the largest source of radiation exposure resulting from human activity. However, recent data (National Commission of Radiation Protection and Management 2007) reveal that medical sources may currently exceed 50% of all exposure. In contrast, background radiation is only 3–3.6 mSv/yr.

Two major advances have the potential to lower the radiation dose of plain radiographs and fluoroscopy: **pulsed fluoroscopy and digital imaging**. With pulsed fluoroscopy, the patient is exposed to 30 to 50% less radiation because of the change from continuous to intermittent fluoroscopy (i.e. 7.5 frames/sec). Digital imaging results in significant radiation dose reduction, but there is an increase in image noise—resulting in lower image quality. Images obtained are of diagnostic quality. Not only can digital technology permit dose reduction, it also reduces repeated patient exposure, because of post-processing availability.

CT delivers large doses of ionizing radiation, and one CT examination gives a dose of 35 mSv. Typically paediatric doses should be 2 to 8 mSv.

It is important to utilize techniques with minimal ionizing radiation in all paediatric imagings.

The ALARA (as low as reasonably achievable) concept should be adhered to:

- Screening examination using radiation: Is the examination necessary?
- High exposure examination should be reviewed and appropriate examination selected. MRI should be substituted for CT. This should be done with discussion with the referring physician.

- Consultation to obtain proper tests. The test being performed should have good sensitivity in diagnosis.
- Prescribing the proper protocols (technical factors) for:
  - Radiographs
  - Fluoroscopy
  - Computed tomography (CT)

Multi-slice CT has greater radiation dose than single slice tomography.

Minimizing the radiation to children requires attention and often meticulous technique.

The goal is to achieve a diagnostic image, not the most beautiful. Further research into ways of reducing dose to paediatric patients is crucial. By avoiding an inappropriate examination or changing to a non-radiation-producing modality, the radiation dose is reduced.[1]

IMAGING TECHNIQUES AVAILABLE

Conventional Radiography/X–rays

Portable X-ray machines are using digital technology today, allowing for telediagnostics, if need be. X-ray machines emit ionizing radiation, which requires adequate radiation protection for patients and staff.

Plane X-ray of chest and abdomen continue to be used as primary imaging technique for diagnosis and follow up in most ICU setting.

Ultrasonography can be utilized for diagnostic purposes and in certain interventional procedures.

Portable ultrasound is ideal for bedside examinations and ICU physicians are gaining a certain expertise in point-of-care ultrasound examinations allowing them to follow certain interventions with the assistance of real-time imaging. Diagnostic ultrasound, however, is best performed by radiologist.

Mobile CT and MR are not routinely used, as they are not widely available. CT when performed in the radiology department requires detailed planning of transport logistics for sick ICU patients.

For MRI examinations, there are even more limitations, as only special, MR-compatible equipment has to be used during the procedure.

Plain X-ray with digital technology which includes picture archiving and communication system (PACS) is the backbone of ICU imaging.

Availability, cost-effectiveness and radiation dose are some of the other important factors determining the choice of the imaging modality while investigating various clinical problems. This chapter will discuss the role of conventional radiological procedures vis-à-vis the newer techniques in common clinical situations.

X-ray films should always be viewed on high resolution monitors as important findings can be missed in suboptimal viewing. Never see X-rays in sunlight or hold them up against the window for viewing.

Advantages of computed radiography (CR with PACS):

- Better quality radiographs
- Post-processing
- Rapid transmission of images is available
- Improved diagnostic accuracy and confidence for the radiologist since previous radiographs are easily available with PACS.

However, there is no substitute for daily interaction between radiologist and clinical team.

Thoracic imaging often reveals abnormalities which may not be detected clinically:

- Portable chest radiograph is an integral supplement to physical examination and aids diagnosis and management and monitoring response to therapy. Conditions where this is of great value is in:
  - Malposition of invasive devices.
  - Early detection of new problems, e.g. pneumonia, atelectasis, effusion.
  - Identification of emergency, e.g. pneumothorax and volume loss.
- Abdominal radiographs may be performed for assessment of abdominal distension.
- Plain X-rays of the skull are rarely performed except in Neurosurgery patients specifically with the intention of locating an intraventricular catheter.

Ultrasonography

It has several distinct advantages over other imaging techniques mainly because this technique is non-invasive and free of radiation which makes it especially suitable for imaging children. Technical advances, such as multifrequency transducers and colour Doppler, have enabled greater use of point of care ultrasound. These machines are portable, light weight and have high resolution.[2]

Potential uses of US in the ICU can be diagnostic or therapeutic.

Diagnostic applications of ultrasound are:

- Detection of pleural or pericardial effusion.
- Follow-up focused abdominal sonography (FAST) for trauma patients
- Diagnosis of urinary retention
- Diagnosis of abscess or soft tissue infection
- Hydrocephalus or intraventricular haemorrhage in babies.

Therapeutic applications:

- Placement of vascular access catheters
- Drainage of pleural effusion
- Abdominal paracentesis[2]

Computed Tomography

Obtaining a scan must not obstruct effective resuscitation; rushing the patient to scan before stabilization is a common mistake. Sending images to specialists, through telemedicine/teleradiology is valuable.

IMAGING IN THE INTENSIVE CARE UNIT

Imaging in the ICU can be broadly categorized to cranial, thoracic and abdominal. The mainstay of imaging in the majority of clinical conditions is chest X-rays (portable) and point of care ultrasonography, with or without Doppler imaging.

Common Conditions

Common conditions which demand intensive care in pediatric practice are:

General Conditions

- Poisoning—inhalation injury.
- Polytrauma—for assessment of site and severity of trauma
- Abdominal—sepsis to locate source of infection.
- After tube placement, catheter insertion.
- Burns.

CNS

- Seizures and ICSOL
- Meningitis, brain abscess, otitis media.
- Head trauma—playgrounds, road traffic.

Respiratory System

- Foreign body inhalation
- Croup
- Pneumothorax—trauma, sepsis
- Pneumonia
- Inhalation injuries—burns, poisons
- Asthma
- ARDS

Gastrointestinal System/Abdomen

- Pain abdomen—surgical, non-surgical, like gall-stones, renal stones, constipation
- As part of polytrauma, sepsis, torsion testis
- Intra-abdominal abscess—liver, retroperitoneal haematoma

Radiology evaluation for all abdominal lesions includes fluoroscopy to evaluate airways and diaphragm.

Cardiovascular System

- Pulmonary emboli—due to oral contraceptive.
- Central line occlusion
- Complication of line—thrombosis, arterial or venous
- Check X-ray after tube/pacing wire/catheter insertion

Ventilated Patients

- To look for improvement
- To look for collapse/consolidation
- Post-bronchoscopy to look for clearance of opacity.

Cranial Imaging

Plain X-rays of the skull are rarely performed except in neurosurgical patients specifically with the intention of locating an intraventricular catheter.

Common emergencies in the ICU setting which require head and neck imaging are:

- Seizures and ICSOL (intracranial space occupying lesion)
- Meningitis, brain abscess, otitis media
- Head trauma in—playgrounds or, road traffic

Transcranial Doppler sonography (TCD) can measure mean blood flow velocity, pulsatility index. These indices effectively rule out high probability of vasospasm. TCD studies have a high specificity for the confirmation of intracranial circulatory arrest and brain death. However, one requires highly trained staff for diagnostic monitoring.[3]

Computed tomography is the mainstay and the investigation of choice for all conditions of the head and neck.

Cervical spine imaging recommendations are variable. If a head CT is being performed, the neck should be included. Without a neck CT, plain X-rays (two views) of the spine are taken in patients <5 years and an odontoid peg view is added in those older than 5 years.[4]

The mainstay of all ICU imaging is the plain X-ray of the chest.

Thoracic imaging often reveals abnormalities which may not be detected clinically. Portable chest radiograph is an integral supplement to physical examination and aids diagnosis, management and monitoring response to therapy. Conditions where this is of great value are in:

- Malposition of invasive devices,
- Early detection of new problems, e.g. pneumonia, atelectasis
- Identification of emergency (pneumothorax), volume loss.[5]

Role of chest X-ray and approach to interpreting the portable chest radiograph:

- Technical quality
- Look for all catheters and devices
- Assess cardiovascular status
- Check abnormal parenchyma opacities
- Search for evidence of barotrauma
- Look for pleural effusion
- Comparison with all previous imaging studies is crucial.

INVASIVE DEVICES

Proper positioning is not clinically apparent.[6,7]

Endotracheal Tube

It should be 5 cm above the carina. ET tube is inserted for ventilation of both lungs and to prevent aspiration. It should lie mid-way between larynx and carina, approximately at the level of thoracic vertebra 3 so that injury to either structure or complications, like inadvertent extubation or selective main-stem bronchus intubation are avoided (Fig. 25.1). Selective

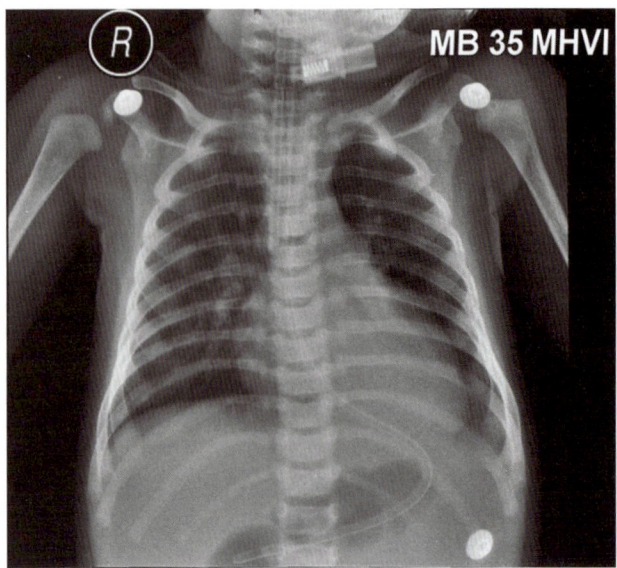

Fig. 25.1. Correct placement of the endotracheal and naso-gastric tubes

intubation can cause collapse of the contralateral lung and, hyperinflation of the ipsilateral lung. An immediate chest X-rays after intubation is warranted to check the correct position of the ET tube. Right or left mainstem intubation can be clinically occult in about 60% of patients and revealed only on chest X-rays (Figs 25.2A and B).[6]

Inadvertent oesophageal intubation is a dreadful complication, which is mostly diagnosed clinically; it

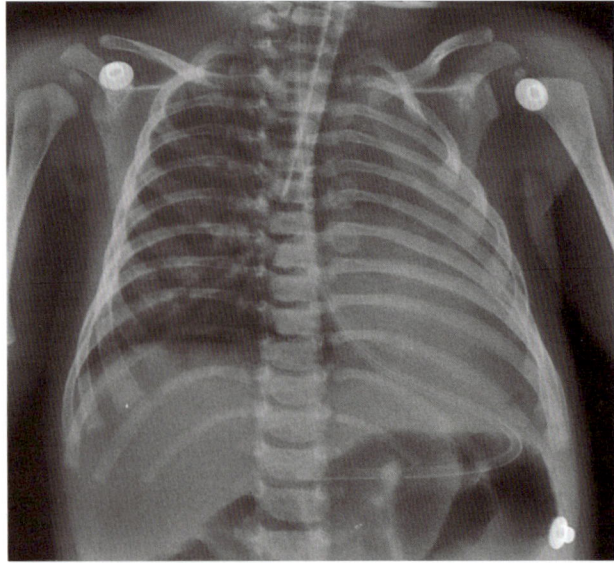

Fig. 25.2A. Placement of the endotracheal tube selectively into the right mainstem bronchus has resulted in collapse of the left lung

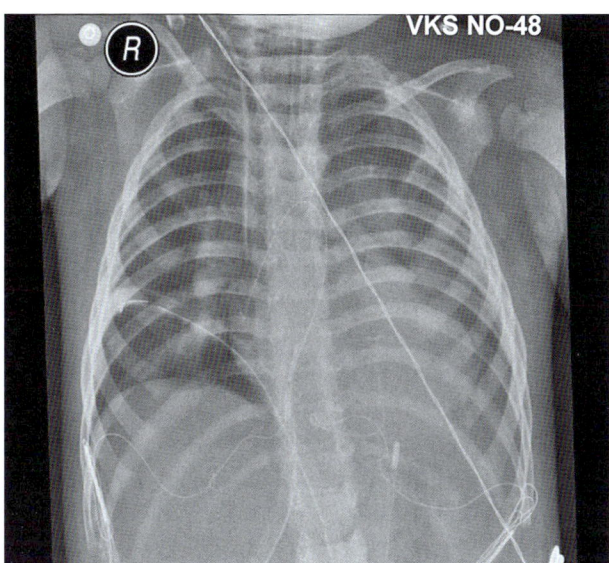

Fig. 25.2B. Chest X-ray after 20 min. The ET tube has been withdrawn to its correct position. Both lungs are well expanded

can be detected radiographically by the presence of an over-distended stomach.

Nasogastric Tube/Feeding Tube

Nasogastric tubes (NG) are used to feed patients or for gastric aspiration in appropriate clinical circumstances. Radiographs are required for accurate placement of NG tubes and are not used except when the patient is unconscious and there is risk of placement of the tube into the bronchial tree. The lower tip of the NG is generally placed in the upper small bowel, which may be confirmed with an abdominal radiograph.

Central Venous Catheters

The tip must be intrathoracic and beyond all venous valves the last of which is at the anterior end of the first rib.

Central venous pressures (CVP) is monitored by central vein catheters placed either through the subclavian or the internal jugular vein; or occasionally via the femoral vein, particularly in babies where access via jugular or subclavian vein is unavailable. These catheters are also used for safe delivery of large volumes of fluids over long periods. Correct placement of the tip of CVP line is important for accurate measurement of central venous pressure. The ideal location of the tip of the CVP line is distal to the last

venous valve, which is located at the junction of internal jugular and subclavian veins. On the chest X-ray, position of the valve corresponds to the inner aspect of the first rib. The venous line should be well positioned in the superior vena cava.

Delayed complications of CVP lines are embolization, obstruction and occasionally vessel perforation.[7]

Thoracostomy Tube

Thoracostomy tubes are often placed into the pleural space to treat a pneumothorax or drain pleural fluid. Post placement; a chest radiograph is obtained to identify its position. It is important to recognize that on a supine AP radiograph, air accumulates anteriorly and fluid gravitates posteriorly. Correct placement of thoracostomy tube is determined by presence of fenestrations within the thoracic cavity. Adequate drainage is possible only if the holes of the drainage tube are within the fluid collection. The hole in a thoracostomy tube can be identified by an interruption in the radio-opaque line.

This interruption in the radio-opaque line should lie within the thoracic cavity, if not and or with evidence of subcutaneous air, a misplaced tube should be suspected. Incorrectly placed tubes for empyemas may delay drainage and result in loculation of the purulent fluid (Fig. 25.4C).[8]

SPECIFIC DISEASE STATES

Specific disease states commonly encountered in the ICU setting are pulmonary oedema, ARDS (acute respiratory distress syndrome), barotrauma, pneumonia, aspiration and pleural effusion.

Pneumonia or air space consolidation is seen as a homogenous opacity in either a segment or lobe of the lung (Fig. 25.3). Often consolidation can be non homogenous or patchy in distribution. Patchy lesions are often due to aspiration or can be due to superadded infection.

Lobar pneumonia is confined to a particular anatomical lobe and usually takes 6–10 days for resolution with adequate therapy. **Aspiration** pneumonias clear rapidly.

Pleural effusion: In the supine patient, the effusion generally is seen as a diffuse haze over the lung bases or right up to the apex (Fig. 25.4A). The telltale sign

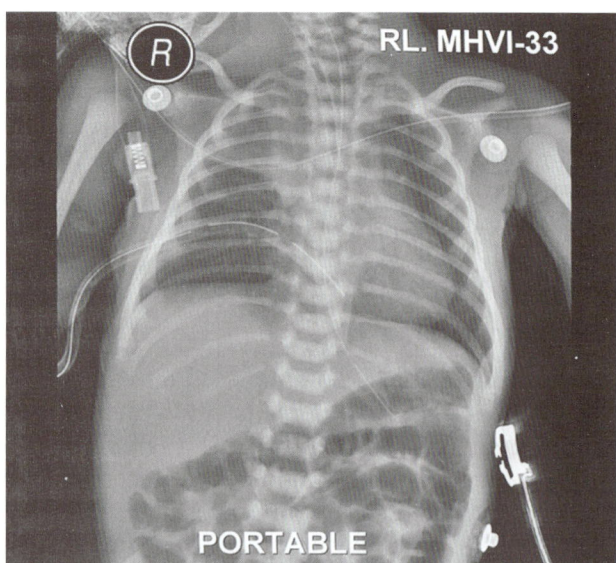

Fig. 25.3. Several support devices, namely ET, NG and thoracostomy tubes are seen. Well-defined homogenous opacity seen in the right upper lobe pneumonia

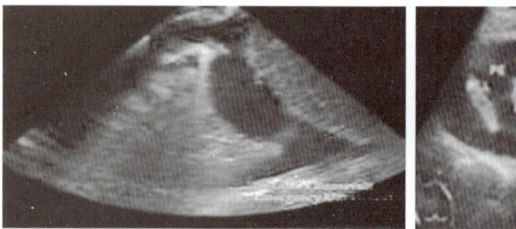

Fig. 25.4B. Ultrasonography of the right thorax shows anechoic pleural effusion

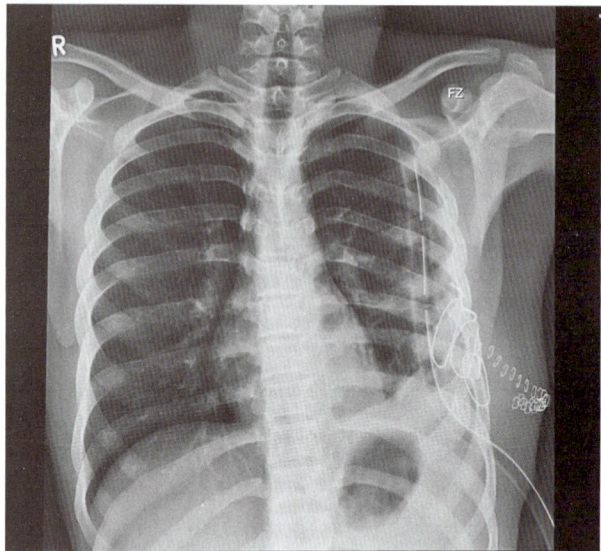

Fig. 25.4C. After thoracotomy, intercostal drainage tube has been inserted into the pleura to drain the residual pus. (**Note** Interruption in the white line of the IC tube is placed within the pleura, indicating correct positioning)

of costophrenic angle obliteration, may or may not be present. Ultrasonography is more sensitive in assessing effusions. Small quantities of fluid are easily detected with US (Fig. 25.4B).

Pulmonary diseases, such as pulmonary oedema and ARDS, can be associated with generalised systemic illness. Pulmonary oedema is typically divided into cardiogenic (acute left ventricular failure), non-cardiogenic (from capillary leak) and due to fluid overload which is secondary to renal causes or other iatrogenic lesions.

In the clinical scenario, these distinctions are not always clear and PE may develop from mixed aetiologies.

Cardiogenic PE is generally not encountered in children. Occasionally, it may be seen secondary to myocarditis.

Noncardiogenic PE is commonly seen with aspiration pneumonia, drowning, hydrocarbon/smoke poisoning and drug reaction. Chest X-ray will reveal indistinct or fuzzy vascular or bronchial walls, Kerley's lines and thickened fissures. Pleural effusion is generally not seen in non-cardiogenic pulmonary oedema.

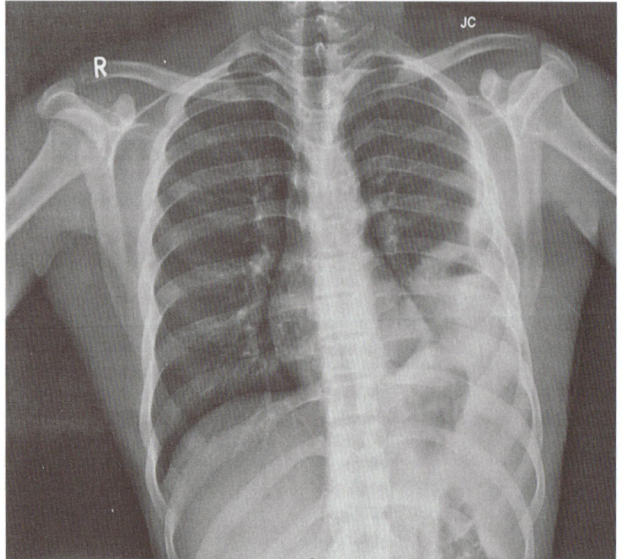

Fig. 25.4A. Chest X-ray in this 8-year-old child reveals left-sided pleural effusion. On ultrasonography, this was thick, confirming the diagnosis of empyema

Alveolar oedema manifests when air in the alveoli is replaced by fluid. Typically, this happens within hours and is quite sudden. X-ray findings are variable. Initially multiple fluffy air space opacities are seen all over the lungs. These opacities may become confluent over time. Air bronchogram is visible as consolidation progresses. Acute alveolar oedema is central and generally confined to the hilar and perihilar region and seen as a "butterfly pattern" in distribution (Fig. 25.5).[8]

ARDS is usually encountered in shock, hypotension, and multiple injuries and with severe respiratory infection.

Acute (acute respiratory distress syndrome) lung injury results in increased permeability, and hence PE. Surfactant dilution and inactivation, alveolar filling and decreased lung compliance result in hypoxaemia. Imaging findings in ARDS depend upon timing from injury or insult. Initially, the chest X-ray is normal, and later focal or diffuse lesion may be seen.

Lesions may clear over a period of time with adequate support or alveolar oedema may progress to respiratory failure and may be fatal.

Pneumothorax (air collection in the pleural cavity) resulting from barotrauma is a life-threatening emergency in ventilated patients (Fig. 25.6). Diagnosis of pneumothorax is often missed on X-rays as apical accumulation of air is uncommon in supine films. In the supine position, air accumulates in the anteromedial or the subpulmonic recess.

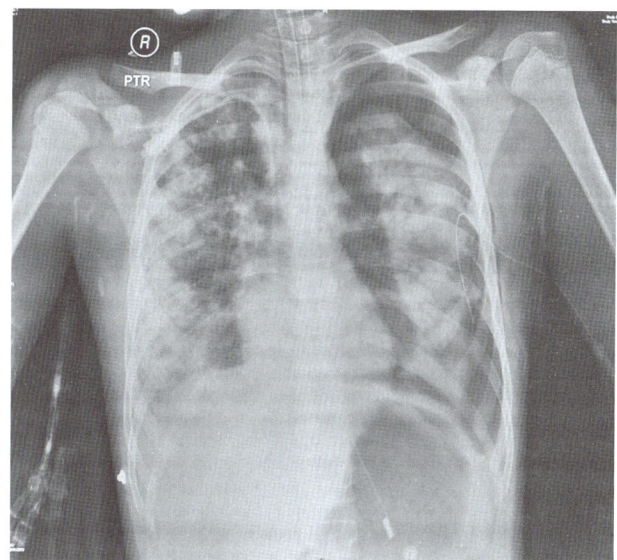

Fig. 25.6. ARDS on ventilator. Increased ventilated pressure has resulted in barotrauma and left-sided pneumothorax. The alveolar oedema has progressed to frank bilateral consolidation

Atelectasis occurs in intubated patients as well as those breathing spontaneously. Small opacity which clears quickly or fluctuates (in hours) is more typical of atelectasis.

The left lower lobe is the commonest site affected followed by right lower lobe.

Chest CT has many advantages over plain X-rays as CT is more sensitive in the evaluation of all disease processes. The drawback of increased radiation and difficult patient transport are a deterrent for routine use of CT in paediatric patients.

IMAGING-GUIDED INTERVENTION

Central venous catheter placement with ultrasound guidance reduces complications of central venous annulation, specially for internal jugular vein, however, this is not so efficacious for subclavian vein catheterization.[9]

Central vein catheter occlusion and thrombosis is common in ICU settings. Occlusion can be partial or complete and due to mechanical reasons versus thrombosis. Clinical diagnosis is unreliable, and other clinical signs may be absent. Contrast venography is the gold standard for diagnosis of occlusion.

However, this is invasive. US is a viable alternative especially with the advent of Doppler, it is easy to locate large thrombi in sizable structures, like the inferior vena cava.[2,9]

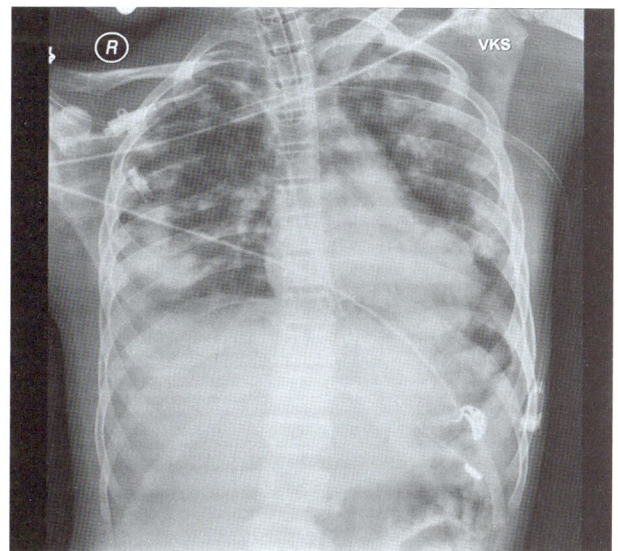

Fig. 25.5. ARDS in a 16-year-old boy with transverse myelitis. Multiple fluffy alveolar infiltrates are seen in both lung fields

CONCLUSION

Imaging has a vital role in management of critically ill patients, both for diagnostic and therapeutic purposes.

However, it is imperative that a trained radiographer is available in the PICU at all times and a daily review of all radiological evaluations be done by an experienced radiologist.

Care must be taken to follow all regulations and take precautions against radiation exposure of the personnal involved.

REFERENCES

1. Slovis TL, Frush DP, Berdon WE, Hall Eric J. Biologic effects of radiation in children. In: Slovis (Ed). Caffeys Pediatric Diagnostic Imaging, 11th edn. Mosby Elsevier 2008; p 6–10.

2. Habib FA, Mckenney MG. Performed US in the ICU setting. Surg Clin N Am 2004;84:1151–1179.

3. Wartenberg KE, Schmidt JM, Stephen MA. Multimodality monitoring in Neurocritical care. Crit Care Clin 2007; 23:507–538.

4. Lutman D, Peters J Mark. Trauma and Transport. In: Bingham, Lloyd Thomas (Eds). Hatch and Sumner's Textbook of Pediatric Anesthesia, 3rd edn. London. Hodder Arnold 2008; p 637.

5. Rubinowitz Ami N, Siegel Mark D, Tocino I. Thoracic Imaging in the ICU. Crit Care Clin 2007;23:539–573.

6. Jain SN. A pictorial essay: Radiology of lines and tubes in the intensive care unit. Indian J Radiol Imaging. 2011; 21(3):182–190.

7. Jacobs BR. Central venous catheter occlusion and thrombosis. Crit Care Clin 2003;19:489–514.

8. Khan NA, Jahdali AL, Ghanam S-AL, et al. Reading chest radiographs in the critically ill (part 1 and 2), Radiography of lung pathologies common in the ICU patient. Annals of Thoracic Medicine 2009;4(3):p. 14–157.

9. Liu L, Gropper MA. Overview of anesthesiology and critical care medicine. In: Ronald D Miller (Ed). Miller's Anesthesia, 7th edn. Philadelphia: Churchill Livingstone, 2010; p. 2863.

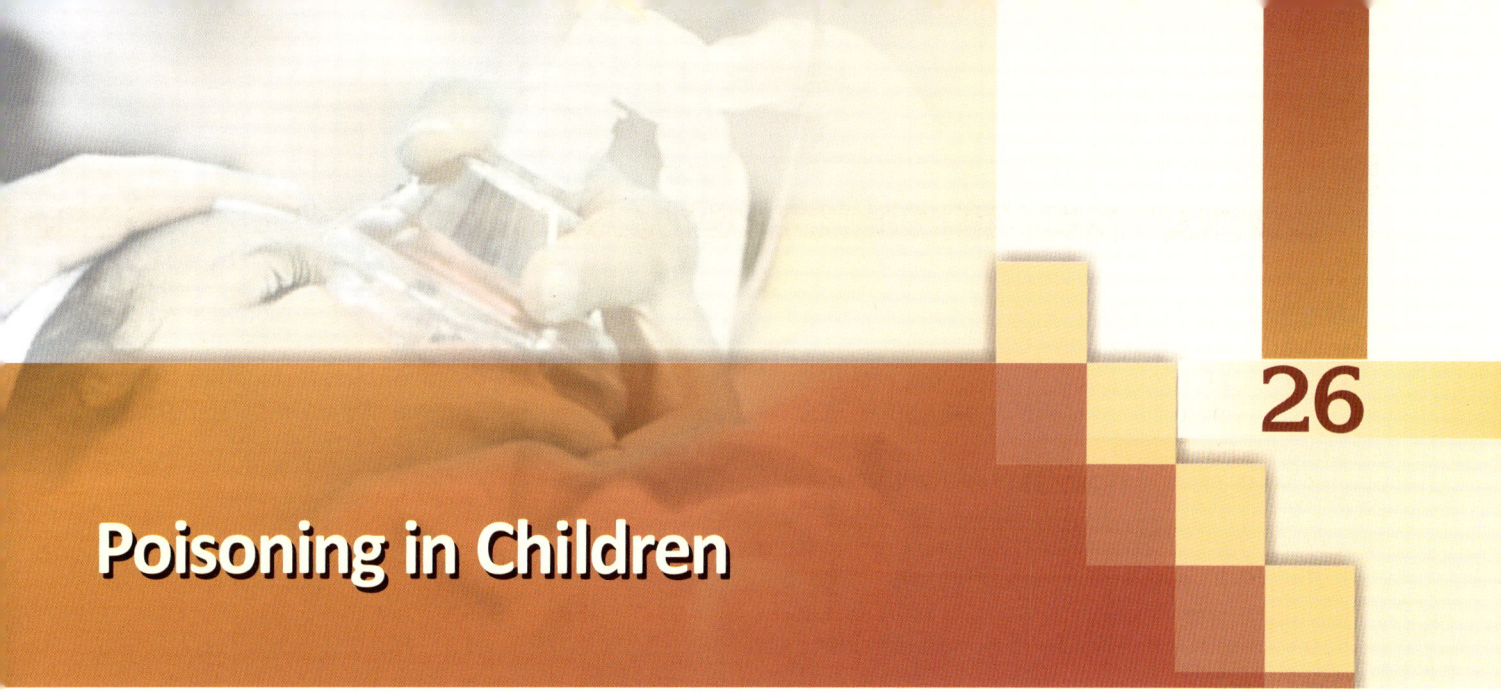

26

Poisoning in Children

Asha Tyagi

- **Epidemiology**
- **Risk factors**
- **Diagnosis**
- **General principles of management**
- **Elimination of poison**
- **Antidotes**
- **Prevention of re-exposure**

INTRODUCTION

Poisonings in childhood shows a biphasic pattern of presentation with regard to age of the patient. The two peaks include occurrence at age lesser than 5 years and a later one during adolescence. In India, the commonest cause of poisonings in children includes accidental intake of pesticides, insecticides and kerosene. With such toxic causative agents, the poisoning may prove to be fatal. Certain drugs available at home and consumed accidentally by a child may also result in potentially lethal toxicity, and extended release preparations may cause delayed presentations mandating long periods of observation. In adolescents, suicidal poisonings and drug abuse are common. Such a scenario for poisonings in childhood mandates involvement of the intensivist for stabilization and resuscitation, monitoring, supportive care or specific treatment.

EPIDEMIOLOGY

As per literature from western countries, majority of poisonings in children are seen in less than 5–6 years age group,[1–3] and are benign, with a low mortality and brief periods of hospitalization.[1,2] In last four decades, the mortality dropped by almost 85% in these cases with up to 75% patients discharged home either immediately or within 24 hours of admission, and only 1.5% of cases, mainly adolescent girls who attempted suicide admitted to intensive care unit.[2,4] Most exposures involved oral ingestion (76%), occurred in the home (93%), and were unintentional (more than 80%).[3] Amongst various drugs responsible for childhood poisonings, the most toxic ones are iron, antidepressants, hypoglycaemics, cardiovascular drugs, salicylates, anticonvulsants, and illicit drugs.[5]

In developing countries, like India, the epidemiology of poisonings in childhood appears to be in contrast to developed nations. While similar to the developed countries, majority of patients (up to 90%) are in the less than 5–6 years age group with a male predominance,[6,9] most admissions are reported to be symptomatic (up to 70%) with almost 11% requiring intensive care in certain databases.[6,8] The mortality due to poisoning in children is also higher, ranging from 3 to 11.6%[6,7,9,10] in various publications. The probable reason for higher mortality is the inherent toxicity of the substances implicated, in sharp contrast to developed countries, where common non-toxic household products are the common poisons.[6] As per World Health Organization (WHO), the rate of fatal poisoning is noted to be four times higher in low-income and middle-income countries than the high-income countries.[11] Fatality of poisoning is strongly related to low socioeconomic strata, whether within or beyond a political boundary. Poisoning in children constituted 2.1% of the total paediatric admissions and 1.2% of total hospital deaths,[10] and was identified to cause 6% of unnatural deaths in population less than 19 years of age.[12]

A distinct pattern of suicidal poisonings, and those due to substance abuse is recognized in older children, typically adolescents. In the Indian scenario also, while almost all (97.2%) poisonings in younger age group were accidental in nature, in the 12–18 years group, majority (80.9%) were found to be suicidal.[10]

The nature of poisons consumed also varies between developed and developing countries.[11] In developed countries, most childhood poisonings are due to consumption of household products or medications available at home.[1] Non-toxic compounds, such as shampoo, ink, nail polish, cleaners and disinfectants, are well-known causes. Less common ones may include iatrogenic causes, such as delivery of mistaken medications at home or in health care facility, or as a part of Munchausen syndrome. In contrast, non-medicinal insecticides, pesticides and kerosene have consistently been the commonest causes of poisoning in children in India (up to 69.2%), with some geographical variations.[6,7,9,10]

RISK FACTORS

The risk factors for poisoning in young children and adolescents are different.[11] In young children, the hand-to-mouth reflex and their natural curiosity predisposes to accidental ingestion of household products. Their less well-developed physiology as compared to adults may make them more predisposed to effect of poisonings. In adolescents, alcohol or drug abuse and over dose due to risk-taking behaviour and experimentation due to peer-pressure may result in poisoning despite being aware of the consequences. Boys have higher rates of poisoning than girls in all geographic regions.

Besides the risk factors dependent on subjects, certain factors are related to the poison itself:[11] toxicity, nature, physical appearance and storage; as well as season and weather conditions; policies, standards and laws governing the manufacture, labelling, distribution, storage and disposal of poisoning agents; and access to quality health care for treatment.

DIAGNOSIS

The history, presentation as well as laboratory tests aid in diagnosis of poisoning.[1,13,14]

History: A strong index of suspicion is warranted in a previously healthy child presenting with unexplained loss of consciousness or sudden organ dysfunctions. In suspected cases of poisoning, a history should be taken to establish the probable mode (usually ingestion), timing and quantity of the poison consumed, even if these are approximations at best.

Presentation: The presentation of most poisons remains non-specific and the nervous system is most commonly involved. The signs and symptoms usually occur in a constellation of signs and symptoms and have been termed toxic syndromes,[14] e.g. the cholinergic state seen with organophosphates. Both anticholinergic and adrenergic syndromes may present with tachycardia, dilated pupils, hyperthermia, agitation and hallucinations. While the skin is typically dry with anticholinergic states it is diaphoretic with an adrenergic presentation. A cholinergic syndrome presents with bradycardia, constricted pupils, normal temperature, fasciculations, increased lacrimation and salivation, wheezing and respiratory distress. Hypoventilation with constricted or dilated pupil is typical with narcotics and sedatives, respectively. Co-ingestion of products with divergent effects may prevent one single toxic syndrome on presentation. The patient's mental status, vital signs, pupil reactivity, skin moisture and colour, and bowel sounds should also be noted.[15]

Urine examination: A macroscopic physical assessment and analytical tests of urine specimen are useful in poisonings. Urine sample turning smoky dark green in colour on standing is seen with phenol poisoning; presence of ketones with acetone, salicylate or isopropyl alcohol poisoning; oxalate crystals with ethylene glycol; and ferric chloride testing producing red colour with salicylates, or purple green with phenothiazines, or violet with phenol poisoning.

Blood tests: Blood tests for organ dysfunction are indicated as in cases of adult poisoning. An arterial blood analysis can assist in assessment of acid-base and ventilation status.

Toxicologic screening: Without clinical suspicion or suspected access to illicit drugs, toxicologic screens are not usually useful in guiding treatment.[16]

GENERAL PRINCIPLES OF MANAGEMENT

The management depends on severity of poisoning and the clinical progress.[1,13,17] The clinical course of patient can result in discharge from emergency itself if asymptomatic, or require admission in intensive care on the other extreme. While caring for an asymptomatic child with suspected toxin ingestion, monitoring for a longer period should be considered, if there is a suspicion of ingestion of a delayed-action medication.[16]

Irrespective of nature of toxin, the essential steps in managing any poisoning include:

1. Initial stabilization and resuscitation, with special emphasis on the airway, breathing and circulation.
2. Supportive care to maintain the homeostasis; prevent and treat complications.
3. Attempts to confirm the diagnosis.
4. Preventing further absorption of the poison.
5. Increasing elimination of the poison.
6. Use of specific antidote, if applicable.
7. Preventing re-exposure.

Initial Stabilization and Resuscitation

Besides stabilization of respiration and circulation, the symptoms of hypoglycaemia and blood sugar reading should be sought (less than 80 mg/dl). In presence of signs or symptoms, intravenous dextrose (5 ml/kg of 10% formulation) should be infused.[15,16] In case of difficulty with establishing an intravenous access, 1.0 mg of intramuscular glucagon may be given as a temporizing measure.[18]

Admission to an intensive care unit is warranted, if there is severe poisoning, intake of life-threatening dose, requirement of continued antidote, haemodynamic instability, need for invasive monitoring, coma, GCS <6, convulsions, prolonged QTc or arrhythmias, pH <7.2, respiratory compromise, or an indication for intubation or ventilatory therapy.

Monitoring that may be required in these patients includes an ECG in those who have ingested cardiotoxic medications or other potent medications. Continuous cardiovascular monitoring, i.e. ECG and blood pressure, should be instituted, if any abnormalities are noted or suspected.[19] Invasive monitoring may be required, if patient develops haemodynamic instability. Pulse oximetry is helpful in assessing all patients, especially those with impaired mental or respiratory status.[15] Although altered mental status in a child may be presumed to be from poisoning, traumatic head injury should also be considered.

Preventing Absorption

The usual route of poisoning in childhood is oral ingestion. For preventing further absorption, potential therapies have included emesis, cathartics, gastric lavage, activated charcoal administration and whole-bowel irrigation.

Emesis and cathartics are no longer recommended for in-hospital treatment of poisonings.[16]

The original enthusiasm for using gastric lavage has given way to its guarded use, under specific circumstances only. The American Academy of Clinical Toxicology and European Association of Poison Centres and Clinical Toxicologists discourage the routine use of gastric lavage in the emergency department, unless performed by well-practiced physicians within one hour of the ingestion.[20] Reasons for a shift from recommending it ubiquitously include lack of evidence to prove improvement in outcome following mild and moderate poisonings, risk of aspiration pneumonitis, inability to remove ingested tablets, increased propulsion of contents into duodenum and traumatic complications.[18,20] It should be used for potentially lethal poisons consumed within last 1 hour. Various fluids, such as normal saline, half-normal saline and water, have been recommended for the lavage. Using potable tap water (1–2 ml/kg, up to maximum of 15 ml/kg) till clear fluid appears to be a popular choice to prevent electrolyte imbalances. For a satisfactory lavage, patient should be turned on his or her left side, head slightly lower than the feet and the largest orogastric tube that can be easily passed should be used. Before instilling any lavage fluid, contents must be aspirated. Attempts to retrieve entire instilled volumes should be made. Whenever used, protection of airway should be ensured. It is contraindicated in hydrocarbon, petrochemical and corrosive poisonings.

Activated charcoal remains a more efficacious method then emesis or gastric lavage for prevention of absorption. It has been called a "universal antidote" since it absorbs a wide array of poisons. Combining it with other methods of gastric decontamination does not increase the efficacy, and also increases the complications. Although it is the most effective method of gastrointestinal decontamination, it does not improve clinical outcome. Activated charcoal should be used only for severe poisonings and that too within the first hour of ingestion. It is most effective, if given within an hour of ingestion, and is ineffective after 2 hours of ingestion.[17,18,21] It remains contraindicated for cyanide, metallic, acid, alkali and corrosive poisoning; as well as in presence of ileus, intestinal haemorrhage and unprotected airway. It is crushed made into slurry and administered orally or via nasogastric tube. If given orally, orange juice or sugar syrup has been used to make it palatable, but risks decreasing the surface area and hence the efficacy.[15] The dose varies between 1 and 2 gm/kg depending on severity of poisoning. Repeat dose therapy using 0.25 – 0.5 gm/kg at 4–6 hourly interval after initial dose may be used for lethal poisoning with substances having delayed gastric emptying or significant enterohepatic circulation, such as phenytoin, carbamazepine, phenobarbital, theophylline, salicylates, dapsone and quinine.

Whole-bowel irrigation has a limited use for ingestion of sustained release drugs, such as crack vials or body packs. It is administered using polyethylene glycol (250–500 ml/hr) orally or by nasogastric tube, till rectal effluent becomes clear (usually 2–6 hours).

In India, poisoning with pesticides is commoner than with pharmaceutical products thus skin decontamination may also be required. It involves removing clothes, if soiled with the pesticides. Contaminated areas should be washed with abundant water and soap. Using lubricants can cause the pesticides to further stick to the skin and should be avoided.

INCREASED OR ENHANCED ELIMINATION

This refers to use of techniques, such as forced diuresis, alkalinization of urine, haemodialysis or haemoperfusion in an attempt to eliminate the poison to a greater degree. Usually enhanced elimination is applied to poisonings only if methods to decrease absorption are contraindicated or have failed, or if the period at presentation is too long for their application.

Forced diuresis has no role in current scenario.

Alkalinization of urine may be tried for salicylate poisoning by using 1–2 mEq/kg IV of sodium bicarbonate, titrating the urinary pH between 7 and 8. It is contraindicated in impending or established renal failure. Hypokalaemia can interfere with the alkalinization so should be treated.

Haemodialysis can be used for small molecules with low protein bindingae, such as ethanol, methanol, ethylene glycol, salicylates and lithium. Incorporation of an activated charcoal filter during dialysis, i.e. hemoperfusion is useful for phenytoin, carbamazepine, phenobarbital and theophylline poisonings. It is ineffective for alcohols and heavy metal poisonings.

Exchange transfusion may be used for poisonings associated with red blood cell damage, such as arsenic toxicity or during methaemoglobinaemia.

Elimination of heavy metals requires chelation.

Carbon monoxide poisoning may respond to hyperbaric oxygen therapy.

ANTIDOTES

Antidote acts either as physiologic antagonist or by neutralizing the poison. Its use decreases the morbidity and mortality associated with poisoning. However, not all poisons have antidotes. Specific antidotes are available for certain poisonings only. Although pesticide and kerosene poisonings are commoner in India than drug-induced accidental exposures, from amongst them antipyretics, antiepileptics and phenothiazines have been implicated more commonly.[7] In adolescents, substance abuse is more likely. Antidotes of some common poisons are presented in Table 26.1.

PREVENTION OF RE-EXPOSURE

In children, access to potentially toxic substances has to be prevented. In adolescents, psychological counselling may be of paramount importance in preventing further suicidal attempts or substance abuse.

To conclude, the epidemiology of poisoning in children is slightly different in India as compared to developed countries. While it remains common in less

Table 26.1 Specific antidotes to common poisonings in Indian scenario

Poison	Antidote	Dose[1,17]
Organophosphates	Atropine	0.05–0.1 mg/kg IM or IV in children, and 2–5 mg in adolescents, repeat every 10–15 min until signs of atropinization.
	Pralidoxime	25–50 mg/kg IV over 30 minutes; repeat in 1 hour PRN, then every 6–8 hours for 24–48 hours. If as an infusion: after the loading, 1% at 500 mg/hr in adolescents and 10 mg/kg/hr in children.
Paracetamol	N-acetylcysteine	150 mg/kg IV over 1 hour; then 12.5 mg/kg/hr for 4 hrs, then 6.25 mg/kg/hr; enteral: 140 mg/kg then 70 mg/kg every 4 hours.
Anticholinergics	Physostigmine	0.02 mg/kg slow IV; may repeat after 15 min till desired effect; subsequent doses every 2–3 hours PRN.
Methaemoglobinaemias	Methylene blue	1–2 mg/kg (1%) IV slow over 5–10 min if severe cyanosis or levels >40%.
Benzodiazepines	Flumazenil	0.01 mg/kg IV over 30 seconds; can be repeated every 1-minute up to 3 mg.
Cyclic antidepressants	Sodium bicarbonate	1–2 mEq/kg (IV) to achieve and maintain QRS width <100 ms.
Isoniazid	Pyridoxine	Gram-per gram equivalent dose to what was ingested. If ingested dose not known, start with 5 gram and repeat every 5–20 minutes, if needed. Overdose may cause neuropathy.
Narcotics	Naloxone	0.1 mg/kg in <5 years; 0.1–0.8 mg/kg in older children.
Methanol and ethylene glycol	Ethanol; fomipezole	10 ml/kg of 10% solution loading over 1 hour; 0.15 ml/kg/hr infusion; titrated to blood ethanol level of 100 mg%. Fomipezole preferred; 15 mg/kg; maintenance of 10 mg/kg every 12 hours (4 doses), then 15 mg/kg every 12 hours.
Arsenic/mercury/gold/lead	Chelating agent (BAL)	3–5 mg/kg/dose deep IM every 4 hours for 2 days, every 4–6 hours for additional 2 days, then every 4–12 hours for up to 7 more days.
Iron	Deferroxamine	5–15 mg/kg/hr IV; use higher doses for severe symptoms and decrease dose as patient recovers.

than 6 years old, is commoner in boys and usually accidental, the causes and outcome are dissimilar. More toxic insecticides, pesticides and kerosene are the commonest causes in India as compared to innocuous household compounds or pharmaceutical products available at home. The outcome thus appears poorer in the Indian context. The principles for management of poisonings in children are similar to those in adults. Due care must be taken of the physiologic differences in younger age group. In adolescents, poisoning is usually suicidal or secondary to substance abuse.

SUMMARY

- The principles for management of poisonings in children are similar to those in adults.

- Due care must be taken of the physiologic differences in younger age group.

- Essential steps are to be considered during treatment which include attempts to establish the diagnosis, initial stabilization and resuscitation, supportive care and decontamination, prevention of absorption, enhancing elimination, and prevention of re-exposure.

- Intensive care management of these patients may be indicated for monitoring, stabilization, supportive care as well as specific treatment.

REFERENCES

1. Tibbalis J. Paediatric poisoning. In: Bersten AD, Soni N (Eds). Oh's Intensive Care Manual, 4th edn. Philadelphia: Butterworth Heinemann Elsevier 2009;p. 1179–1188.

2. Lamireau T, Llanas B, Kennedy A, et al. Epidemiology of poisoning in children: a 7-year survey in a paediatric emergency care unit. Eur J Emerg Med 2002;9:9–14.

3. Watson WA, Litovitz TL, Rodgers GC (Jr), et al. Annual report of the American Association of Poison Control Centers Toxic Exposure Surveillance System. Am J Emerg Med 2005;23:589–666.

4. Penny L, Moriarty T. Poisoning in children. Contin Educ Anaesth Crit Care Pain 2009;9:109–113.

5. Hoffman R, Osterhoudt KC. Evaluation and management of pediatricpoisonings. Pediatr Case Rev 2002;2:51–63.

6. Bhat NK, Dhar M, Ahmad S, Chandar V. Profile of poisoning in children and adolescents at a North Indian tertiary care centre. Journal, Indian Academy of Clinical Medicine 2011;13:37–42.

7. Dutta AK, Seth A, Goyal PK, et al. Poisoning in children: Indian scenario. Indian J Pediatr 1998;65:365–370.

8. Kohli U, Kuttiat VS, Lodha R, Kabra SK. Profile of childhood poisoning at a tertiary care centre in North India. Indian J Pediatr 2008;75:791–794.

9. Ram P, Kanchan T, Unnikrishnan B. Pattern of acute poisonings in children below 15 years—a study from Mangalore, South India. J Forensic Leg Med 2014;25: 26–29.

10. Gupta S, Govil YC, Misra PK, Nath R, Srivastava KL. Trends in poisoning in children: experience at a large referral teaching hospital. Natl Med J India 1998;11: 166–168.

11. www.who.int/violenece_injury_prevention/child/injury/world_reportPoisoning accessed on 27.6.15.

12. Debata PK, Deswal S, Kumath M. Causes of unnatural deaths among children and adolescents in northern India—a qualitative analysis of postmortem data. J Forensic Leg Med 2014;26:53–55.

13. Menon P Ramesh. Poisonings, injuries and accidents. In: Vinod K Paul, Arvind Bagga (Eds). Ghai Essential Pediatrics, 8th edn. New Delhi: CBS Publishers & Distributors Pvt. Ltd. 2013;697–707.

14. Kenneth K. Initial management of ingestions of toxic substances. N Engl J Med 1992;326:1677–1681.

15. Riordan M, Rylance G, Berry K. Poisoning in children 1: General management. Arch Dis Child 2002;87:392–396.

16. McGregor T, Parkar M, Rao S. Evaluation and management of common childhood poisonings. Am Fam Physician 2009;79:397–403.

17. Osterhoudt KC, Ewald MB, Shannon M, Henretig FM. Toxicologic emergencies. In: Fleisher GR, Ludwig S (Eds). Textbook of Pediatric Emergency Medicine, 6th edn. Philadelphia: Lippincott Williams and Wilkins; 2010; p. 1171–1223.

18. Barry JD. Diagnosis and management of the poisoned child. Pediatr Ann 2005;34:937–946.

19. Morse SB, Hardwick WE Jr, King WD. Fatal iron intoxication in an infant. South Med J 1997;90:1043–1047.

20. Vale JA, Kulig K, for the American Academy of Clinical Toxicology; European Association of Poisons Centres and Clinical Toxicologists. Position paper: gastric lavage. J Toxicol Clin Toxicol 2004;42:933–943.

21. Lapus RM. Activated charcoal for pediatric poisonings: the universalantidote? Curr Opin Pediatr 2007;19:216–222.

Index